Sensory Blending

Sensory Blending

On Synaesthesia and Related Phenomena

EDITED BY

Ophelia Deroy

OXFORD
UNIVERSITY PRESS

OXFORD
UNIVERSITY PRESS

Great Clarendon Street, Oxford, OX2 6DP,
United Kingdom

Oxford University Press is a department of the University of Oxford.
It furthers the University's objective of excellence in research, scholarship,
and education by publishing worldwide. Oxford is a registered trade mark of
Oxford University Press in the UK and in certain other countries

First Edition published in 2017

Published in the United States of America by Oxford University Press
198 Madison Avenue, New York, NY 10016, United States of America

British Library Cataloguing in Publication Data
Data available

Library of Congress Control Number: 2016954547

ISBN 978–0–19–968828–9

Contents

Part III. Boundaries of Synaesthesia: Unconscious, Acquired, and Social Varieties of Sensory Unions

List of Figures

List of Tables

List of Contributors

André J. Abath, Department of Philosophy, Federal University of Minas Gerais

Malika Auvray, Institut des Systemes Intelligents et de Robotique, Centre National de la Recherche Scientifique, Paris

Berit Brogaard, Brogaard Lab for Multisensory Research, University of Miami

Jonathan Cohen, Department of Philosophy, University of California, San Diego

Ophelia Deroy, Institute of Philosophy, University of London and Munich Centre for Neuroscience, Ludwig Maximilian University, Munich

Mirko Farina, Department of Philosophy, King's College, University of London

Yasmina Jraissati, Department of Philosophy, American University of Beirut

Roi Cohen Kadosh, Department of Experimental Psychology, University of Oxford

David P. Luke, Department of Psychology & Counselling, University of Greenwich

Lawrence E. Marks, Department of Psychology, Yale University

Mohan Matthen, Department of Philosophy, University of Toronto

Myrto Mylopoulos, Department of Philosophy and Institute of Cognitive Science, Carleton University, Ottawa

Casey O'Callaghan, Department of Philosophy, Washington University, Saint Louis

Tony Ro, Department of Psychology, City College & The Graduate Center, CUNY

Noam Sagiv, Centre for Cognition and Neuroimaging, Brunel University

Monika Sobczak-Edmans, Centre for Cognition and Neuroimaging, Brunel University

Michael Sollberger, Department of Philosophy, University of Fribourg

Charles Spence, Department of Psychology, University of Oxford

Devin B. Terhune, Department of Experimental Psychology, Goldsmiths, University of London

Frédérique de Vignemont, Institut Jean-Nicod, Paris

Adrian L. Williams, Brunel University, Centre for Cognition and Neuroimaging

Introduction

Ophelia Deroy

When she was sixteen, Patricia Duffy and her father were reminiscing about how, as a child, she learned to write all of the letters very quickly except for the letter 'R'. She said to her father that this lasted 'until one day, I realized that to make an "R" all I had to do was first write a "P" and then draw a line down from its loop. And I was so surprised that I could turn a yellow letter into an orange letter just by adding a line'. 'Yellow letter? Orange letter?' her father wondered, 'what do you mean?' 'Well, you know, "P" is a yellow letter, but "R" is an orange letter. You know, the colours of the letters.' 'The colours of the letters?' her father replied.

It is at that moment, when seeing her father's bewildered reaction, that Patricia realized that the whole world might not share these perceptions. As far as she remembered, each letter of the alphabet would automatically appear with a specific colour, and remain invariably the same, time after time. However, until then, it never came up in any discussion that she saw yellow Ps, orange Rs, or purple Vs. Had it appeared before, she would still have thought such a statement to be as ordinary as saying that apples are red and leaves are green. At that time, Patricia had never heard of synaesthesia, a condition in which ordinary stimuli elicit unordinary experiences. She suddenly realized that perception could be something individuals did not share, although most assumed they did: Could perception, she wondered, be 'something that put them on a private island, mysteriously separated from others'?[1]

Patricia's reaction at the discovery of synaesthesia will certainly be shared by everyone learning about the strange 'sensory blending' that seems to affect her, along with 4 to 6 per cent of the population. While most cases of synaesthesia are similar to Patricia's experience of coloured graphemes, some also consist in visualizing colours when hearing certain musical notes, others in experiencing a taste when reading the names of famous individuals or subway stations, or feeling shapes when eating specific foods. What these cases have in common is not just their oddity, but also their involuntary character: synaesthetes are not able to turn off the eruption of

[1] Duffy, 2001: 5.

additional experiences, like they would do for other forms of mental imagery. Whereas a piece of music, for instance, might lead us to imagine a landscape or some moving lines, it still leaves us with the possibility to stop this visual imagery, or eventually control its content. Synaesthetes who have colour experiences when they hear musical notes cannot stop them from occurring, nor can they decide to modulate the colour which these sounds bring to mind. Even training has almost no power on the content of these additional experiences.[2]

Cases of synaesthesia such as coloured graphemes or colour hearing do not easily fit within our usual way of carving conscious experiences: They are vivid, automatic, and consistent like perceptual experiences, and yet they do not seem to represent objective properties of objects, or to arise from the same route as normal percepts. They could be assimilated to cases of mental imagery if it was not for the lack of control that characterizes their induction and content. Explaining how the content of synaesthetic experiences is determined is no less difficult than finding their place within our usual taxonomy of experiences: they do not seem absolutely random, as synaesthetic repertoire sometimes obeys a form of regularity, within or across individuals, and yet remains highly idiosyncratic; the association does not seem to be innately determined, as synaesthetic monozygotic twins will not associate the same colours to the same sounds or letters; nor does it seem to come from past experience, and respond to exposure to new associations.

What makes synesthesia so interesting to consider is that it is a separate kind of mental state, and—what is pretty rare—a positive symptom. In other words, it is defined by the presence of additional experiences, rather than by the absence of a function. Synaesthesia is not associated with any other particular pathology or general cognitive or perceptual dysfunction, although it can co-exist with other conditions, like savantism and autism, for instance.[3] In other words, besides their synaesthesia, synaesthetes are in all respects similar to non-synaesthetes. This avoids some of the concerns one can have when generalizing from atypical to typical cases, where key differences might exist beyond the symptom at stake.

Questions remain as to what the general lessons of synaesthesia should be. What do synaesthetes' experiences, and the capacity for the synaesthetic brain to generate such experiences, reveal beyond fascinating idiosyncrasies? In recent years, synaesthesia has started to be used as a model to think about more widespread cases of sensory interactions, making sensory blending a broad characteristic of our sensory systems and experiences. As synaesthetes come closer to non-synaesthetes, new questions arise as to whether these arbitrary sensory pairings should not, after all, join up with our concepts of perception, mental imagery, or learned associations, or whether the category of synaesthetic association should not be extended to phenomena previously labelled under different names. At this stage it is important to see that

[2] See Deroy and Spence, 2013 for a discussion of some recent training studies.
[3] E.g. Baron-Cohen et al., 2007.

the problem is not terminological, but conceptual. Sorting mental phenomena in the same or different categories has implications for the way we think about the mind and its relation to the brain as well as the external world. This is what the philosophers and cognitive neuroscientists in this volume address.

Most of the scientific efforts have for a long time been concentrated on establishing the reality of the reports given by a few individuals. The patient work of key researchers, such as Richard Cytowic, Lawrence Marks, Vilyanur Ramachandran, Simon Baron-Cohen, Jamie Ward, David Eagleman, and many others, has provided researchers with a battery of psychophysical tests and neuro-imagery criteria to show how the behavioural responses and brain activity of synaesthetes differ from control groups. This increased evidence, however, has not made theoretical questions disappear: the problem here is not merely that synaesthetes' experience is different from that of others, but that it is at odds with reality: the orange shade experienced by a coloured-hearing synaesthete when she hears a certain note is not a sign that the note out there is really orange. What can this experience be about, then? Does it attribute an illusory colour property to the sound? Does it have any representational content at all? Synaesthetic experiences, as we begin to understand, do not easily fit into the dominant representationalist framework. More recent studies, though, give us new reasons to look at synaesthesia as a source of objections to standard theories of perception and mental processes.

I.1 Beyond minority reports

Philosophers and cognitive neuroscientists mostly base their accounts of synaesthesia on coloured graphemes, which remain the most frequent kind of synaesthesia. Many other forms of synesthesia exist, however, with inducers as diverse as flavours, swimming movements, or proper names. The additional experiences generated by the presentation of these objects may involve colour, but also all sorts of sensory or non-sensory contents: digits can be associated to certain locations in space, words can induce taste sensations in the mouth, tastes can trigger tactile shape sensations. In cases of personification, numbers or days of the week are associated with personality traits, emotions, or gender.

These peculiar experiences, despite their variety, still have much in common regarding their aetiology, duration, and range of manifestations: atypical conscious manifestations were experienced from a very early age, when a stimulus was presented or imagined in a certain sensory modality, and they continue to do so automatically and in a highly consistent way in adulthood. Congenital cases, in this respect, remain the most investigated and discussed form of synaesthesia. Still, there are other cases where the stimulation of one sensory stream coincides with the involuntary activation of another unstimulated stream, to which the synaesthetic label could apply. There are cases where the activation in the unstimulated stream remains non-conscious, but might still interfere with the processing of information in the stimulated one; there are transient drug-induced experiences where hearing sounds also leads to experiencing visual concurrents while one's eyes are closed; 'visual experiences' can also emerge after the onset of blindness, and individuals might feel pain when they see someone else in pain.

Deciding to count these cases as related to synaesthesia not only makes it more frequent and widespread, but also potentially universal. If the occurrence of a conscious concurrent is not necessary, or if the occurrence of a thought is sufficient to count as synaesthesia, then the surprising intuitive connections we all make between sensory attributes, such as high pitch and high spatial elevation or low pitch and darkness, become potential candidates to join the synaesthetic crowd. But should we classify all sorts of surprising, or at least unpredicted, conscious experiences as synaesthesia—independently of the content of the experience? Should we restrict the name synaesthesia to the idiosyncratic forms of sensory blending, or extend it to other regular forms of cross-talk across sensory channels? If only some forms of synaesthesia are conscious, doesn't consciousness at least make a difference? These questions come with normative constraints, asking us to go beyond superficial similarities between a large variety of phenomena, to see whether they share some relevant commonality, or where the differences are.

I.2 Revising our definitions of perception

These questions raise new challenges for philosophers, who have to accept that they need to move beyond the quasi-idealized version of synaesthesia they have held over the last decades.[4] The assumption that synaesthetic experiences behave exactly like a perceptual experience, except for being anomalous and non-veridical, made them too quickly look like another kind of illusion or hallucination. The specific as well as the general lessons of synaesthesia might have been lost in this assimilation.

Isn't the systematic correlation with the external world sufficient to consider synaesthetic experiences as perceptual? The insistence on veridicality after all can be bargained for a set of accuracy conditions, which can relate the experience of, say, the colour yellow to the occurrence of a middle C. The fact that the synaesthetic colour comes hand in hand with the experience of the musical note, and perhaps as an enrichment of its content,[5] means that the synaesthete can eventually use it as further evidence that the note was played, and to form the true belief that they heard middle C.

Not being shared is certainly not a reason to consider a certain kind of experience as non-genuinely perceptual, or illusory. Take the case of taste perception: due to genetic determinants, certain perceivers (super-tasters) have an experience that very few other tasters share, and taste intense bitterness where others taste nothing. It has been argued that flavour perception, because of this genetic and other acquired

[4] E.g. Auvray and Deroy, 2015 for a review and discussion. [5] Deroy, 2015.

differences, makes us all live in 'different taste-worlds'[6] similar to the 'private islands' that Patricia Duffy describes in her opening story. In a more conceptual fashion, the so-called 'inverted spectrum' thought experiment[7] presses the same point: if the qualitative experience an individual has when they see ripe apricots, oranges, and mandarins is similar to the ones the rest of us have when seeing limes or leaves, and vice-versa, the individual, unique character of their experience doesn't rule out that they are having a perception. Likewise, the idiosyncratic difference exhibited by synesthetic experiences is not sufficient to say that they are not perceptual.

More generally, the definitions and descriptions of synaesthesia given in the scientific literature all seem to converge on its inclusion as perception—for criteria which seem to be to do with the underlying mechanism. Synesthesia is defined as 'the stimulation of one sensory modality reliably caus[ing] a perception in one or more different senses' (Cytowic, 1997) or as an 'anomalous sensory perception' (Asher et al., 2009). One way to think of synesthesia might be as a case of 'indirect stimulation' occurring when 'stimulation of one sensory modality automatically triggers a perception in a second modality, in the absence of any direct stimulation to this second modality' (e.g., Baron-Cohen et al., 2007). An important question to ask, then, is whether we should insist on the difference between direct and indirect stimulation (Cohen, Chapter 3 of this volume) or welcome cases of non-retinal vision as instances of 'phantom perception', as proposed by Pearson and Westbrook (2015).

I.3 Accepting arbitrariness and missing control

New questions need to be answered before we can decide how conscious cases of synaesthesia compare to other cases of multisensory interactions, notably cases where one automatically forms a mental image in a non-stimulated sensory modality. Is the difference to be found in the fact that synesthetic experiences really present themselves like perceptual experiences, whereas mental images remain subjectively distinguishable from perceptual experiences? Is this indistinguishability sufficient to consider synaesthetic experiences as perceptual?

An important question to consider here concerns the mechanisms that differentiate between sensations that are under voluntary and involuntary control. Is there a distinct mechanism that explains why we have the sensation of voluntarily inducing or changing a mental image, and could such a volitional mechanism also be present during synaesthesia, but missed by synaesthetes who would then feel the mental image to be involuntary? The latter possibility shows that synaesthesia might have to do with a failure not of control, but of being metacognitively aware of such control.

Of all the neural accounts of synaesthesia that are currently available—i.e., disinhibition of feedback, a breakdown of modularity, enhanced neural connectivity, or

[6] Bartoshuk et al., 1996. [7] Block, 1978.

neural cross-talk[8]—none makes a strong prediction regarding such discontinuity between the synaesthetic and non-synaesthetic brain. If the available evidence seems to point to there being a critical period for the development of synaesthesia, probably only in those with a genetic predisposition to develop the condition, this does not rule out the existence of transient or weaker forms of synaesthesia in the rest of the population.[9]

But how weak can the effects of a connection between sensory areas or sensory domains be to still count as synaesthesia? What if these connections make no difference to the conscious experience we have, or to the categorizations or discriminations we make? Is the apparently arbitrary character of the association, which is characteristic of both the conscious and unconscious cases, sufficient to be defined as synaesthesia?

I.4 Redrawing the distinction between the senses

If it is possible to hear colours or experience colours as a result of auditory stimulation, synesthesia suggests that the senses are not as separated as we commonly think and cannot be individuated by pairs of characteristic stimuli and experiences. It is therefore a challenge to modularity and the individuation of the senses.[10]

If pairs of stimuli and experiences start to appear as far too simple, shall we not look further into the sensory pathways that are activated during non-synaesthetic and synaesthetic experiences? Brain imaging studies have revealed that synaesthetic experiences often involve increased activation in primary sensory brain areas. For instance, when synaesthetes hear an auditory inducer that triggers colours for them, there is increased activity in the area in the fusiform gyrus known as V4 or V8; that is, the brain areas involved when non-synaesthetes perceive colours. Interestingly, such increased activation does not occur in non-synaesthetes trained to associate sounds with colours and who are subsequently asked to visually imagine the corresponding colour when hearing the sound. Other—not strictly sensory—areas of the brain (i.e., parietal and frontal regions) also show specific patterns of activation in some synaesthetes. Synaesthesia is likely to be characterized more broadly as an increased cortical connectivity between various sensory brain regions, either directly or indirectly (via the mediation of non-sensory processing). Further questions then arise as to whether the increased connectivity comes from a lack of inhibition or from an abnormal increase in connectivity. Localization of the activity might also end up playing a less crucial role than finer structural or functional differences in terms of the neural correlates of synaesthesia.

[8] See Rouw et al., 2011. [9] See Martino and Marks, 2001; Simner, 2012.
[10] E.g. Deroy, 2015 ; Segal, 1997; Keeley, 2013.

More recently, doubts have also arisen as to whether shared localization in V4/V8 from bold activity means that the same kinds of neurons are active in synaesthetic colour-enriched auditory experience and non-synaesthetic colour experiences. A study by Van Leeuwen et al. (2010) revealed that the neurons involved in synaesthetic experiences do not show the same patterns of suppression through repetition as the ones involved in typical perception, concluding that 'the neural correlates of synaesthetic colour experience and real colour experience are not fully shared'.[11]

A cautious note is needed here, given the obvious need for further exploration and empirical research, but also the dependence between the neuroscientific investigation and the conceptual questions highlighted before: if it is not clear that there is a unified condition called 'synaesthesia', which is the same in coloured-grapheme, coloured-hearing, and taste-words synaesthetes, and which also includes mirror-touch phenomena or spatial-number cases, the underlying mechanisms of synaesthesia might be much more varied and complex than expected.

I.5 Overview

As the range of sensory blending documented as synaesthetic becomes wider, researchers like Lawrence Marks (Chapter 1) admit spending 'much time and energy chasing down the elusive creature known as synesthesia'. 'Early in this quest', Marks reflects, 'I thought I'd caught up with it: I was poised, ready to snare it—only to watch it get away. Apparently, my first synesthesia-catcher was too small, and insufficiently flexible, to capture a critter at once so large and agile'.

Saying that synaesthesia is getting larger is almost a euphemism: some, like Jonathan Cohen (Chapter 3), consider that synaesthesia might be a pervasive trait of sensory processing, where one sense modality draws on the information present in another sensory stream. The challenge raised by Cohen in this respect is not to accept that atypical cases of coloured graphemes or coloured hearing might present distinctive characters, but to question why they should not be seen as continuous with typical cases of sensory integration.

However, the extension of the list of synaesthetic phenomena also depends how synaesthesia is assessed and measured, as discussed by Yasmina Jraissati (Chapter 4). Crucially, extending the list of synaesthetic phenomena also depends on whether one thinks that synaesthesia blurs into perception, something which is at the centre of the debate between Casey O'Callaghan (Chapter 2), Mohan Matthen (Chapter 8), and Michael Sollberger (Chapter 9). As Merleau-Ponty noted, and as discussed by André Abath (Chapter 7), the same question might arise for a broader range of less conscious synaesthetic effects, which might come to play an unnoticed role in everyday perception.

[11] See also Hupe et al., 2012.

Obviously, though, the occurrence of anomalous, arbitrary conscious experiences is still the sore point which raises questions for our theories of consciousness (as discussed by Myrto Mylopoulos and Tony Ro, in Chapter 5) and our models of perceptual circuitry (as detailed by Berit Brogaard, in Chapter 6). It is perhaps the systematic and involuntary character of the conscious experience, more than its unusual content, which makes synaesthesia so special, as Charles Spence and I argue in Chapter 10.

What then of the boundaries of synaesthesia? Pharmacological agents, in particular serotonin agonists, have consistently been shown to produce synaesthesia-like experiences, but whether such experiences are associated with the same behavioural markers as genuine synaesthesia remains unknown. Associative training, notably under hypnosis or following the loss of sight, is also accompanied by more or less transient forms of synaesthetic experiences, with black shapes or sounds starting to elicit colour experiences. What would be the marker of synaesthesia that could decide on whether these phenomena are continuous with the more canonical developmental cases? This is discussed in Chapters 11 and 12 respectively by Devin Blair Terhune, David P. Luke, and Roi Cohen Kadosh; and Malika Auvray and Mirko Farina.

Even developmental cases and non-transient cases raise new questions: in mirror-touch or mirror-pain cases, for instance, individuals experience a conscious tactile or painful sensation on the same body part as the person they observe being touched or hurt. Is this 'synaesthesia', or is the connection not arbitrary enough to count as such? Would the idea of vicarious experience do a better job, as suggested by Frédérique de Vignemont in Chapter 13? The question is not terminological and asks which cases we should see as related; it arises acutely when considering cases of blendings which are more frequent in synaesthetes, but not specific to them, like the tendency to attribute genders or personality traits to inanimate objects—a case of personification with which Noam Sagiv, Monika Sobczak-Edmans, and Adrian L. Williams conclude in Chapter 14. These series of cases question the function of such apparently arbitrary conscious experiences—i.e. whether they arise out of certain learning conditions or subserve a social or memory function.

Overall, these contributions stress the increased relevance synaesthesia has for our understanding of the mind. They also show why this relevance depends on philosophical and neuroscientific issues being addressed together: the lessons of synaesthesia depend on the definition and extension that the category takes, and how one chooses to draw the boundaries of the condition, or individuate its various forms. Functionalist and physicalist criteria, and *a priori* distinctions between perception and mental imagery, are all challenged by the cases discussed here. Synaesthesia in this respect might be unique in having offered, since its very first discussions in the early decades of the nineteenth century, a forum where the criteria for individuating psychological kinds have always come into tension, and generated opposite solutions. What it shows now, more than ever, is how conceptual and empirical challenges need to be addressed together.

Acknowledgements

I am very grateful to the Arts and Humanities Research Council and the University of London for sustained support for the research that has led to this volume. Many colleagues, collaborators, and postdoctoral students have been an inspiration and a source of instruction on this path, and their contribution to the present volume, as well as their patience all through its completion, are the best testimonies of the intellectual friendship that academic life can create. I would particularly like to thank Malika Auvray and Charles Spence, who were my first interlocutors and collaborators on the topic of sensory blendings. Additional thanks should go to Amir Amedi, Paul Boghossian, Ned Block, Yi-Chuan Chen, Sam Coleman, Paul Coates, Tim Crane, Merle Fairhurst, Chris Frith, Vittorio Gallese, Vincent Hayward, Ron Kupers, Anthony Marcel, Peter Momtchiloff, Bence Nanay, Matthew Nudds, Daniel Ospina and the Crossmodalists,David Papineau, Christopher Peacocke, Maurice Ptito, Joelle Proust, David Rosenthal, Nick Shea, Dan Sperber, and the members of the NASH, Ana Tajadura-Jimenez, and Manos Tsakiris, for the rich discussions that have formed the background to this volume. Among the most precious friendships and sources of support and intellectual stimulation to have blended with this volume is the one I have had the pleasure to share at the Centre for the Study of the Senses with Barry Smith.

References

Asher, J. E., Lamb, J. A., Brocklebank, D., Cazier, J. B., Maestrini, E., Addis, L., Sen, M., Baron-Cohen, S., and Monaco, A. P. (2009) A whole-genome scan and fine-mapping linkage study of auditory-visual synesthesia reveals evidence of linkage to chromosomes 2q24, 5q33, 6p12, and 12p12. *American Journal of Human Genetics*, 84(2), 279–85.

Auvray, M. and Deroy, O. (2015) Synaesthesia: How synaesthetes experience the world, in Matthen, M. (2015) *Oxford Handbook of Philosophy of Perception*, Oxford: Oxford University Press.

Bargary, G. and Mitchell, K. J. (2008) Synaesthesia and cortical connectivity. *Trends in Neuroscience*, 31(7), 335–42.

Baron-Cohen, S., Bor, D., Billington, J., Asher, J., Wheelwright, S., and Ashwin, C. (2007) Savant memory in a man with colour form-number synaesthesia and Asperger syndrome. *Journal of Consciousness Studies*, 14(9–10), 237–51.

Bartoshuk, L. M., Duffy, V. B., Reed, D., and Williams, A. (1996). Supertasting, earaches and head injury: Genetics and pathology alter our taste worlds. *Neuroscience & Biobehavioral Reviews*, 20(1), 79–87.

Block, N. (1978) Troubles with functionalism. In C. W. (ed.), *Minnesota Studies in the Philosophy of Science*, vol. IX. Minneapolis: University of Minnesota Press. Repr. in N. Block (ed.), *Readings in Philosophy of Psychology* (pp. 268–305). Cambridge, MA: Harvard University Press.

Cytowic, R. E. (1997) Synesthesia: Phenomenology and neuropsychology. In S. Baron-Cohen (ed.), *Synesthesia: Classic and Contemporary Readings* (pp. 17–39). Oxford: Blackwell.

Deroy, O. (2013) Synaesthesia: An experience of the third kind? In R. Brown (ed), *Consciousness Inside and Out: Phenomenology, Neuroscience, and the Nature of Experience. Studies in Brain and Mind* (pp. 395–407). Amsterdam: Springer Press.

Deroy, O. (2015) Synaesthesia as enriched experience, in Coates, P. and Coleman, S. (eds.), *Phenomenal Qualities: Sense, Perception, and Consciousness* (pp. 376–399). Oxford: Oxford University Press.

Deroy, O. and Spence, C. (2013) Training, hypnosis, and drugs: Artificial synaesthesia, or artificial paradises? *Front. Psychol.*, 4, 660.

Duffy, P. L. (2001) *Blue Cats and Chartreuse Kittens: How Synaesthetes Color their World.* New York: Times Books.

Hupé, J. M., Bordier, C., and Dojat, M. (2012) The neural bases of grapheme–colour synesthesia are not localized in real colour-sensitive areas. *Cerebral Cortex*, 22(7), 1622–33.

Keeley, B. L. (2013) What exactly is a sense? In J. Simner and E. Hubbard (eds), *The Oxford Handbook of Synaesthesia.* Oxford: Oxford University Press.

Leeuwen (van), T. M., Petersson, K. M., and Hagoort, P. (2010) Synaesthetic colour in the brain: Beyond colour areas. A functional magnetic resonance imaging study of synaesthetes and matched controls. *PLoS ONE*, 5(8), e12074.

Martino, G. and Marks, L. E. (2001) Synesthesia: Strong and weak. *Current Directions in Psychological Science*, 10(2), 61–5.

Pearson, J. and Westbrook, F. (2015) Phantom perception: Voluntary and involuntary nonretinal vision. *Trends in Cognitive Sciences*, 19(5), 278–84.

Rouw, R., Scholte, H. S., and Colizoli, O. (2011). Brain areas involved in synaesthesia: a review. *Journal of Neuropsychology*, 5(2), 214–42.

Segal, G. (1997) Synaesthesia: Implications for the modularity of mind. In S. Baron-Cohen and J. E. Harrison (eds), *Synaesthesia: Classic and Contemporary Reading* (pp. 211–24). Oxford: Basil Blackwell.

Simner, J. (2012) Defining synaesthesia. *British Journal of Psychology*, 103(1), 1–15.

Ward, J. (2013) *Synesthesia. Annual Review of Psychology*, 64, 49–75.

PART I

Defining and Measuring Synaesthesia

1

Synesthesia, Then and Now

Lawrence E. Marks

Over a good part of my scientific career, I've spent much time and energy chasing down an elusive creature known as synesthesia.[1] Early in this quest, I thought I'd caught up with it: I was poised, ready to snare it—only to watch it get away. Apparently, my first synesthesia-catcher was too small, and insufficiently flexible, to capture a critter at once so large and agile.

When I began to study synesthesia (Marks, 1975, 1978b), the topic had already been a matter of inquiry for roughly a century, with scores of articles and books already written about it. Many of these early works discussed colored hearing (*audition colorée*, *Farbenhören*), the evocation of color sensations or color images by sounds (e.g., Bleuler and Lehmann, 1881; Flournoy, 1893), or colored graphemes, the evocation of color sensations or images by (achromatic) numbers, letters, or digits (e.g., Galton, 1880, 1883; Flournoy, 1893; Calkins, 1895). The term synesthesia, however, is itself not quite so old. Flournoy (1893) was apparently the first to use *synesthésie* in its modern sense, applying it not only to colored hearing, colored graphemes, and other examples of visual synesthesia or synopsia, but also to the anomalous arousal of sensations and images of all modalities: auditory, tactile, gustatory, and olfactory, as well as visual. Synesthesia, in one form or another, is relatively uncommon, being found in about 4 percent of the population, according to the most recent and most authoritative study of its prevalence (Simner et al., 2006). Flournoy used *synopsie* to designate the topic of his own research, which focused on the evocation of visual (optic) synesthesia. But *esthesis* casts a wider net than *opsis*, and the term *synesthesia* has stuck.

At first, I viewed synesthesia primarily from the perspective of sensory processing (Marks, 1975, 1978b), fully expecting that an understanding of sensory processes would help elucidate the mechanisms of synesthesia. At the same time, recognizing that perceptual processing involves multisensory as well as unisensory mechanisms

[1] This chapter is abridged and revised from: Lawrence E. Marks, Synesthesia, Then and Now, originally published in *Intellectica* (2011), 51, 47–80, copyright by the Association pour la Recherche Cognitive and published here by permission.

(Marks, 1978a), I had hoped that a better understanding of synesthesia might, in turn, shed further light on mechanisms of sensory information processing, especially multisensory processing. My prototype for synesthesia at the time was visual hearing—the ways that, in a very small fraction of people, acoustic stimuli produce not only auditory percepts of sound but visual sensations as well: Speech may evoke colors, or melodies may evoke moving patterns or shapes.

A fruitful approach to begin studying human sensory processing in general is psychophysical: the systematic investigation of the ways that basic perceptual attributes, such as the pitch, loudness, and timbre of sounds, depend on pertinent aspects of the physical stimulus, such as acoustic spectrum. Extending this psychophysical perspective to synesthesia, it is possible to ask how the hue and brightness, the shape and motion, of a synesthetic visual response depend on the temporal and spectral distributions of an inducing sound's acoustic spectrum. A striking outcome of this psychophysical approach is the simple mapping, in several instances, between nonsynesthetic and synesthetic psychophysical relations. To a first approximation, both the nonsynesthetic perception of auditory pitch and the synesthetic perception of visual lightness and brightness are monotone increasing functions of sound frequency (Marks, 1975).[2] This outcome implies, in turn, that synesthetic lightness and brightness relate directly to auditory pitch (see Marks, 2011: 48–50 for detailed discussion).

The psychophysical relation between the brightness of induced color and the pitch of inducing sound serves to quantify a principle first suggested by Bleuler and Lehmann (1881) and Flournoy (1893), dubbed in both cases a *law of brightness* (*Helligkeitsgesetz, loi de clarté*). Findings of this sort appeared especially compatible with the view that sensory processes underlie synesthesia. Even if sensory processes do provide an underpinning to synesthesia, however, synesthesia can also reveal itself in higher-level cognitive processes, especially to the extent that these higher-level processes capitalize on lower-level sensory information, as information from synesthetic perception is made available to more abstract cognitive systems, such as language.

A broad, inclusive account of synesthesia would embrace both its functions in perception and its manifestations in cognition. After all, sensory and perceptual processes themselves play a substantial role in cognitive processing—*nihil est in intellectu quod non prius fuerit in sensu*. So it is not surprising that synesthesia plays a role in both the senses and the intellect. This approach to the study of synesthesia rests on the heuristic principle that sensation and cognition are

[2] Technically, brightness applies to the perception of luminous objects, varying along a dimension that runs from dim to bright. Lightness applies to the perception of reflecting surfaces, varying along a dimension that runs from dark to light—in the case of achromatic surfaces, from black to white. In visual-auditory synesthetes, and in the perception of similarity in nonsynesthetes, visual brightness and lightness both correlate closely with auditory pitch, although only brightness but not lightness correlates closely with loudness.

continuous and contiguous processes, connected and overlapping; as Alexander Pope (*An Essay on Man*) suggested, 'Remembrance and reflection how allied/What thin partitions sense from thought divide.'

1.1 Synesthesia and the 'unity of the senses'

The theoretical framework for understanding synesthesia that I described nearly forty years ago is neatly characterized by the expression 'the unity of the senses' (Marks, 1978b)—a term borrowed from Hornbostel (1925) and Werner (1934), who both used it to emphasize the argument, considered heterodox early in the twentieth century, that sensory systems act in concert and not in isolation, dependently and not independently. As both asserted, the senses of sight, hearing, touch, taste, and smell interrelate and interact. Borrowing again, this time from Charles Baudelaire's poem *Correspondances*, we might say that the senses speak a common language—in the poet's words, '*les parfums, les couleurs et les sons se répondent.*' From my vantage point in 1978, synesthesia in perception represented a dramatic example of sensory unity, an extension and elaboration of the broader view that synesthesia is importantly—indeed, fundamentally—a sensory phenomenon (see also Cytowic, 1989).

The conceptual framework captured in the expression 'unity of the senses' rests, in large measure, on a *Weltanschauung* often found in science, especially in physics; an approach to understanding the world that seeks to discern uniformities and coherence in apparent diversity, an approach that Isaiah Berlin (1953) famously associated with hedgehogs as opposed to foxes—attributing to Aristarchus the remark that 'the hedgehog knows one great thing while the fox knows many little things.' By this account, the cadre of hedgehogs includes Sensory Unitarians. And to a Sensory Unitarian, synesthesia can be paradigmatic. Striking in this regard is the evidence that analogous psychophysical principles can characterize both the perception of those relatively few individuals who experience vivid synesthetic perception and the perception and cognition of the vast majority of individuals, who may show synesthetic tendencies, but who do not experience synesthesia *per se*. Evidence of widespread, perhaps universal, synesthetic tendencies in perception and cognition suggests that synesthesia may rest substantially on mechanisms of sensory processing that are found in everyone, not just synesthetes (Marks, 1978b; see also Ward et al., 2006).

1.2 Synesthetic perception

Synesthesia commonly refers to the curious experiences reported by a small fraction of the population, in whom, to give one example, sounds may reliably, consistently, and automatically induce visual sensations, images, or qualities. To a person with auditory-visual synesthesia, music or voices may evoke colors or shapes, as when the composer Rimsky-Korsakov reported 'seeing' music in the key of A-major as yellow

(Myers, 1911). These induced sensations, images, or qualities are vivid and can sometimes interact with the processing of nonsynesthetic perceptual information, for example in perceptual grouping (Ramachandran and Hubbard, 2001; Kim et al., 2006) and in synesthetic analogs to Stroop interference. In a task requiring subjects to identify the colors of digits printed in red and green ink, a person with digit-color synesthesia who sees 3 as synesthetically red or 5 as synesthetically green may find it relatively difficult to quickly and accurately identify a green 3 or a red 5, due to interference from the synesthetic colors (e.g., Mills et al., 1999; Dixon et al., 2000; Mattingley et al., 2001).

Synesthesia is multifaceted, in part because it assumes so many forms. Synesthetes may experience a gamut of hues and shapes when they hear music or voice, or they may experience different hues when they view achromatic printed letters or numbers. Synesthetes may see colors in pains, or taste flavors in words. Or they may see sequences of numbers, days of the week, or months of the year as laid out in space, each number, day, or month having its location in a one-dimensional, two-dimensional, or even three-dimensional array (e.g., Eagleman, 2009). Many neuroscientists in particular limit the domain of synesthesia proper to these phenomena, which I have elsewhere called *vivid synesthesia* (Marks, 2009). There is mounting evidence that the experience of vivid synesthesia is correlated with patterns of neural activity in the brain that differ from the patterns observed, under comparable stimulus conditions, in the brains of nonsynesthetes (e.g., Nunn et al., 2002; Hubbard et al., 2005; Hubbard and Ramachandran, 2005) and that synesthesia, long known to run in families, has a genetic component (Baron-Cohen et al., 1996; Barnett et al., 2008; Asher et al., 2009).[3]

1.3 Synesthetic tendencies in perception

Sometimes, synesthesia is also taken to refer to a set of much more common, and much less idiosyncratic, perceptual experiences than those evidenced in vivid synesthesia. These *synesthetic tendencies*, to use the terminology of Osgood (1960), encompass several well-grounded and widespread perceptual similarities between and among sensory experiences in different modalities. Much as the color aqua is more similar phenomenologically to cerulean than to pink, the flavor of lime more similar to lemon than to banana, so too are low notes played on a bassoon or an organ more like dark colors such as brown or black than bright colors such as yellow or white, while the higher notes played on a clavier or flute resemble yellow or white more than brown or black.

[3] The evidence applies to what has been called idiopathic or developmental synesthesia. It is also possible that there are specific neural correlates to acquired forms of synesthesia, for example to synesthesia resulting, say, from brain injury, disease, or ingestion of psychoactive drugs—entailing, of course, an underlying neuroanatomical substrate having its own genetic basis.

Few people are vividly synesthetic. Most of us do not see colors or shapes when we hear voices or when we listen to music. Nevertheless, most of us do recognize or appreciate similarities between sensory experiences in different modalities. When asked, 'which is brighter, a cough or a sneeze?', most of us readily acknowledge that sneezes are brighter—perhaps because sneezes are more compact in terms of the distribution of energy over time, 'sharper,' if you will, and generically higher in pitch. So the connection between brightness and pitch does not typify vivid perceptual synesthesia alone, but also typifies synesthetic tendencies. And synesthetic tendencies, in turn, may be universal, or nearly so.

Many of the principles that characterize synesthesia—in particular, many of the rules of cross-sensory correspondence in individuals with auditory-visual synesthesia—also characterize synesthetic tendencies in individuals who lack synesthesia. Nonsynesthetic subjects systematically set higher frequencies to match surfaces with greater luminous reflectance, for example, implying a correspondence between auditory pitch and visual lightness, analogous to the correspondence observed in auditory-visual synesthesia (e.g., Marks, 1974; T. Hubbard, 1996; Ward et al., 2006; for additional examples, see Marks, 2011).

Auditory-visual correspondences are commonly found in several domains: between pitch and brightness/lightness (higher-pitched sounds induce brighter responses in synesthetes and are judged by nonsynesthetes to be more similar to brighter than dimmer/darker colors); between loudness and brightness (louder sounds induce brighter responses in synesthetes and are judged by nonsynesthetes to be more similar to brighter lights); between pitch and size (higher-pitched sounds induce smaller-sized visual images in synesthetes and are judged by nonsynesthetes to be more similar to smaller sizes); and between pitch and shape (higher-pitched sounds induce more angular and pointed visual images in synesthetes and are judged by nonsynesthetes to be similar to more angular and pointed shapes). A possible example of this last principle is the well-known pair of abstract figures that Köhler (1947) constructed, an angular figure that people readily matched to the name 'takete', with it high-pitched consonants and vowels, and a rounded figure that people readily matched to the lower-pitched 'maluma' (a finding replicated by Ramachandran and Hubbard, 2001, who used similar figures and the names 'kiki' and 'bouba'; for review, see Spector and Maurer, 2009).

1.4 Synesthesia versus synesthetic tendencies

All of this said, synesthesia and synesthetic tendencies are far from being identical. Synesthesia and synesthetic tendencies differ phenomenologically, of course, in that synesthetes report actually experiencing sensory transfers—to an auditory-visual or grapheme-color synesthete, sounds or letters of the alphabet actually evoke color experiences. Evidence from neuroimaging studies shows activity in regions of the brains of synesthetes that are also specifically activated by optic stimuli—for instance, reports of synesthetic colors correlate with activity in regions, such as V4, that are activated by chromatic visual stimuli. Evidence of this sort, discussed further at the end of this chapter, lends additional credence to the phenomenal reports. Nevertheless, it is possible, as also considered later, that the difference between perception in synesthetes and in nonsynesthetes is a matter of degree rather than kind.

Be this as it may, there appear to be a couple of crucial differences between the transfers or translations of sensory quality experienced in vivid synesthesia and the cross-modal similarities or correspondences between qualities revealed in synesthetic tendencies: These differences reside in the extent to which synesthesia and synesthetic tendencies are absolute versus relative, and rigid versus malleable.

First, synesthetic tendencies are largely relativistic. The level of a sound's pitch or loudness that people judge to be most similar to the brightness of a visual stimulus depends strongly on the stimulus context; for instance, on the range of possible stimulus levels. When people who do not report experiencing vivid synesthesia compare sounds and lights, they tend to match the brightest light to the highest-pitched and loudest sound of the stimulus ensemble, regardless of their absolute levels (Marks, 1989). Vivid synesthesia, on the other hand, appears more absolute. People with auditory-visual synesthesia show much more precise and consistent matches of colors with sounds than do people who do not report synesthesia (Ward et al., 2006; but see also Arnold et al., 2012). Indeed, long-term consistency is a hallmark of vivid synesthesia, and is used by many as a 'test of genuineness' (Baron-Cohen et al., 1987), a criterion for validating the presence of synesthesia (e.g., Rich et al., 2005; Simner et al., 2006; Barnett et al., 2008). This said, we still do not know just how absolute or relative synesthesia itself may be: To what extent do the psychophysical properties of vivid synesthetic experience depend on stimulus context? To the best of my knowledge, no studies to date have quantified whether and how, for example, the brightness, color, size, or shape of vividly experienced visual synesthesia depends on the context of the inducing acoustic events.

Second, where the cross-modal transfers of sensory quality that characterize vivid synesthesia are generally rigid and often automatic, cross-modal similarities observed in synesthetic tendencies are much more flexible (e.g., Marks, 1974, 1989; see also Gertner et al., 2009). It is perfectly possible, for instance, to instruct a person to match stimuli in a manner that contravenes the rules of cross-modal similarity; for example, to match bright colors to low-pitched or soft sounds rather than high-pitched or loud ones. This capacity reveals a kind of flexibility to cross-modal similarity that vivid synesthetic perception lacks. Cross-modal similarity is controlled, or can be controlled, by relatively high-level cognitive mechanisms that can operate on abstract representations of sensory dimensions, a property that also characterizes metaphor. It may also be sensitive to cultural conventions. As Gardner (1974) wrote, 'Which particular line, face, description, etc., is metaphorically linked to loudness is a communal decision dependent, in part, on the alternatives available and the nature of the surrounding context' (85).

1.5 Synesthetic tendencies in children

Cross-modal similarities (synesthetic tendencies) reveal themselves in the perceptual behavior of young children and infants. So, for example, children as young as four years of age readily match the higher-pitched of two tones to the brighter of two lights (Marks et al., 1987). Indeed, there are even reports that infants as young as one month will implicitly 'match' greater loudness to greater brightness (Lewkowicz and Turkewitz, 1980) and that infants at two to three months of age will respond preferentially to dynamic sounds and visual stimuli that change congruently, increasing in pitch with rising spatial position or increasing figural angularity (Walker et al., 2010), dynamic change being critical (Jeschonek et al., 2012).

Some intersensory similarities, such as those between pitch and brightness and between loudness and brightness, are probably 'hard-wired,' although not all may be. Marks et al. (1987) found that most young children (4–5 years of age), like most adults, matched both the higher-pitched of two equally loud sounds and the louder of two equal-pitch sounds to the brighter of two lights. But most 4–5-year-olds did not match the lower-pitched of two sounds to the larger of two visual images; pitch-size matching did not become consistent until about age eleven. It is possible, for example, that the inverse similarity relation between pitch and size (lower pitch corresponding to larger size) is learned through experience, in particular through experience with the resonance properties of objects, as several investigators have suggested (e.g., Osgood et al., 1957; but see Mondloch and Maurer, 2004, for evidence that children as young as three years can recognize pitch-size similarity). For extended discussion, see Marks (2011: 55–9).

There is an ecological association between lower sound frequency and larger size, based in principles of physics. Given objects constructed of the same material, the larger objects will have greater mass and consequently will resonate at lower sound frequencies than will smaller ones (Osgood et al., 1957; Marks et al., 1987). Children are generally smaller than adults, with smaller vocal apparatus and higher-pitched voices, a relation that young children doubtless come to recognize. In reciting to a child the story of 'The Three Bears' (*Les Trois Ours*), a parent is likely to assume a deep voice for *le grand ours*, with increasingly higher-pitched voices for *le moyen ours* and *le petit ours*.

Even if a few intersensory relationships are learned, as some undoubtedly must be, it is plausible that several are 'built into' the nervous system, perhaps reflecting overlapping neural codes, in different modalities, for sensory dimensions such as pitch, loudness, and brightness (Marks and Bornstein, 1987; see also Walsh, 2003). If so, then it is also plausible to infer, despite the phenomenological difference between synesthesia and cross-modal similarity, that both share, at least in part, a core of common mechanisms of sensorineural coding. That is, it is plausible that common codes for pitch and brightness manifest themselves in a small portion of the population as auditory-visual synesthesia, and in the vast majority of the population as similarity—although the precise nature of the underlying coding mechanisms need to be clarified.

1.6 Synesthetic tendencies in language and metaphor

Synesthesia is sometimes taken to refer not only to the experiences of vivid perceptual synesthesia but also to certain tropes of language, to 'the perception, or *description of the perception* [italics mine], of one sense modality in terms of another' (Preminger, 1974: 839). Synesthetic cognition, a short-hand for the cognitive expression of synesthetic tendencies, includes the construction and comprehension of cross-modal metaphors found in many languages—often in well-worn expressions of daily life, such as 'loud colors.' Synesthetic cognition also includes the far more esoteric synesthetic metaphors of poetic language, as when the poet Conrad Aiken, in *The House of Dust*, contrasts 'violins . . . weaving a weft of silver' to 'horns . . . weaving a lustrous brede of gold' or when Wallace Stevens, in *Parochial Themes*, describes how 'The wind blows. In the wind, the voices/Have shapes that are not yet fully themselves,/Are sounds blown by a blower into shapes,/The blower squeezed to the thinnest *mi* of falsetto.'

Synesthetic cognition is closely linked to synesthetic tendencies in perception, and therefore to synesthesia. This is especially clear in the evidence that the rules of cross-modal correspondence or similarity hold in language much as they do in perception. Where people with vivid synesthesia report that loud or high-pitched sounds induce bright images, and where most (nonsynesthetic) people note a perceptual resemblance between bright lights and relatively loud or high-pitched sounds, so do most people interpret cross-modal metaphors along similar lines: Words or phrases referring to acoustic events that are judged as soft or low in pitch are also judged as dim, whereas words or phrases referring to acoustic events judged loud or high in pitch are also judged as bright; conversely, words or phrases referring to optic events described as dim (or bright) are also judged as low-pitched and soft (or high-pitched and loud) (Marks, 1982; Marks et al., 1987).

The close connection between synesthetic tendencies in perception (cross-modal similarity) and in language (cross-modal metaphor) is also evident in children, albeit with one important caveat: Synesthetic tendencies are much stronger, or at least more prevalent at a given age, when measured in perceptual tasks compared to verbal tasks (Marks et al., 1987). Synesthetic tendencies observed in language lag behind analogous tendencies observed in perception, and this outcome is consistent with the hypothesis that the cross-modal similarities arise in perception itself, then become available to higher-level, cognitive mechanisms, such as language. In his review of the ways that adjectives in a given language transfer their meanings over time, from one sense modality to another—that is, 'synesthetically'—Williams (1976) suggested the possibility that common principles operate in various Indo-European languages and in Japanese; Shen and Aisenman (2008) provided related evidence for a common principle of semantic transfer, from 'lower' to 'higher' senses, in Hebrew, Arabic, Chinese, Japanese, and Indonesian, as well as English. Perhaps there is a general principle: that semantic changes in various languages reflect, at least in part, perceptual similarities that are available to cognitive mechanisms (see Shen and Aisenman, 2008).

The close relation between synesthetic tendencies in perception and language fits well within the framework of the unity of the senses, in which synesthesia is interpreted as largely a sensory phenomenon that expresses intrinsic similarities in the coding of sensory information in different modalities. Although nonsynesthetic individuals do not share the vivid experiences of synesthetes, nonsynesthetes have linguistic access to the same cross-modal similarities, several of which may arise directly from sensory coding mechanisms. These similarities express themselves initially in perception, from which they become available, through development, to more abstract representations in language. For further discussion of these synesthetic tendencies in perception and language, and relations to metaphor, see Marks (2011).

1.7 The puzzle of synesthesia

There is little doubt that sensory processes can play an important role in synesthesia. To interpret synesthesia within the framework of the unity of the senses entails a critical assumption: that sensory processes play a leading role and not a supporting one. But this interpretation also rests on a second, implicit, assumption—as, I suspect, do most theories in science—namely, that certain pieces of evidence are important to the theory and need to be incorporated into it and explained, while other pieces of evidence should be ignored, either because they are relatively unimportant or, more crucially, because they will ultimately turn out to be irrelevant.

When I first began investigating synesthesia, I felt like a character in the well-known fable of the blind men and the elephant, trying on the basis of limited information to comprehend synesthesia in all of its diversity and complexity. Eventually, it became clear that there is a better metaphor for understanding synesthesia than integrating multiple views (or 'feels') of a pachyderm; namely, solving what might be called a *decoyed jigsaw puzzle*. A standard, run-of-the-mill jigsaw puzzle is clearly defined, in that all of the pieces belong to the puzzle: Put all of the pieces into their proper locations and orientations relative to one another, and the picture is complete, the puzzle solved. A decoyed puzzle, however, contains, as its name implies, not only all of the pieces of a standard puzzle but several extra pieces as well: a bunch of decoys, each of which looks, at first glance, as if it might fit the puzzle. But the decoys don't fit, because they don't belong.

To solve a decoyed puzzle, therefore, one must ignore or discard the extra pieces. But to do this, one must know which pieces are decoys—obvious once the puzzle is solved, but not during the solving. And solving scientific puzzles is made especially difficult because Nature often seems ingenious both at spawning decoys and at concealing until the very end exactly what the completed puzzles will look like.

Lacking predefined algorithms with which they can search for decoys and discard them, scientists typically find themselves engaging, willy-nilly, in practical, bootstrapping strategies, trying to fit together as many pieces as possible, creating tentative hypotheses to decide which pieces of information are likely to be decoys, then setting these pieces to the side, leaving the option of bringing them back into the puzzle-solving game if and when the hypotheses change.

1.8 Varieties of synesthesia

Which pieces matter to the puzzle of synesthesia? And which pieces matter most?

By its etymology, *synesthesia* should be a sensory-perceptual phenomenon. After all, the very name derives from Greek terms denoting a union or combination (*syn*) of sensations or perceptions (*esthesis*)—evident in traditional definitions, such as Warren's (1934): 'a phenomenon characterizing the experiences of certain individuals, in which certain sensations belonging to one sense or mode attach to certain sensations of another group and appear regularly whenever a stimulus of the latter type occurs' (270). Flournoy (1893) was apparently the first to use the term synesthesia (*synesthésie*) in this modern sense. Two millennia earlier, in discussing friendship (*Eudemian Ethics*, *Nicomachean Ethics*), Aristotle used its root, the Greek verb *sunaisthanesai*, in a rather different way. To Aristotle, *sunaisthanesai* 'in all likelihood designated a "feeling in common," a perception shared by more than one [person]' (Heller-Roazen, 2004: 36). Speaking etymologically, we might say that before synesthetic sensation perhaps came synesthetic empathy.

Synesthesia, in its modern sense, comes in an astonishing variety. This would not necessarily pose a problem to sensory accounts if synesthetic responses depended mostly, or most of the time, on relatively low-level sensory features associated with inducing stimuli, such as the pitch and loudness of an auditory inducer. But less and less this seems the case, suggesting that sensory accounts of synesthesia are incomplete. Synesthesia sometimes relies on sensory features of the inducing stimulus. But not always. So it is necessary to consider the range and variety of the pieces to the puzzle, the range and variety of both synesthesia-inducing stimuli and synesthetic responses.

To be sure, there are several different ways to classify or categorize the phenomena that currently fall under the rubric of synesthesia. Flournoy (1893) suggested a pair of terms to denote synesthetic stimuli and responses, which he called *inducteurs* and *induits*; I'll call them *inducers* and *inductants*. Both are diverse. Auditory inducers range widely, from environmental noises and animal sounds to single musical notes, melodies, and human voices, including spoken numbers and words. Visual inducers range from printed numbers and letters to words, but also, notably, may include examples of brief events or episodes—such as the sight of another person being touched (in what has been called *mirror-touch synesthesia*: Blakemore et al., 2005). And inducers include pains, odors, and flavors—flavors themselves being examples *par excellence* of multisensory stimuli. Flavor perceptions result from integrated responses to gustatory, olfactory, and somatosensory signals produced by food stimuli, sometimes influenced also by sound (e.g., food being chewed) and sight (e.g., the color of a food, seen before taking it into the mouth).

In his treatment of synopsia, where all of the inductants are visual, Flournoy (1893) divided inducers into two subcategories, which he designated as *sensorielle* and *psychique*. The first is clearly *sensory*. But Flournoy expressed unhappiness with the second term, as he noted that sensations too, and not only abstract ideas, are *psychique*. Given that Flournoy described mental inducers as 'abstract' and given that his mental inducers included days of the week, numbers, and names, it is reasonable to characterize Flournoy's second subcategory of inducers as *cognitive*. In any case, as Flournoy and others long ago recognized, inducers need not be explicitly sensory, which is to say that synesthetic responses often correlate better with an inducing stimulus's meaning than with its sensory or perceptual qualities.

Synesthetic inductants or responses too can be diverse. Although they often consist of simple colors, inductants, like inducers, can also be more complex. For instance, inductants may be flavors—flavors being, as already noted, multisensory representations of food stimuli. And inductants may be affective responses, feelings of liking or disliking, or personifications, attributes normally associated with people and their personalities, as Flournoy (1893) and others (e.g., Galton, 1880; Calkins, 1895) reported more than a century ago.

It is convenient, therefore, to classify inducers and inductants as perceptual, cognitive, or affective—taking 'perceptual' to include sensory features. And, at the risk of sounding like a character in an operetta by Gilbert and Sullivan who 'knows the scientific names of perceptions *synestheticus*,' as a matter of further convenience I shall classify each variety of inducer-inductant synesthesia by labeling it, for instance, *perceptual-perceptual*, *cognitive-perceptual*, or *cognitive-affective*. The summary that follows is by no means exhaustive, but instead selects a few examples that seem critical to solving the puzzle of synesthesia. Indeed, there are other ways of slicing the synesthetic pie, for example by classifying, where possible, inducers and inductants as cross-dimensional (same modality) or cross-modal (different modalities). Word-color synesthesia, for example, is cross-dimensional when the color is induced by an achromatic visual word, but cross-modal when induced by a spoken word. Just as significant, however, is the extent to which words operate as inducers because of their perceptual characteristics (constituent letters or phonemes) or cognitive ones (semantic content).

1.9 Perceptual-perceptual synesthesia

Perceptual-perceptual synesthesia includes two main subgroups: cross-modal and cross-dimensional. Cross-modal synesthesia includes not only colors, shapes, and other visual characteristics synesthetically induced by sounds, but also colors (and other visual characteristics) induced by pains, touches, tastes, and smells, shapes induced by touches, and so forth. Synesthesia has been, and still often is, defined as a cross-modal phenomenon, in terms of the arousal, by a single sensory stimulus, of sensations or images in two (or more) modalities, and auditory-visual synesthesia surely fits this bill. But the fact of the matter is that cross-modal synesthesia is relatively uncommon, even among synesthetic individuals. In the best study to date of synesthesia's prevalence, Simner et al. (2006) systematically and thoroughly tested 500 university students and found that roughly 4 percent of them (twenty-two in all) showed at least one form, a considerably higher prevalence than earlier research had suggested. Of the twenty-two synesthetes confirmed by evidence of high consistency over time, only one of them showed cross-modal, perceptual-perceptual synesthesia, this being music-color (auditory-visual).

Even when inductants depend on low-level sensory features of the inducer, such as pitch and loudness in auditory-visual synesthesia, the synesthetic responses often, perhaps typically, depend also on the inducer's learned perceptual or cognitive features. This is clear in auditory-visual synesthesia, where speech and music are often the most potent inducers of visual responses, whereas environmental noises generally are not. Speech and music are meaningful constructions of a culture. To be sure, the brightness of a synesthetically evoked color can vary systematically with the pitch of a vowel phoneme or with the pitch height of a musical note—but the synesthetic hue itself depends on the sound perceived as a phoneme of the language or on the note as encoded on a familiar musical scale.

In this regard, music-color synesthesia may have something in common with absolute pitch perception: To a typical music-color synesthete, a given note, such as C or F-sharp, will consistently have its own hue; the brightness of the synesthetic color may vary with the register of the note, but the hue remains constant (e.g., C may be sky blue, brighter in high octaves and dimmer in low ones). To the extent that every musical note is 'named' (identified) by its synesthetic hue, synesthesia confers a degree of 'absoluteness' to pitch perception. Be this as it may, both musical notes and phonemes, like the names of colors, are learned within frameworks defined by a particular culture—its musical scale and its language. Both exemplify perceptual categories that are absorbed through experience in a particular culture (Ward and Simner, 2003), constituting what Marks and Odgaard (2005) called 'cultural artifacts'.

Although some instances of perceptual-perceptual synesthesia are heteromodal, it turns out that many are homomodal, taking place within a single modality. The prototype here is grapheme-color synesthesia, in which achromatically printed letters or numbers, presented visually, evoke color. Grapheme-color synesthesia was first reported more than a century ago (Galton, 1880, 1883; Flournoy, 1893; Calkins, 1893). Because grapheme-color synesthetes are relatively numerous, much current research focuses on this form of synesthesia.

Many of the instances of synesthesia uncovered in the systematic study by Simner et al. (2006) were homomodal, with visual stimuli (letters and/or numbers) inducing colors in ten of the twenty-two synesthetes. Of the ten, eight had colors induced by both letters and number, one by letters alone, and one by numbers alone. Sometimes, at least, synesthetic colors depend on relatively low-level sensory processes. Thus, for example, Hubbard et al. (2006) found that the colors induced in a grapheme-color synesthete depended strongly on the contrast level in the visual stimulus. In a related vein, Ramachandran and Hubbard (2001) reported that induced color could vary with the retinal location of the grapheme inducer much as the color of a chromatic visual stimulus can; they also showed effects of other perceptual processes in the synesthetic responses, such as masking and grouping. Lastly in this regard, a recent study by Nikolić et al. (2007) reported evidence of opponent-color processing in grapheme-color synesthesia. In vision, opponent effects can appear early in the processing of color, evident in responses of retinal neurons (e.g., ganglion cells). Color-opponent cells derive information from wavelength-selective photoreceptors and recode the information into chromatically opponent subsystems, one subsystem coding red versus green colors and the other blue versus yellow colors (for review, see Martin, 1998). Given that opponent-color processing is itself sensory, and given that synesthetic color responses reveal effects of opponent processing, it is plausible to infer that synesthesia can involve sensory processing.

Results such as these do not mean, however, that variations in synesthetic responses must, or must always, reveal sensory or perceptual processing, or that the very same synesthesia cannot reveal both sensory and higher-level cognitive processes. It is useful in this regard to keep in mind a distinction that Garner (1970) made between what he called state limitations and process limitations to human information processing. Consider the ability to make rapid responses to different stimulus events in the face of distraction. Performance may be better or worse depending on the ability of the person to attend selectively and ignore the distracting stimulus (process limitation), but performance may also be better or worse depending on stimulus properties, such as energy or contrast, that affect the ability to detect or discriminate the different events (state limitation), independent of the capacity to attend selectively.

1.10 Cognitive-perceptual and perceptual-cognitive synesthesia

Cognition has long been implicated in synesthesia, where it can play at least two distinctive roles. On the one hand, it is often the meaning of an inducing stimulus that determines the synesthetic response, as in those instances of digit-color synesthesia in which the induced hue depends on the concept of the number. On the other hand, cognition may also be a kind of beneficiary, as when personifications serve to enrich the meaning of numbers by adding animate characteristics. Wheeler (1920) and Wheeler and Cutsforth (1922a) studied sensory, perceptual, and cognitive processes in a blind synesthete, identified in the articles as Cutsforth, who had lost his sight in an accident at age eleven. Despite focusing on the sensory constituents of the synesthetic experiences, especially their color, Wheeler and Cutsforth (1922a, 1922b) argued that synesthesia is not just a sensory or perceptual phenomenon but a cognitive one as well. As they wrote, 'Synaesthesis in our reagent [subject] is not confined to the field of perception; it is a cognitive process per se, pervading his entire life as far as it has been studied; functionally, it differs in no respect from any process of meaning. Synaesthesis is a process of meaning' (Wheeler and Cutsforth, 1922a: 102). Notable was Wheeler and Cutsforth's (1922b) claim that the development of synesthesia plays an important role in perceptual development, and in particular in the development of new systems of meaning, a claim that, although based primarily on introspective evidence, fits comfortably with recent findings (e.g., Simner et al., 2009; Simner and Haywood, 2009).

A related theme was later promulgated by Odbert et al. (1942) and Karwoski et al. (1942). Karwoski and Odbert (1938) had found evidence that the sensory experiences in colored-music synesthesia play a role in cognition, in both representing and augmenting musical meanings. Odbert et al. and Karwoski et al. then showed how the perception of analogous, cross-modal perceptual similarities (synesthetic tendencies) play a comparable role in the cognition of nonsynesthetic individuals.

Recent investigations have asked, experimentally, whether, when, and how synesthetic responses depend on cognitive processes. It has long been known that some grapheme-color synesthetes report colors not only when they look at printed letters or numbers, but also when they think about them. Dixon et al. (2000) showed, in a digit-color synesthete who perceived the number 7 as yellow, that the sum of 5 + 2 also produced yellow. The implication is that the synesthesia is induced, or can be induced, at least in part, conceptually, by the meaning of the number. In some digit-color synesthetes, colors may be evoked by both Arabic and Roman numerals (Ramachandran and Hubbard, 2001), albeit perhaps more strongly by the more familiar Arabic, suggesting that synesthetic responses can be governed by a relatively high-level conception of quantity, rather than low-level sensory or perceptual properties of the inducing stimulus. Cohen Kadosh and Henik (2006) came to a similar conclusion by using a color-interference paradigm to study the effect of varying numeric (conceptual) distance in a digit-color synesthete. It is possible, of course, that some synesthetic inducers gain their power intrinsically or primarily from sensory or perceptual features, while others are intrinsically or primarily cognitive. Ramachandran and Hubbard (2001) offered a distinction between 'lower' and 'higher' forms of synesthesia, roughly corresponding to forms of synesthesia evoked by relatively low-level, perceptual mechanisms and by relatively high-level, cognitive ones (also Grossenbacher and Lovelace, 2001; Cohen Kadosh et al., 2007).

In a related vein, Simner and her colleagues (e.g., Ward and Simner, 2003; Simner and Ward, 2006) have explored extensively what they call *lexical-gustatory* synesthesia—although this form of synesthesia is more precisely designated as lexical-*flavor*; in the chemosensory sciences, 'gustatory' refers to sensory signals that encode only the qualities sweet, sour, salty, bitter, and (perhaps) savory or 'umami,' mediated primarily through the chorda tympani and glossopharyngeal nerves, whereas 'flavor' refers to multisensory signals that make it possible to identify foods and beverages. Flavor percepts integrate gustatory, olfactory, somatosensory, auditory, and visual signals arising from food. In lexical-flavor synesthesia, a form noted more than a century ago (e.g., Pierce, 1907), words evoke specific flavors. In the synesthesia of Pierce's young female subject, the name 'Edith,' for example, evoked the flavor of potato soup, 'Francis' the flavor of baked beans. The findings of Simner and Haywood (2009) suggest a sequence of events in the development of lexical-flavor synesthesia: Flavors come first to be connected to the names of the foods that evoke the flavors, then spread to other words that are connected to the food names, either semantically or phonetically. These findings place language learning at the core of this particular form of synesthesia. Results such as these do not mean, however, that synesthesia must, or must always, involve linguistic (or other cognitive) processing.

1.11 Perceptual-affective and cognitive-affective synesthesia

Two variants of synesthesia are especially curious. One of these is among the longest known forms of synesthesia, the others among the most recent. I shall designate both as *affective*.

More than a century ago, Flournoy (1893) and Calkins (1893, 1895) included within their framework for synesthesia the reports of *personifications*. Calkins described, for example, the ways that letters or numbers could evoke feelings of 'liking' or 'disliking,' and, notably, the physical or psychological characteristics of people. To give an example, one synesthete reported especially disliking the numbers 11, 13, and 17: 'I suppose,' she said, 'because they are prime' (Calkins, 1893: 454). And another noted that 'Ts are generally crabbed, ungenerous creatures. U is a soulless sort of thing. 4 is honest, but mathematically angular and ungraceful. 3 I cannot trust, though it is fairly good-looking in personal appearance. . . . 9 is dark, a gentleman, tall and graceful, but politic under his suavity' (454). The title of a recent article by Smilek et al. (2007) provides two additional examples: 'When "3" is a jerk and "E" is a king.' Simner and Holenstein (2007) reported that personification—the attribution of animate qualities, such as personality traits or genders to letters, numbers, days of the week, and months of the year—shows many of the same characteristics found in other forms of synesthesia (e.g., being consistent and automatic), and that personification can interact with these other forms, from which the authors concluded that personification should therefore be considered as a form of synesthesia.

That personification and (other forms of) synesthesia show similar properties, and indeed can interact, does not prove, of course, that the one is a subset of the other. Is personification a decoy? Or is it one of the pieces critical to solving the puzzle of synesthesia? In designating personification as affective, it should not be assumed that personification is not also cognitive, for personifications certainly contribute to the meaning of the overall experience. But first and foremost, personification expresses dynamic properties, revealing evaluative and emotional attributes that have long been associated, by some investigators, with synesthesia. Notable among these investigators is Werner (1957), who proposed that perceptual processing is, in the beginning (considered both ontogenetically and microgenetically), holistic, syncretic, synesthetic, and physiognomic. To Werner, it is a physiognomic property of visual perception that a willow tree looks 'sad' or that yellow may be a 'happy' color. Personifications would presumably partake of such physiognomic properties, and physiognomic perception, putatively a universal property of basic perceptual responses, provides part of the substrate to Werner's (1934) conception of a 'unity of the senses.' From this perspective, personification would not only be appropriately considered a form of synesthesia, but would in fact be a paradigmatic form.

Where the vintage of personification is old, dating from the nineteenth century, the vintage of *mirror-touch synesthesia* is distinctly modern, dating from the twenty-first. Blakemore et al. (2005) described a young woman who reported that the sight of another person being touched evoked tactile sensations in an equivalent region of her body—on the same side, when the person was next to her, but on the opposite (mirrored) side, when the person faced her. The subject reported having several family members with grapheme-color synesthesia, and had experienced it herself in the past, though not at the time of testing. Neuroimaging suggested that the mirror-touch sensations were accompanied by correlated activity in pertinent regions of the brain, including somatosensory cortex.

Banissy and Ward (2007) subsequently showed, in a group of ten mirror-touch synesthetes, that mirror-touch sensations could interact with nonsynesthetic tactile sensations produced by a mechanical stimulus. Perhaps most significantly, the mirror-touch synesthetes evidenced greater *empathy* on one of three measures (emotional reactivity, but not cognitive empathy or social skills). The authors concluded that, 'experiencing aspects of affective empathy may particularly depend on shared interpersonal representations. This supports the notion that empathy is multifaceted and that the tactile mirror system may modulate some, but not all, aspects of this ability' and that 'the differences in empathic ability reported here appear consistent with the hypothesis that we understand and empathize with others by a process of simulation' (816).

It is probably fortuitous that Banissy and Ward's interpretation of mirror-touch synesthesia so strikingly resembles the distinctly non-modern way, mentioned earlier, that Aristotle, perhaps presciently, used the Greek root *sunaisthanesai* to refer to common perceptions among friends (Heller-Roazen, 2004). In any case, these recent revelations of mirror-touch synesthesia raise the possibility of some connection between empathy and synesthesia. Once more, we may have another piece to the puzzle of synesthesia—or another decoy.

If mirror-touch perception in particular and empathy more generally turn out to be important pieces in the puzzle of synesthesia, then it may be useful to consider other examples of empathy that, at first glance, share at least a few general characteristics with synesthesia. One case in point is *empathic pain*, where the sight of, or other information about, another person's pain or distress may, quite automatically, consistently, and reliably produce discomfort or even pain.[4] The findings of several neuroimaging studies converge in revealing a distinctive cluster of neural correlates to empathic pain. Especially noteworthy is the finding that direct pain produced in a person by delivering noxious stimulation (e.g., pinprick) and indirect, empathic pain induced when the person sees someone else receiving noxious stimulation have common neural correlates in the brain. Regions of the anterior cingulate cortex, anterior insula, and cerebellum are activated by both direct pain and empathic pain (e.g., Singer et al., 2004; Jackson et al., 2005). Jackson et al. noted further that activity in the anterior cingulate correlated strongly with the participants' ratings of the pain in others. These regions of the brain are themselves associated with the affective dimension of pain, but not with its purely sensory component.[5] Evidence from functional magnetic resonance imaging indicates that sensory responses may be limited to directly stimulated pain but not indirect pain (Singer et al., 2004); evidence from event-related cortical potentials, however, suggests that empathic pain too may be associated with activation of sensory pain mechanisms (Bufalari et al., 2007).

As with mirror-touch perception, we may ask: Is empathic pain a variant of synesthesia? If so, then what about other possibly related conditions, such as the *couvade syndrome*? The couvade syndrome refers to a set of empathic symptoms, including nausea, toothache, backache, and abdominal pain, that are sometimes observed in 'expectant partners'—partners of women during pregnancy and shortly after childbirth.[6] Although the syndrome's name may be unfamiliar, the syndrome itself (or at least one component of it) is reported fairly often. An epidemiological study by Lipkin and Lamb (1982) of husbands of pregnant women in Rochester, NY reported a prevalence of the couvade syndrome (defined by the husband reporting at least one symptom) of 22 percent. Unlike synesthesia, which is a 'long-haul' phenomenon, the couvade syndrome is generally limited to the time period during

[4] I experience a version myself, the induced sensation being a 'queasy feeling in my stomach.'

[5] As is well known, Aristotle did not include pain in his enumerations (*De Anima*, *De Sensu*) of the five senses, omitting it from the qualities of touch. Instead, Aristotle identified pain among the 'passions of the soul.' Omitting/ignoring the sensory component, Aristotle zeroed in on pain's affective nature.

[6] The term *couvade* likely derives from the French *couver*, to brood or hatch. Tylor (1865) was apparently the first to name and describe the *couvade ritual*, with variants found in many cultures. In the couvade ritual, the male partner of a pregnant woman takes to bed, as if he too were pregnant.

and just after pregnancy. Even if, as seems likely, it does not itself represent a form of synesthesia, the couvade syndrome may well share mechanisms with empathic forms of synesthesia.

1.12 Boundaries of synesthesia

There are lots of potentially useful ways to slice the synesthetic pie—according to broad characteristics of the inducers and inductants (both of which may operate largely, significantly, or primarily at any of several levels, including the perceptual, cognitive, and affective); according to narrower characteristics of the inducers and inductants (for instance, according to sensory modality); and according to various other schemes. To mention three: Ramachandran and Hubbard (2001) distinguished between lower and higher synesthesia—similar to the distinction between perceptual and cognitive inducers in synesthesia. Dixon et al. (2004) distinguished between projection and association synesthesia—between inductants projected into the external space of the inducer, as when the color is seen in the inducing grapheme, and inductants perceived 'in the mind's eye' (but see Ward et al., 2007, for a different interpretation). And Martino and Marks (2001) distinguished between strong and weak synesthesia—related to the distinction made in the present chapter between synesthesia and synesthetic tendency.

Further, it is not always clear exactly what constitutes an example or type of synesthesia and what does not. Personification has long been included among the types of synesthesia (Calkins, 1895), but tradition is not infallible. Number forms share many characteristics with other types of synesthesia (Sagiv et al., 2006), a finding that is also suggestive but not conclusive. And if mirror-touch perception is a type of synesthesia, then perhaps we should also give serious consideration to other reported examples of empathetic perception, such as empathic pain, and maybe even to instances of couvade syndrome in which there are clear inducers as well as inductants. Alternatively, some of these examples may constitute intermediate cases, not being paradigmatic of synesthesia, but examples of synesthesia nonetheless.

Analogous questions arise with regard to other synesthesia-like phenomena, such as strong visual imagery in response to music (Karwoski et al., 1942), which might fall somewhere between synesthesia and synesthetic tendency. It has become a common practice, in recent research on synesthesia, to rely on a high level of consistency in inducer-inductant relations over time as a measure of 'genuineness' (Baron-Cohen et al., 1987), to require consistency to classify a given person as synesthetic. Every grapheme, for instance, should induce the same color, each word a flavor, not only automatically but also repeatedly, over long intervals of time (e.g., months; consistency has even been observed over decades: Simner and Logie, 2007). Participants who report having synesthetic experiences but who do not pass a test of consistency as a matter of convenience are commonly excluded from the experimental cohort of synesthetes. Yet Ward and Mattingley (2006) have cautioned against using consistency in the definition of synesthesia, and it is possible that at least some people who report experiencing synesthesia but do not show long-term consistency differ in important ways from those who do not even report synesthesia. Where, and how, to set boundaries is central to eliminating decoys from the puzzle of synesthesia. Perhaps synesthesia is simply not conducive to a single, overarching, comprehensive theoretical formulation (for suggestions along related lines, see Harrison, 2001; Mattingley et al., 2001; Marks and Odgaard, 2005).

1.13 Monism, dualism, pluralism

Several formulations of synesthesia have been offered over the years, and in a recent review (Marks, 2009), I tried to encapsulate many of them by distinguishing among what I called monistic, dualistic, and pluralistic viewpoints. To summarize: Synesthetic *monism* posits a single category of perception and behavior, with vividly experienced synesthesia represented at one end of a perceptual-behavioral continuum. Synesthetic *dualism* posits two broad categories of perception and behavior, one corresponding to synesthesia (in all of its vividly experienced forms and varieties) and the other to nonsynesthesia. And synesthetic *pluralism* posits three (or more) categories: nonsynesthesia and at least two categories of synesthesia.

Figure 1.1 compares the three viewpoints schematically, with monism on the left, pluralism in the center, and dualism on the right. The aim here is not to be exhaustive and catalog all possible varieties of synesthesia or formulations of monism, pluralism, and dualism. Instead, the aim is to point out the main characteristics of each viewpoint, focusing on a handful of critical examples. These examples include (a) vivid synesthetic perception, as when musical notes, achromatic letters or numbers, or pains induce what a small number of people report as sensations of color; (b) cross-modal imagery, as when music leads to visual images of colors or patterns, but not necessarily either automatically or with great consistency; (c) cross-modal similarity in perception, where people who report neither vivid synesthesia nor cross-modal imagery nevertheless perceive, for example, that drum notes resemble black and brown colors, while violin notes resemble white and yellow; and, finally, (d) cross-modal similarity in language, where people who report neither vivid synesthesia nor cross-modal imagery nevertheless metaphorically interpret the words 'squeak' and 'sneeze' to connote brightness, the words 'thunder' and 'cough' darkness.[7]

As it is represented in Figure 1.1, monism essentially abolishes any distinct boundary separating synesthesia from quasi-synesthetic perception or synesthetic tendencies, positing instead what is essentially a continuous dimension (or multidimensional space) of synesthesia-ness, with minimally synesthetic perception and behavior represented at the top and maximally synesthetic perception and behavior at the bottom.

[7] In this respect, Hornbostel (1925) noted that the German 'hell,' or 'bright,' originally referred to high pitch.

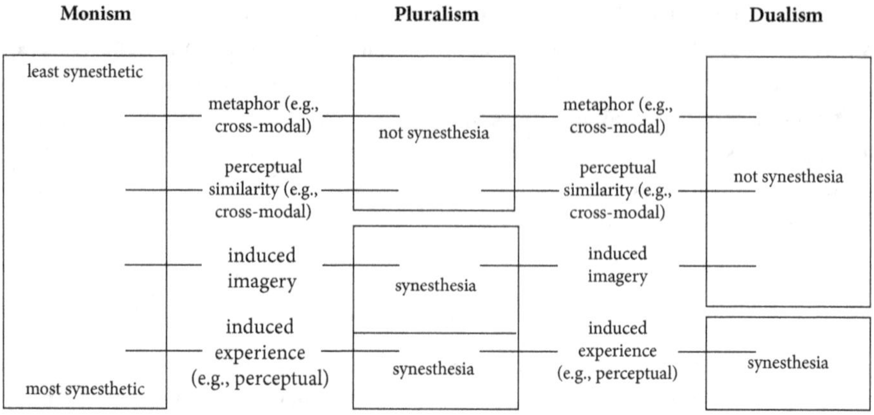

Figure 1.1. Schematic representations of monism, which treats synesthesia as the end-point on a continuous spectrum of perception; dualism, which distinguishes sharply between synesthetic perception and nonsynesthetic perception; and pluralism, which, like dualism, distinguishes between synesthetic perception and nonsynesthetic perception, but also distinguishes subcategories within the broad category of synesthesia.

Several explicitly or implicitly monistic views of synesthesia (e.g., Glicksohn et al., 1992; Hunt, 2005) point to the centrality of physiognomic or affective properties in perception (cf. Werner, 1957; Lindauer, 1986), and the experience of vivid synesthesia may involve in an important way affective or emotional as well as sensory *qualia*. Cytowic (1989) has indicated, for example, that one of the defining characteristics of synesthesia (viewed narrowly) is being laden with affect (see also Cytowic and Eagleman, 2009). Recent research into what has been called mirror-touch synesthesia, discussed earlier, points to its likely connection to empathy (Banissy and Ward, 2007).

By way of contrast, both dualism and pluralism sharply distinguish synesthesia from synesthetic tendencies, which bear some similarities to synesthesia but which dualism and pluralism exclude from that category. But dualists and pluralists may not agree as to what constitutes synesthesia and what does not. Dualism typically limits synesthesia to perceptions that occur vividly, automatically, and consistently, and thereby excludes cross-modal imagery, which sometimes is not vivid, sometimes comes under voluntary control, and sometimes is inconstant.[8] Pluralism, however, may (although it need not) include cross-modal imagery as a subcategory of synesthesia. As to other putative forms of synesthesia, such as personification, number forms, and mirror-touch perception, dualists and pluralists alike must apply appropriate theoretical criteria to decide which, if any, to include within the global category of synesthesia. If a dualist classifies both personification and number

[8] These distinctions too are not always sharp. Mulvenna (2012), for example, reported evidence of voluntary control in grapheme-color synesthesia.

forms as synesthesia, then both would fall within that single category. If a pluralist classifies both as synesthesia, however, they could fall within different categories of pluralism.

Clearly, the three perspectives on synesthesia need not translate in a simple or straightforward fashion from one to another. Pluralism is not just an elaboration of dualism, dividing synesthesia-as-a-dualist-sees-it into two or more subunits. Instead, pluralists and dualists can disagree as to whether certain phenomena are examples of synesthesia at all. Many contemporary researchers use consistency as a rule-of-thumb criterion for assessing whether a particular person has 'genuine' synesthesia (e.g., Rich et al., 2005; Simner et al., 2006; Barnett et al., 2008). The high level of test-retest consistency shown by certain individuals, often over long periods of time, is remarkable, and surely is suggestive; but, from a pluralistic point of view, it does not 'prove' that those who fail to show this kind of consistency therefore lack synesthesia—assuming that one has some other criteria to establish and define synesthesia.

1.14 Dualism's common denominators

Distinguishing among monistic, pluralistic, and dualistic views leads, almost inexorably, to the question: What are the criteria for deciding what constitutes synesthesia? Synesthesia involves inducers and inductants, although these can be diverse and hard to characterize—inducers can be external stimuli, such as sounds or words, but they can also be stimuli that arise within the body, such as the sources of stimulation that produce internal pain. Further, inducers can be abstract—for instance, conceptualized or imagined stimuli. From the perspective of dualism, which pervades current research in synesthesia, the search for criteria has been, to a great extent, a search for still-elusive *common denominators*, the set of properties that could serve to define and distinguish synesthesia.

This perspective is especially compatible with a reductionistic approach, which seeks to discover the genetic, neuroanatomical, and neurophysiological mechanisms responsible for idiopathic (developmental) synesthesia. The process of discovery, the process of solving the puzzle of synesthesia, is a dynamic one: As we learn more about the mechanisms, we better understand the common denominators, and thereby sharpen the boundaries of synesthesia, better defining it; at the same time, as we better define synesthesia, we may better understand its mechanisms. Uncovering the mechanisms, in turn, should help us decide what is and is not synesthesia. A deeper understanding of the pertinent mechanisms will presumably make it possible to answer the question why, for instance, inducers and inductants can vary so widely.[9]

[9] A deeper understanding may also help to answer one of the gnawing questions about synesthesia, namely why it exists at all. Synesthesia does not confer an obvious Darwinian advantage, nor must it. Yet it is possible that a biological advantage does emerge either from synesthesia itself or, more likely, from one of the putative correlates of synesthesia, such as creative cognition (Mulvenna, 2007).

There is already a large body of evidence, gleaned mainly from neuroimaging, that points to neural substrates for certain forms of synesthesia, especially grapheme-color (e.g., Hubbard and Ramachandran, 2005; Hubbard et al., 2005). There is also considerable evidence pointing to a genetic propensity to develop synesthesia (e.g., Barnett et al., 2008; Asher et al., 2009). We are still far, however, from identifying the genes, the anatomical neural networks, and the neurophysiological processes that may help define synesthesia.

What might we learn by uncovering the pertinent genetic, anatomical, and neurophysiological mechanisms? For one, discovering the mechanisms should help us develop a plausible account of the diversity of inducers and inductants. Even if there are specific biological propensities toward developing idiopathic synesthesia, the forms of synesthesia that develop in a given individual may depend substantially on experiential and environmental factors—broadly speaking, on gene-environment (e.g., epigenetic) interactions, for example the activation of particular genes by environmentally triggered biochemical events. Such a supposition is consistent with the evidence at hand and suggests a possible basis for the diversity in the forms of synesthesia among family members (e.g., Barnett et al., 2008). By implication, the same genetic predisposition may develop into any of several forms of synesthesia. Consider the hypothetical case of children born with a genetic propensity for synesthesia but raised in a non-literate society, with no opportunity to develop grapheme-induced or word-induced synesthesia. If one potential outlet for synesthesia is lacking, will synesthesia not appear? Or will it take on other forms? Perhaps the different forms of synesthesia that arise over different timeframes or periods in development are influenced, or determined, by timetables in the unfolding of gene-environment interactions.

In this regard, recent findings of Asher et al. (2009) suggest the existence of several genes that confer susceptibility to developing synesthesia, as well as the possibility that these genes may act in concert (oligogenic inheritance). Might these genes combine their effects? If so, then one outcome could be gradations in the probability that synesthesia will appear or, when it does appear, gradations in measures of its strength (e.g., its vividness or consistency). The most vivid or highly consistent instances of synesthesia—perhaps prototypical instances—may, therefore, be associated with the presence of multiple genes. These genes could affect neuroanatomy and neurophysiology by influencing the degree and nature of neural connectivity (for a recent review, see Cytowic and Eagleman, 2009).

Neuroanatomical and neurophysiological theories relate synesthetic experiences, broadly speaking, to neural traffic between brain regions that lack such neural traffic in nonsynesthetic experience. The difference between the experiences of synesthetes and nonsynesthetes may reflect differences in neuroanatomy. It is possible that grapheme-color synesthetes and nonsynesthetes differ because the synesthetes have neural connections between ensembles of neurons responsible for processing graphemes and ensembles processing color (Ramachandran and Hubbard, 2001).

And synesthetes and nonsynesthetes may differ in their neuroanatomy because synesthetes are born with, or are programmed to develop, hyperconnectivity, whereas nonsynesthetes are not. Alternatively, it is possible that the neural connections between ensembles exist in synesthetes and nonsynesthetes alike, but the neural traffic between ensembles is (or comes to be) inhibited in nonsynesthetes but not inhibited, or disinhibited, in synesthetes (Grossenbacher and Lovelace, 2001). A third possibility is that all infants are born with hyperconnections between neural ensembles, and during infancy and childhood these hyperconnections are pruned or inhibited in nonsynesthetes, but persist in synesthetes (Maurer and Mondloch, 1996, 2005; for a thorough recent review and consideration of the implications of Maurer's theory, see Spector and Maurer, 2009).[10] In principle, specific genes might be associated with any of these hypothesized neural mechanisms (for a review of plausible genetic and neural mechanisms of synesthesia, see Bargary and Mitchell, 2008).[11]

1.15 Pluralism's prototypes

Dualistic views of synesthesia fit comfortably with the notion that synesthesia will ultimately come to be characterized through a set of common denominators, likely to be represented themselves through neural, genetic, and epigenetic structures and mechanisms. This is to say that synesthesia would be defined in terms of a *conjunction* of properties, processes, or mechanisms. Pluralistic views of synesthesia, on the other hand, characterize it in terms of a broad category containing several subcategories, and therefore not in terms of a conjunction but a *disjunction* of overlapping properties, processes, or mechanisms. Perhaps synesthesia has remained a puzzle for so long because, at least in part, it is disjunctive rather than conjunctive.[12]

[10] Maurer's theory could help to explain another puzzle: cross-modal similarity. Why, for example, should high-pitched sounds resemble bright colors, while low-pitched sounds resemble dark or dim colors? This puzzle has two parts: How does similarity transcend the difference in modalities? And why do high and low pitch resemble bright and dark, respectively? Marks and Bornstein (1987) suggested an answer to the second part in terms of common mechanisms for coding pitch and brightness. By hypothesizing inborn connections across sensory modalities, Maurer's theory can help answer the first as well.

[11] As we come to understand more about the genetics, neuroanatomy, and neurophysiology of synesthesia, it should be possible to ask—and answer!—several important questions that, so far, have only occasionally been asked or suggested (cf. Ramachandran and Hubbard, 2001; Hubbard and Ramachandran, 2005). Let me list a few of them. First, how much neural activation is necessary to have a synesthetic experience? If synesthetic colors are experienced when the cross-activation of neural networks includes responses in, say, area V4, what is the threshold for this experience? If synesthesia reflects hyperconnectivity, how many 'additional' neural connections are needed? How much 'extra growth' or 'reducing pruning' will suffice to provide the necessary neural substrate? Or if synesthesia reflects disinhibition of neural cross-activation, how much disinhibition suffices? These questions obviously have broad implications for the deep and long-standing issue that Fechner (1860) called inner psychophysics: the neural substrate of consciousness.

[12] Disjunctive categories have long been known to pose special cognitive demands. In their seminal work on concept attainment, Bruner et al. (1956) showed the difficulty that people have in discovering concepts that are defined by disjunctions of features. In a nine-fold universe of blue, red, and green circles,

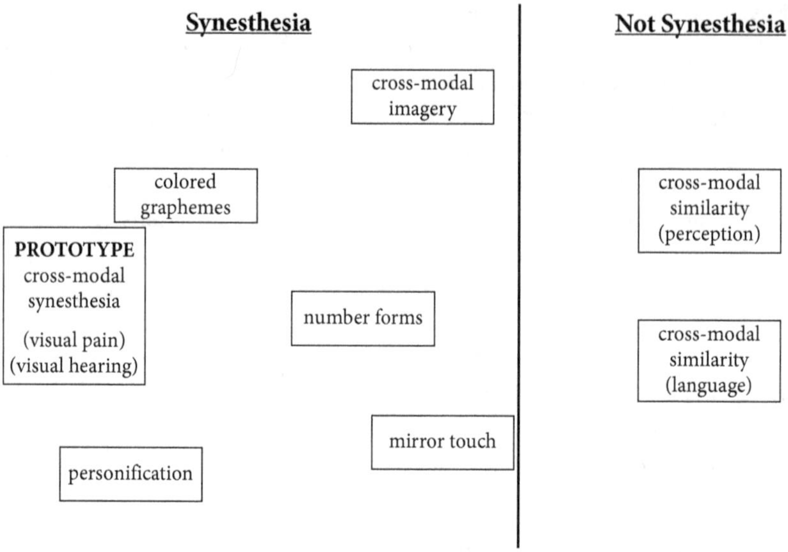

Figure 1.2. An example of a pluralistic model of synesthesia, in which cross-modal synesthesia is prototypical, with other kinds of synesthesia falling close to the prototype (e.g., cross-dimensional synesthesia, such as colored graphemes) or farther from the prototype (e.g., mirror touch, induced cross-modal imagery).

From this pluralistic perspective, the broad category of synesthesia consists of one or more prototypes, plus other subcategories that may fall near to or far from the prototype, depending on the extent to which the other subcategories share the pertinent properties, processes, or mechanisms that define the prototype. These properties might include, for example, experience of perceptual *qualia* and automaticity in inducing them, but the properties themselves would be specified through an explicit theory. Figure 1.2 sketches a scheme in which cross-modal perceptual synesthesia constitutes a prototype. As in Figure 1.1, cross-modal similarity in both perception and language (metaphor) falls outside the realm of synesthesia, whereas cross-modal imagery falls within it, although relatively far from the prototype (visual imagery and vivid forms of synesthesia may show substantial differences in neural activation: Rich et al., 2006). As represented in Figure 1.2, the prototype embraces the many forms of synesthesia in which both the inducer and inductant are perceptual and heteromodal. Visual hearing, including both colored and patterned hearing, falls

triangles, and squares, it is much easier to discover the conjunctive concept 'blue triangle' than the disjunctive one 'blue or triangle.' Note, however, that in their discussion of conjunctive and disjunctive concepts in science, Bruner et al. do not give very compelling examples of disjunction, pointing out instead how disjunctions in science often give way, in the end, to the discovery of the conjunctions or common denominators.

within the prototype, as do colored touches, tastes, smells, and pains, as well as other forms of perceptual synesthesia.

Figure 1.2 implicitly attributes three major, albeit not equally important, properties to the prototype for synesthesia: First of all is phenomenal experience. To experience synesthesia is to experience induced *qualia*. Lacking these experiences, there is no synesthesia, which is why cross-modal similarity lies outside the realm. Second, prototypical synesthesia is automatic (largely involuntary), reliable, and consistent. Although phenomenal experiences (*qualia*) are present in induced cross-modal imagery, cross-modal imagery is not always automatic, reliable, or consistent (or presumably less so than prototypical synesthesia)—and, consequently, cross-modal imagery falls relatively far from the prototype. And third, prototypical synesthesia involves abstract and seemingly arbitrary relations between inducer and inductant. Drawing an analogy to different kinds of memory, prototypical synesthesia is akin to semantic memory rather than episodic memory (Tulving, 1972). It is this property that largely distinguishes cross-modal imagery (semantic relations) from memory images (episodic relations, as in the so-called 'Proust phenomenon,' in which an external stimulus, commonly olfactory, evokes a strong, detailed memory image of an earlier scene or experience: Chu and Downes, 2000), and that distinguishes prototypical (semantic) synesthesia from mirror-touch (episodic) synesthesia.

To call prototypical synesthesia 'semantic' is to acknowledge the benefit of synesthesia to cognition. In a long tradition of research in synesthesia, Wheeler and Cutsforth (1922a, 1922b), Karwoski and his colleagues (Karwoski and Odbert, 1938, Karwoski et al., 1942; Odbert et al., 1942), and Osgood and his colleagues (e.g., Osgood, 1960; Osgood et al., 1957) all concluded that synesthesia comprises a system of meanings, operating much in the same way that semantic systems do in non-synesthetes. Osgood in particular argued that the meanings inherent in auditory-visual synesthesia (sound-induced colors, shapes, and patterns) are connotative, as are the corresponding metaphorical meanings in language.

The example in Figure 1.2 brings us by a *commodius vicus* of recirculation back to the notion that cross-modal synesthesia serves as a prototype (Marks, 1975, 1978b)—despite the fact that cross-modal synesthesia is far from the most common form. To assert that cross-modal synesthesia is prototypical is not to claim that most synesthesia is cross-modal; instead, it is to posit that cross-modal processes play a pivotal role in synesthesia's development.

This version of pluralism is especially compatible with Maurer's (Maurer and Mondloch, 1996, 2005) hypothesis regarding the development of synesthesia, recently elaborated by Spector and Maurer (2009), and the remaining discussion derives largely from Maurer's work. In brief, Maurer has hypothesized: first, that because of innate connections (hyperconnectivity) between and among sensory centers, young infants essentially perceive the world synesthetically, or quasi-synesthetically; second, that the neural apoptosis or pruning that occurs during development in most infants and children eliminates (or inhibits) pathways that could subserve synesthetic perception later in childhood and adulthood; and third, that this pruning does not occur in a small number of children, who thereby maintain their synesthesia, or retain a capacity to develop it.[13]

It is difficult to know whether infants actually have synesthetic experiences; that is, whether they experience two or more sensory *qualia* from a single stimulus. That they can readily 'match' or 'transfer' experiences across modalities (e.g., Lewkowicz and Turkewitz, 1980; Walker et al., 2010; Jeschonek et al., 2012) suggests that infants do not easily discriminate stimuli presented in different modalities, such as sounds and lights. But as Maurer and Mondloch (2005) point out, it is not possible to determine, in infants, whether visual stimuli actually induce auditory sensations, and auditory stimuli induce visual sensations (strong version of the hypothesis of neonatal synesthesia), or whether visual and auditory stimuli are only poorly discriminated, hence by implication perceptually similar (weak version of neonatal synesthesia). Either way, perception in infancy clearly reveals strong links across sensory modalities, presumably subserved by neural connections from which adult synesthesia could subsequently emerge.

The hypothesis that the perceptual world of infants and young children is synesthetic was articulated strongly half a century ago by Werner (1957). Werner characterized perceptual experiences in infancy and early in childhood as largely *syncretic*; that is, functionally undifferentiated, and as *physiognomic*; that is, imbued with expressive and affective properties (see Schlessinger, 1980; Lindauer, 1986), as well as synesthetic. Syncretic and physiognomic characteristics are interrelated, and often show up in (adult) synesthesia. Werner noted a relation between physiognomic perception and the development of personification. These views are closely associated with his arguments for a 'unity of the senses' (Werner, 1934): Werner argued that synesthetic perception precedes nonsynesthetic perception, both ontogenetically and microgenetically. As perception develops ontogenetically, infants perceive the world synesthetically before they develop abstract, discrete nonsynesthetic perception. And as a single percept unfolds (in adults) microgenetically, the initially undifferentiated, physiognomic, and synesthetic response to the stimulus eventually gives way to discrete perceptual qualities, which take time to unfold. Indeed, more recent microgenetic theories assert that at least some kinds of perceptual stimuli may initially be processed holistically, as 'blobs,' with this early holistic processing followed by more discrete, dimensional analysis (e.g., Lockhead, 1972), although these processes need not recapitulate perceptual development of early childhood.

The multifarious forms of idiopathic synesthesia that are observed in adults typically develop during childhood, but have their roots in neural mechanisms that

[13] Marks and Odgaard (2005) criticized this view on the grounds that pruning occurs very early in infancy, whereas synesthesia typically develops much later, often through experience with 'cultural artifacts,' as mentioned earlier. As Simner and Hubbard (2006) pointed out, however, pruning may occur over protracted periods of time, so Maurer's hypothesis remains plausible.

are undoubtedly present in early infancy. It is possible that infants too experience some kind of synesthesia, but if they do, the range of synesthesia in infants is undoubtedly much narrower than the range in adults. Most inducers of synesthesia in adults are letters, numbers, words, days of the week, months of the year, and names—all artifacts of culture (see also Mroczko-Wąsowicz and Nikolić, 2014). To the extent that the perceptual experience of infants may be synesthetic, it presumably resembles the cross-modal perceptual synesthesia observed in that fraction of adult synesthetes in whom low-level sensory properties of stimuli induce low-level properties in another modality. Yet the principles of cross-modal synesthesia pervade perception, in infancy, childhood, and adulthood; they are readily found not just in a tiny number of synesthetes, but also, as cross-modal similarities, in the general population of nonsynesthetes as well. And the mechanisms that underlie prototypical, cross-modal synesthesia may well serve as the wellspring for the development of synesthesia's diverse other forms.

References

Arnold, D.H., Wegener, S.V., Brown, F., & Mattingley, J.B. (2012). Precision of synesthetic color matching resembles that for recollected colors rather than physical colors. *Journal of Experimental Psychology: Human Perception and Performance*, 38, 1078–84.

Asher, J.E., Lamb, J.A., Brocklebank, D., Cazier, J.-B., Maestrini, E., Addis, L., Sen, M., Baron-Cohen, S., & Monaco, A.P. (2009). A whole-genome scan and fine-mapping linkage study of auditory-visual synesthesia reveals evidence of linkage to chromosomes 2q24, 5q33, 6p12, and 12p12. *American Journal of Human Genetics*, 84, 279–85.

Banissy, M.J., & Ward, J. (2007). Mirror-touch synesthesia is linked with empathy. *Nature Neuroscience*, 10, 815–17.

Bargary, G., & Mitchell, K.J. (2008). Synaesthesia and cortical connectivity. *Trends in Neurosciences*, 31, 335–42.

Barnett, K.J., Finucane, C., Asher, J.E., Bargary, G., Corvin, A.P., Newell, F.N., & Mitchell, K.J. (2008). Familial patterns and the origins of individual differences in synaesthesia. *Cognition*, 106, 871–93.

Baron-Cohen, S., Burt, L., Smith-Laittan, F., Harrison, J., & Bolton P. (1996). Synaesthesia: Prevalence and familiality. *Perception*, 25, 1073–9.

Baron-Cohen, S., Wyke, M.A., & Binnie, C. (1987). Hearing words and seeing colours: An experimental investigation of a case of synaesthesia. *Perception*, 16, 761–7.

Berlin, I. (1953). *The hedgehog and the fox: An essay on Tolstoy's view of history*. London: Weidenfeld & Nicolson.

Blakemore, S.-J., Bristow, D., Bird, G., Frith, C., & Ward, J. (2005). Somatosensory activations during the observation of touch and a case of vision-touch synaesthesia. *Brain*, 128, 1571–83.

Bleuler, E., & Lehmann, K. (1881). *Zwangmässige Lichetempfindungen durch Schall und verwandte Erscheinungen* [Induced light sensations from sound and related phenomena]. Leipzig: Fues' Verlag.

Bruner, J.S., Goodnow, J.J., & Austin, G.A. (1956). *A study of thinking*. New York: John Wiley.

Bufalari, I., Aprile, T., Avenanti, A., Di Russo, F., & Aglioti, S.M. (2007). Empathy for pain and touch in the human somatosensory cortex. *Cerebral Cortex*, 17, 2553–61.

Calkins, M.W. (1893). A statistical study of pseudo-chromesthesia and mental-forms. *American Journal of Psychology*, 5, 439–64.

Calkins, M.W. (1895). Synaesthesia. *American Journal of Psychology*, 7, 90–107.

Chu, S., & Downes, J.J. (2000). Long live Proust: The odour-cued autobiographical memory bump. *Cognition*, 75, B41–B50.

Cohen Kadosh, R., Cohen Kadosh, K., & Henik, A. (2007). The neuronal correlate of bi-directional synesthesia: A combined event-related potential and functional magnetic resonance imaging study. *Journal of Cognitive Neuroscience*, 19, 2050–9.

Cohen Kadosh, R., & Henik, A. (2006). Color congruity effect: Where do colors and numbers interact in synesthesia? *Cognition*, 42, 259–63.

Cytowic, R.E. (1989). *Synesthesia: A union of the senses*. New York: Springer.

Cytowic, R.E., & Eagleman, D.M. (2009). *Wednesday is indigo blue: Discovering the brain of synesthesia*. Cambridge, MA: MIT Press.

Dixon, M.J., Smilek, D., Cudahy, C., & Merikle, P.M. (2000). Five plus two equals yellow. *Nature*, 406, 365.

Dixon, M.J., Smilek, D., & Merikle, P.M. (2004). Not all synaesthetes are created equal: Distinguishing between projector and associator synaesthetes. *Cognitive, Affective, and Behavioral Neuroscience*, 4, 335–43.

Eagleman, D.M. (2009). The objectification of overlearned sequences: A new view of spatial sequence synesthesia. *Cortex*, 45, 1266–77.

Fechner, G.T. (1860). *Elemente der Psychophysik* [Elements of psychophysics]. Leipzig: Bretikopf und Härtel.

Flournoy, T. (1893). *Des phénomènes de synopsie* [Phenomena of synopsia] Paris: Alcan.

Galton, F. (1880). Visualised numerals. *Nature*, 21, 252–6, 494–5.

Galton, F. (1883). *Inquiries into human faculty and its development*. London: Macmillan.

Gardner, H. (1974). Metaphors and modalities: How children project polar adjectives onto divers domains. *Child Development*, 45, 84–91.

Garner, W.R. (1970). The stimulus in information processing. *American Psychologist*, 25, 350–8.

Gertner, L., Henik, A., & Cohen Kadosh, R. (2009). When 9 is not on the right: Implications from number-form synesthesia. *Consciousness and Cognition*, 18, 366–74.

Glicksohn, J., Salinger, O., & Roychman, A. (1992). An exploratory study of syncretic experience: Eidetics, synaesthesia and absorption. *Perception*, 21, 637–42.

Grossenbacher, P., & Lovelace, C.T. (2001). Mechanisms of synesthesia: Cognitive and physiological constraints. *Trends in Cognitive Sciences*, 5, 36–41.

Harrison, J. (2001). *Synaesthesia: The strangest thing*. New York: Oxford University Press.

Heller-Roazen, D. (2004). Company. *October*, 117, 35–43.

Hornbostel, E.M. von (1925). Die Einheit der Sinne [The unity of the senses]. *Melos, Zeitschrift für Musik*, 4, 290–7.

Hubbard, E.M., Arman, A.C., Ramachandran, V.S., & Boynton G.M. (2005). Individual differences among grapheme-color synesthetes: brain-behavior correlations. *Neuron*, 45, 975–85.

Hubbard, E.M., Manohar, S., & Ramachandran, V.S. (2006). Contrast affects the strength of synesthetic colors. *Cortex*, 42, 184–94.

Hubbard, E.M., & Ramachandran, V.S. (2005). Neurocognitive mechanisms of synesthesia. *Neuron*, 48, 509–20.

Hubbard, T.L. (1996). Synesthesia-like mappings of lightness, pitch, and melodic interval. *American Journal of Psychology*, 109, 219–38.

Hunt, H. (2005). Synaesthesia, metaphor and consciousness. *Journal of Consciousness Studies*, 12, 6–45.

Jackson, P.L., Meltzoff, A.N., & Decety, J. (2005). How do we perceive the pain of others? A window into the neural processes involved in empathy. *NeuroImage*, 24, 771–9.

Jeschonek, S., Pauen, S., & Babocsai, L. (2012). Cross-modal mapping of visual and acoustic displays in infants: The effect of dynamic and static components. *European Journal of Developmental Psychology*. Retrieved at: doi:10.1080/17405629.2012.681590

Karwoski, T.F, & Odbert, H.S. (1938). Color-music. *Psychological Monographs*, 50, 222, 1–60.

Karwoski, T.F, Odbert, H.S., & Osgood, C.E. (1942). Studies synesthetic thinking. II. The role of form in visual responses to music. *Journal of General Psychology*, 26, 199–222.

Kim, C,-Y., Blake, R., & Palmieri, T.J. (2006). Perceptual interaction between real and synesthetic colors. *Cortex*, 42, 195–203.

Köhler, W. (1947). *Gestalt psychology* (2nd Edition). New York: Liveright.

Lewkowicz, D.J., & Turkewitz, G. (1980). Cross-modal equivalence in early infancy: Auditory-visual intensity matching. *Developmental Psychology*, 16, 597–607.

Lindauer, M.S. (1986). Perceiving, imaging, and preferring physiognomic stimuli. *American Journal of Psychology*, 99, 233–55.

Lipkin, M. Jr, & Lamb, G.S. (1982). The couvade syndrome: An epidemiologic study. *Archives of Internal Medicine*, 96, 509–11.

Lockhead, G.R. (1972). Processing dimensional stimuli: A note. *Psychological Review*, 79, 410–19.

Marks, L.E. (1974). On associations of light and sound: The mediation of brightness, pitch, and loudness. *American Journal of Psychology*, 87, 173–88.

Marks, L.E. (1975). On colored-hearing synesthesia: Cross-modal translations of sensory dimensions. *Psychological Bulletin*, 83, 303–31.

Marks, L.E. (1978a). Multimodal perception. In E.C. Carterette and M.P. Friedman (Eds.), *Handbook of perception*. Vol. 8. *Perceptual coding* (pp. 321–39). New York: Academic Press.

Marks, L.E. (1978b). *The unity of the senses: Interrelations among the modalities*. New York: Academic Press.

Marks, L.E. (1982). Bright sneezes and dark coughs, loud sunlight and soft moonlight. *Journal of Experimental Psychology: Human Perception and Performance*, 8, 177–93.

Marks, L.E. (1989). On cross-modal similarity: The perceptual structure of pitch, loudness, and brightness. *Journal of Experimental Psychology: Human Perception and Performance*, 15, 586–602.

Marks, L.E. (2009). Synaesthesia across the spectrum. In M.J. de Córdoba, E. Hubbard, D. Riccò, and S.A. Day (Eds.), *Proceedings of the Third International Congress on Synesthesia, Science and Art*. Granada, Spain: Ediciones Fundación Internacional Artecittà (DVD).

Marks, L.E. (2011). Synesthesia, then and now. *Intellectica*, 55, 47–80.

Marks, L.E., & Bornstein, M.H. (1987). Sensory similarities: Classes, characteristics, and cognitive consequences. In R.E. Haskell (Ed.), *Cognition and symbolic structures: The psychology of metaphoric transformation* (pp. 49–65). Norwood, NJ: Ablex.

Marks, L.E., Hammeal, R.J., & Bornstein, M.H. (1987). Perceiving similarity and comprehending metaphor. *Monographs of the Society for Research in Child Development*, 52, 1–100 (Whole No. 215).

Marks, L.E., & Odgaard, E.C. (2005). Developmental constraints on theories of synesthesia. In L.C. Robertson and N. Sagiv (Eds.), *Synesthesia: Perspectives from cognitive neuroscience* (pp. 214–36). New York: Oxford University Press.

Martin, P.R. (1998). Colour processing in the primate retina: Recent progress. *Journal of Physiology*, 513, 631–8.

Martino, G., & Marks, L.E. (2001). Synesthesia: Strong and weak. *Current Directions in Psychological Science*, 10, 61–5.

Mattingley, J.B., Rich, A.N., Yelland, G., & Bradshaw, J.L. (2001). Unconscious priming eliminates automatic binding of colour and alphanumeric form in synaesthesia. *Nature*, 410, 580–2.

Maurer, D., & Mondloch, C. (1996). Synesthesia: A stage of normal infancy? In S. Masin (Ed.,), *Fechner Day 96: Proceedings of the 12th meeting of the International Society for Psychophysics* (pp. 107–12). Padua: ISP.

Maurer, D., & Mondloch, C.J. (2005). Neonatal synesthesia: A reevaluation. In L.C. Robertson and N. Sagiv (Eds.), *Synesthesia: Perspectives from cognitive neuroscience* (pp. 193–213). New York: Oxford University Press.

Mills, C.B., Boteler, E.H., & Oliver, G.K. (1999). Digit synaesthesia: A case study using a Stroop-type test. *Cognitive Neuropsychology*, 16, 181–91.

Mondloch, C.J., & Maurer, D. (2004). Do small white balls squeak? Pitch-object correspondences in young children. *Cognitive, Affective, & Behavioral Neuroscience*, 4, 133–6.

Mroczko-Wąsowicz, A., & Nikolić, D. (2014). Semantic mechanisms may be responsible for developing synesthesia. *Frontiers in Human Neuroscience*, 8 (doi: 10.3389/fnhum.2014.00509).

Mulvenna, C.M. (2007). Synaesthesia, the arts and creativity: A neurological connection. In J. Bogousslavsky and M.G. Hennerici (Eds.), *Neurological disorders in famous artists—part 2* (pp. 206–22). Basel: Karger.

Mulvenna, C.M. (2012). *On creativity in synaesthetes: Roles of neural connectivity, cognitive control, and perceptual correspondence.* Doctoral thesis, University College London.

Myers, C.S. (1911). A case of synaesthesia. *British Journal of Psychology*, 4, 228–38.

Nikolić, D., Lichti, P., & Singer, W. (2007). Color opponency in synaesthetic experience. *Psychological Science*, 6, 481–6.

Nunn, J.A., Gregory, L.J., Brammer, M., Williams, S.C.R., Parslow, D.M., Morgan, M.J., Morris, R.G., Bullmore, E.T., Baron-Cohen, S., & Gray, J.A. (2002). Functional magnetic resonance imaging of synaesthesia: Activation of V4/V8 by spoken words. *Nature Neuroscience*, 5, 371–5.

Odbert, H.S., Karwoski, T.F., & Eckerson A.B. (1942). Studies synesthetic thinking: I. Musical and verbal associations of color and mood. *Journal of General Psychology*, 26, 153–73.

Osgood, C.E. (1960). The cross-cultural generality of visual-verbal synesthetic tendencies. *Behavioral Science*, 5, 146–69.

Osgood, C.E., Suci, G.J., & Tannenbaum, P.H. (1957). *The measurement of meaning.* Urbana, IL: University of Illinois Press.

Pierce, A.H. (1907). Gustatory audition: A hitherto undescribed variety of synaesthesia. *American Journal of Psychology*, 18, 341–52.

Preminger, A. (Ed.). (1974). *Princeton encyclopedia of poetics*. Princeton, NJ: Princeton University Press.

Ramachandran, V., & Hubbard, E.M. (2001). Synaesthesia—a window into perception, thought and language. *Journal of Consciousness Studies*, 8, 3–34.

Rich, A.N., Bradshaw, J.L., & Mattingley, J.B. (2005). A systematic, large-scale study of synaesthesia: Implications for the role of early experience in lexical-colour associations. *Cognition*, 98, 53–84.

Rich, A.N., Williams, M.A., Puce, A., Syngeniotis, A., Howard, M.A., McGlone, F., & Mattingley, J.B. (2006). Neural correlates of imagined and synaesthetic colours. *Neuropsychologia*, 44, 2918–25.

Sagiv, N., Simner, J., Collins, J., Butterworth, B., & Ward, J. (2006). What is the relationship between synaesthesia and visuo-spatial number forms? *Cognition*, 101, 114–28.

Schlessinger, L.B. (1980). Physiognomic perception: Empirical and theoretical perspectives. *Genetic Psychology Monographs*, 101, 71–97.

Shen, Y., & Aisenman, R. (2008). 'Heard melodies are sweet, but those unheard are sweeter': Synaesthetic metaphors and cognition. *Language and Literature*, 17, 107–21.

Simner, J., Harrold, J., Creed, H., Monro, L., & Foulkes, L. (2009). Early detection of markers for synaesthesia in childhood populations. *Brain*, 132, 57–64.

Simner, J., & Haywood, S.L. (2009). Tasty non-words and neighbours: The cognitive roots of lexical-gustatory synaesthesia. *Cognition*, 110, 171–81.

Simner, J., & Holenstein, E. (2007). Ordinal linguistic personification as a variant of synesthesia. *Journal of Cognitive Neuroscience*, 19, 694–703.

Simner, J., & Hubbard, E.M. (2006). Variants of synesthesia interact in cognitive tasks: Evidence for implicit associations and late connectivity in cross-talk theories. *Neuroscience*, 143, 804–14.

Simner, J., & Logie, R.H. (2007). Synaesthetic consistency spans decades in a lexical-gustatory synaesthete. *Neurocase*, 13, 358–65.

Simner, J., Mulvenna, C., Sagiv, N., Tsakanikos, E., Witherby, S.A., Fraser, C., Scott, K., & Ward, J. (2006). Synaesthesia: The prevalence of atypical cross-modal experiences. *Perception*, 35, 1024–33.

Simner J., & Ward J. (2006). The taste of words on the tip of the tongue. *Nature*, 444, 23.

Singer, T., Seymour, B., O'Doherty, J., Kaube, H., Dolan, R.J., & Frith, C.D. (2004). Empathy for pain involves the affective but not sensory components of pain. *Science*, 303, 1157–62.

Smilek, D., Malcolmson, K.A., Carriere, J.S.A., Eller, M., Kwan, D., & Reynolds, M. (2007). When '3' is a jerk and 'E' is a king: Personifying inanimate objects in synesthesia. *Journal of Cognitive Neuroscience*, 19, 981–92.

Spector, F., & Maurer, D. (2009). Synesthesia: A new approach to understanding the development of perception. *Developmental Psychology*, 45, 175–89.

Tulving, E. (1972). Episodic and semantic memory. In E. Tulving and W. Donaldson (Eds.), *Organization of memory* (pp. 381–402). New York: Academic Press.

Tylor, E.B. (1865). *Researches into the early history of mankind and the development of civilization*. London: J. Murray.

Walker, P., Bremner, J.G., Mason, U., Spring, J., Mattock, K., Slater, A., & Johnson, S.P. (2010). Preverbal infants' sensitivity to synaesthetic cross-modality correspondences. *Psychological Science*, 21, 21–5.

Walsh, V. (2003). A theory of magnitude: Common cortical metrics of time, space, and quantity. *Trends in Cognitive Science*, 7, 483–8.

Ward, J., Huckstep, B., & Tsakanikos, E. (2006). Sound-colour synaesthesia: To what extent does it use cross-modal mechanisms common to us all? *Cognition*, 42, 264–80.

Ward J., Li, R., Salih, S., & Sagiv, N. (2007). Varieties of grapheme-colour synaesthesia: A new theory of phenomenological and behavioural differences. *Consciousness & Cognition*, 16, 913–31.

Ward, J., & Mattingley, J.B. (2006). Synaesthesia: An overview of contemporary findings and controversies. *Cortex*, 42, 129–36.

Ward J., & Simner J. (2003). Lexical-gustatory synaesthesia: Linguistic and conceptual factors. *Cognition*, 89, 237–61.

Warren, H.C. (1934). *Dictionary of psychology*. Cambridge, MA: Houghton Mifflin.

Werner, H. (1934). L'unité des sens. *Journal de Psychologie Normale et Pathologique*, 31, 190–205.

Werner, H. (1957). *Comparative psychology of mental development* (rev. ed.). New York: International Universities Press.

Wheeler, R.H. (1920). The synaesthesia of a blind subject. *University of Oregon Publications*, 1, 5, 1–61.

Wheeler, R.H., & Cutsforth, T.D. (1922a). The synaesthesia of a blind subject with comparative data from an asynaesthetic blind subject. *University of Oregon Publications*, 1, 10, 1–104.

Wheeler, R.H., & Cutsforth, T.D. (1922b). Synaesthesia and meaning. *American Journal of Psychology*, 33, 361–84.

Williams, J.M. (1976). Synaesthetic adjectives: A possible law of semantic change. *Language*, 52, 461–78.

2

Synesthesia vs. Crossmodal Illusions

Casey O'Callaghan

2.1 Two opposing perspectives on synesthesia

We can discern two opposing viewpoints regarding synesthesia. On one hand, to borrow from Harrison's (2001) book title, synesthesia is "The Strangest Thing." It is an oddity, an outlier, or a disordered condition. A history of skepticism questions whether it even exists. It has been described as "incredible," "controversial," "mysterious," "unbelievable," and "romantic neurology." On the other hand, synesthesia is touted as pervasive. It is the heart of nearly any distinctively human cognitive achievement. Ramachandran and Hubbard (2001, 2003a,b), for example, suggest that synesthesia helps explain metaphor, creativity, and the origins of language itself.

Which is it? Ultimately, I favor the first perspective, according to which cross-sensory synesthesia is an outlying condition. But the second perspective is not wholly misguided. My discussion has three lessons. First, synesthesia is just one of a variety of effects in which one sense modality causally impacts and reshapes experience associated with another. These effects are utterly common. However, due to their unfamiliarity and their conflict with a widespread conception of the role of the senses in perception and perceptual experience, until recently they have been surprising. Second, synesthesia nevertheless must be distinguished from other intermodal effects that lead to misperception, such as *crossmodal illusions*. Third, synesthesia also may be distinguished from the potentially much broader class of *synesthetic effects*, which could be common across the population and within individuals.

Section 2.2 characterizes synesthesia, section 2.3 characterizes crossmodal illusions, and section 2.4 contrasts synesthesia with crossmodal illusions. Section 2.5 contrasts synesthesia with synesthetic effects and presents a conciliatory take on the two viewpoints concerning synesthesia.

2.2 Cross-sensory synesthesia

Stereotypical synesthesia involves stimulation to one sensory system that gives rise to an experience of a type that is typically associated with another sensory modality. This concurrent experience generally is not a case of veridical perception.

Synesthesia has numerous varieties. Some are familiar. Synesthetes may have color experiences in response to sounds or sound experiences in response to visible colors. They may experience graphemes as colored, or days of the week or months of the year as occupying specific locations in space around the body. Other forms of synesthesia are striking. Some synesthetes have tactual or bodily sensations when hearing sounds, or specific taste experiences in response to visible letters or graphemes. Some experience distinctive textural attributes that are prompted by tastes and flavors. The examples multiply.[1]

Contrary to earlier skepticism, current evidence shows that synesthesia exists, that it sometimes manifests as a conscious phenomenon, and that it may involve robust qualitative phenomenology. For instance, grapheme–color synesthesia can generate Stroop interference. It can also improve response times in visual search tasks. However, search times generally do increase with display complexity, so search remains serial rather than parallel, and the effect is not strong enough to support robust popout. Moreover, synesthetic experiences may require focal attention and thus be incapable of capturing exogenous attention. Nevertheless, the most convincing evidence in support of synesthesia is that synesthetes, when compared with non-synesthetes, are remarkably consistent on matching tasks through a great many trials distributed over long periods of time. Synesthetes more accurately match synesthetic concurrents prompted by a particular stimulus than memory should allow. For instance, time after time, year after year, a synesthete might match just the same shade of blue to the letter "G."[2]

How should we characterize synesthesia? As a first pass, we might say that synesthesia occurs when stimulation to one sensory system causes an experience of a type or with a character that is usually associated with another sensory modality. For instance, according to Harrison (2001), "Synaesthesia is a confusion of the senses, whereby stimulation of one sense triggers stimulation in a completely different sensory modality." Wager (1999: 264) says, "According to the standard definition, synaesthesia is a condition in which stimulation of one sensory modality automatically produces an additional experience typical of another, unstimulated sensory modality." And, according to Harrison and Baron-Cohen (1997: 66), synesthesia occurs, "when stimulation of one sensory modality automatically triggers a perception in a second modality, in the absence of any direct stimulation to this second modality."

[1] For an overview, see, e.g., Baron-Cohen and Harrison (1997); Cytowic (2002); Cytowic and Eagleman (2009). On sound–touch synesthesia, see Beauchamp and Ro (2008).

[2] See, e.g., Eagleman et al. (2007).

Macpherson (2007: 66, note 8) quotes this characterization and observes, "This definition is widely cited in the literature."

There are several things to note about this sort of characterization. First, it assumes that we have a good grasp on what it is for an experience or its character to be *in*, *of*, or *associated with* a given sensory modality. Since my topic is neither the individuation of sensory modalities nor the typing of experiences or their phenomenology by modality, I'll simply presuppose in what follows that an account typing experiences by sensory modality is feasible.

Second, it assumes that the synesthetic concurrent is in or of the unstimulated modality, rather than in or of the stimulated modality, or in or of no determinate modality at all. Auvray and Deroy (2015) provide a valuable discussion of why this assumption is suspect as it stands. Thus, for the sake of discussion, I'll reinterpret the claim that the synesthetic concurrent is in or of the unstimulated modality as the claim that it involves an experience as of a given quality or feature that is of an experiential type whose instances typically occur through stimulation of that modality rather than the inducer.

Third, there is a great deal of variety in how synesthetic experiences manifest—in their intensity and in their qualitative and phenomenological character. To take an example, there is a longstanding debate between researchers who think there are *projectors* and *associators* and those who think there are simply *localizers* and *nonlocalizers*. While this debate concerns the nature of synesthetic experiences, both parties agree that some synesthetes experience qualitative features as located in distal space and that some synesthetes do not.

Given this variety, we may distinguish what I'll dub "philosophical synesthesia" from other sorts of synesthesia. Say that a synesthetically induced experience is a case of *philosophical synesthesia* just in case it is qualitatively indistinguishable from having a typical perceptual experience as of the instantiation of the relevant feature. For instance, philosophical grapheme–color synesthesia might involve having perceptual experiences that are phenomenologically or introspectively indistinguishable from seeing a red "8." Synesthesia need not be philosophical synesthesia. For instance, imagery, vivid or diffuse, may suffice.

Fourth, synesthesia need not involve two distinct sensory modalities. For instance, the stimulus or trigger might not be to a sensory system at all. Thinking about a number could be enough to trigger a color experience, as could an affective or emotional stimulus. Even the familiarity of a face can trigger synesthetic color experiences. Moreover, synesthesia commonly involves only one sense modality. For example, low-level grapheme–color synesthesia involves vision alone, and thus is intra-sensory. So, synesthesia is not necessarily cross-sensory. It has more to do with a lack of stimulation of the appropriate variety.

Hubbard (2007: 193) thus says that synesthesia occurs when "stimulation in one sensory or cognitive stream leads to associated experiences in a second, unstimulated stream." Similarly, Brogaard (2012) says, "Synesthesia is a condition in which stimulation in one sensory or cognitive stream involuntarily, or automatically, leads to associated internal or external (illusory or hallucinatory) experiences in a second unstimulated sensory or cognitive system." Wikipedia (November 27, 2014) even characterizes synesthesia as "a neurological phenomenon in which stimulation of one sensory or cognitive pathway leads to automatic, involuntary experiences in a second sensory or cognitive pathway."

Since I want to contrast synesthesia with other crossmodal effects that involve misperception, I'll simply restrict the discussion that follows to cross-sensory varieties of synesthesia.

2.3 Crossmodal illusions

Consider a related class of effects in which stimulation to one sensory system affects experience that is associated with another sensory modality in a way that leads to illusion. A *crossmodal perceptual illusion* is a case in which activity in one sensory system causally impacts processes associated with another sensory system and thereby generates a non-veridical perceptual experience. Seeing can make you have illusory tactual impressions, and hearing can cause visual illusions. Stimulation to one sense can impact processes and alter experiences associated with another sense. Interactions of this sort are rampant, and they sometimes lead to illusions.

Ventriloquism, for instance, involves an illusory auditory perceptual experience of spatial location that is caused by the visible location of an apparent sound source. Ventriloquism is best known from the case of hearing a puppeteer "throw" a voice, and many people are surprised to learn that ventriloquism does not involve throwing sound. Instead, it involves auditorily experiencing a voice illusorily as coming from the place where a dummy is seen. The ventriloquist effect does not require speech. The minimal flash of a dot can impact where you auditorily experience a concurrent beep to come from. The effect is neither inferential nor cognitive, but results from crossmodal perceptual interactions.[3] Similarly, the *rubber hand illusion* involves visual capture of proprioceptive location. This is a case in which a touch to a rubber hand is felt as a touch to one's own hand. However, the rubber hand illusion also involves a proprioceptive location illusion induced by vision. Seeing a rubber hand, or even a prismatically displaced image of your hand, illusorily shifts where you feel your hand to be.[4]

So, visual stimulation readily leads to illusory spatial experiences that are associated with other sense modalities. However, crossmodal illusions occur for features other than space, and other modalities can affect visual experience. For instance, audition impacts temporal characteristics of visual experience in a way that leads to

[3] See Bertelson (1999); Vroomen et al. (2001).

[4] Hay et al. (1965); Pick et al. (1969). See Botvinick and Cohen (1998) for the illusion of a felt touch on the hand caused by vision.

illusion. The start of a sound can alter when a light seems to switch on, so that the light's onset seems synchronous with the sound's. A sound's duration can alter the apparent duration of a visual stimulus. A quick beep can make a moving visible target appear to freeze. Sound can also alter visually apparent rate and even temporal order.[5] So, the tempting hypothesis that vision wins or dominates whenever there's a conflict is false. In fact, crossmodal illusions are far more widespread, and the combinations defy intuition. In the *parchment skin illusion*, hearing a crinkling sound alters the apparent felt texture of a surface.[6] Crunching sounds can affect the apparent flavor of potato chips.[7] Smell not only alters taste, as in sweetness enhancement, but it even influences vision under conditions of binocular rivalry.[8]

Speech perception presents particularly compelling crossmodal illusions, including the *McGurk effect*.[9] When presented with the sound of the bilabial /ba/, pronounced with the lips together, along with incongruent video of a speaker articulating the velar /ga/, pronounced with the tongue at the back of the palette, many listeners report experiencing clearly the sound of the alveolar /da/, pronounced with the tongue near the front of the palette. The presence of the visible speaker leads to an illusory sound experience. Moreover, one modality can influence causal impressions associated with another. Consider the *motion-bounce effect*.[10] Two disks on a screen that traverse crossing diagonal paths most frequently look to subjects to stream past one another. But a sound played when the disks intersect makes the disks most frequently appear to visibly bounce and rebound from one another. Finally, consider a fascinating crossmodal illusion discovered by Shams et al. (2000, 2002). In the *sound-induced flash illusion*, presenting two beeps along with a single flash causes subjects to perceptually experience not just two beeps but also two flashes: "A single flash accompanied by multiple beeps is perceived as multiple flashes. This phenomenon clearly demonstrates that sound can alter the visual percept qualitatively even when there is no ambiguity in the visual stimulus" (Shams et al., 2002: 152). The sound-induced flash effect involves a phenomenological change to the character of visual experience that is produced by audition. It results from crossmodal perceptual mechanisms. It is a visual perceptual illusion caused by audible sounds.

Crossmodal perceptual illusions involve stimulation to one sensory system that illusorily impacts perceptual experience that is associated with another sensory modality. The effects I've described are just a selection from a rapidly expanding body of experimental research that charts the interactions among the senses. Recent findings from psychophysics and neural science demonstrate that crossmodal effects are widespread and common. These results show that processes connected with one

[5] See, e.g.,Vroomen and de Gelder (2000).

[6] Jousmäki and Hari (1998); Guest et al. (2002).

[7] Zampini and Spence (2004).

[8] See Zhou et al. (2010, 2012). See also Smith (2015) for discussion of other crossmodal effects involving chemical senses.

[9] McGurk and MacDonald (1976).

[10] Sekuler et al. (1997).

sensory system impact processes connected with others. Information from one sense can change how another responds. Such results help establish that the exteroceptive modalities of sensory perception are not causally isolated and informationally encapsulated.[11]

2.4 Synesthesia vs. crossmodal illusions

What is the relationship between synesthesia and crossmodal illusions? Synesthesia belongs to a broad class of effects in which one sense modality causally impacts another. Such findings might be thought to support the point of view according to which synesthesia is pervasive. For instance, both cross-sensory synesthesia and crossmodal illusions occur when stimulation to one sensory system impacts and alters experience associated with another sense modality in a way that leads to illusion or hallucination. As with synesthesia, subjects differ in whether and to what extent they are susceptible to crossmodal illusions. Like synesthesia, crossmodal illusions occur for a variety of features, including space, time, texture, phonemes, number, and sound. Like synesthesia, crossmodal illusions vary in intensity and quality. Some, such as the McGurk effect, are strong and robust; others, such as the sound-induced flash, are fragile, with an elusive quality. Like synesthesia, crossmodal illusions are surprising because they conflict with a widespread conception according to which the senses are explanatorily independent modes of awareness and domains of inquiry. Uncovering such a pattern of crossmodal illusions might be supposed to provide evidence that synesthetic effects are more widespread than otherwise imagined.

I want to deflect this line of thought. It is crucial to distinguish typical crossmodal perceptual illusions and recalibrations from synesthesia and synesthetic effects. Doing so illuminates why synesthesia is an outlier—a kind of experiential quirk—rather than a condition that reveals something fundamental about the nature of multisensory perception. Properly understanding the more typical varieties of crossmodal effects suggests that our interest in synesthesia has been exaggerated. If we hope to understand the types of mechanisms that ground multisensory perception, and what they reveal about the nature and function of perceptual awareness, crossmodal illusions are more revealing.

First of all, synesthesia is rare. Synesthesia that involves rich qualitative sensory phenomenology occurs in roughly one in 2,000 persons, according to Baron-Cohen et al. (1996). Simner et al. (2006) put the rate much higher, at roughly one in twenty. Even at the higher rate, synesthesia is an atypical condition, occurring in a small minority. Crossmodal illusions, however, are utterly common across the population.

[11] See, e.g., Shimojo and Shams (2001).

Within individuals, synesthetic effects are relatively isolated and are usually limited to a small range of specific feature types. Crossmodal perceptual illusions, on the other hand, are widespread across a range of different cases and domains. There are crossmodal effects involving vision, hearing, touch, proprioception, smell, and gustation. These may involve spatial, temporal, numerical, causal, or linguistic features, among others.

More to the point, synesthesia is an experiential quirk that results from highly contingent facts about sensory wiring or a specific subject's environment. It is caused by accidental, uninhibited, or counternormative causal interaction enabled by the connectedness or mere proximity of otherwise functionally distinct brain regions and pathways, or by statistical anomalies in a pattern of stimulation.[12]

In synesthesia, stimulation to one sense generates an experience as of a feature which is of a type that you need not otherwise have experienced. And stimulation to the inducer suffices to generate the concurrent experience. For instance, hearing a sound suffices to generate a color experience without the relevant visual stimulation.

In one important respect, then, synesthetically induced experiences are inappropriate. The triggering stimulus does not provide reliable information about the synesthetically experienced feature. Synesthesia tends to involve no stimulation of a sort that is correlated with the presence of the determinate feature that is experienced as the synesthetic concurrent. The process responsible for synesthesia does not enable synesthetes literally to hear colors or to taste roughness. There is no reliable connection between the colors of things and the colors a synesthete experiences as a result of hearing sounds. Things usually just lack the determinate qualities synesthetic experiences attribute. A sound–color synesthete's color experiences may track the disjunctive property of having color or pitch. But this itself does not enhance the reliability of either color or pitch experience in the absence of further inference.

Crossmodal illusions, however, are not merely aberrations or quirks of processing that stem from accidental interference. In crossmodal illusions, stimulation to one sense alters or reshapes an experience you otherwise would have through a different sense. For instance, the visual stimulus reshapes your auditory experience of a phoneme, and two beeps affect the apparent number of visible flashes you see. But stimulation to one sense alone does not suffice to generate a crossmodal illusion. Seeing a talker does not suffice to auditorily experience a phoneme, and hearing a beep does not suffice to visually experience a flash.

Moreover, in one important respect, crossmodal illusions are appropriate. The triggering stimulus is of a type that generally provides reliable information about the illusorily experienced feature. For instance, vision normally affords good information about the location of your hand. Audition typically is reliable when it comes to the

[12] Beauchamp and Ro (2008) discuss a case of stroke-induced synesthesia. For fascinating discussion of learned grapheme–color synesthesia that conforms to the colors of popular Fisher-Price toy letters, see Witthoft and Winawer (2013).

temporal features of happenings in your environment. Visible mouth movements provide informative clues about vocal gestures. Thus, crossmodal perceptual illusions are intelligible responses to unusual or extraordinary circumstances. The visible source of a sound does not often diverge from where the sound seems to be. Visible events in time usually do correspond in number to their acoustic signs. And visible mouth movements and audible sounds do not typically disagree about the phonemes a speaker utters. Paradigmatic crossmodal recalibrations and illusions thus involve reconciling conflicting information across sensory systems. As a general principle, reconciling conflicting information across the senses is a good strategy. Under unusual conditions, it leads to illusion.

Crossmodal biases and recalibrations in fact do help to improve perceptual responses by making use of information from multiple sensory sources. Under a range of normal conditions, vision's impact on other modalities concerning spatial features serves a variety of purposes. In the first instance, crossmodal processes can help to deal with simple physical facts, such as that the light from an event arrives earlier than the sound waves, or that a neural signal takes longer to reach your brain from your foot than from your eye since it must travel farther. Crossmodal interactions can help reconcile temporally offset signals when it is unlikely that they reflect asynchronous sources. Crossmodal processes thus deal with conflicting information, but they also resolve ambiguity, improve precision, and correct perceptual errors stemming from a given sense modality. Such conflict, ambiguity, imprecision, and error can stem from differences in format, perspective, resolving power, accuracy, or noisiness of sensory stimulation in different modalities. For instance, vision's spatial resolution capacity is an order of magnitude greater than audition's. So, the fact that vision can override audition enhances our capacity to perceive spatial features. Similarly, audition's temporal resolution far exceeds vision's, so the fact that audition can override vision improves perception of temporal characteristics. As a result, crossmodal processes commonly help to avoid illusions, as when vision corrects a front-back confusion in auditory localization, which stems from a limitation inherent to audition. They also improve perceptual accuracy, as when visual information enhances auditory phoneme discrimination.

Crossmodal illusions thus are accidentally illusory. They involve the deployment of perceptual strategies that lead to non-illusory experiences when applied across a wide range of typical circumstances. Such strategies help compensate for and smooth out differences in timing, perceptual ambiguities, and inaccuracies. These strategies sometimes lead to illusions—as when experimenters artificially introduce discrepancies, when perception mistakenly resolves a real-world discrepancy, or when perception leaves intact a discrepancy that should be resolved. But these illusions are intelligible and explicable in accordance with general regularities that enhance perception in multisensory contexts. Crossmodal illusions result from *intermodal* organizing strategies, principles, or rules that regularly help us to get things right. Crossmodal perceptual illusions are principled perceptual responses—in general, they predictably conform to strategies that improve the capacity to perceive for creatures like us in typical environments. For instance, in typical intermodal recalibration, information from different senses is weighted according to the relative reliability of its sources (this is evident in the McGurk effect). Such strategies are straightforwardly intelligible as conferring a perceptual advantage. The leading hypothesis is that crossmodal recalibrations enhance the overall reliability of perception.

> Altogether these findings suggest that in carrying out basic perceptual tasks, the human perceptual system performs causal inference and multisensory integration, and it does so in a fashion highly consistent with a Bayesian observer. This strategy is statistically optimal as it leads to minimizing the average (squared) error of perceptual estimates; however, it results in errors in some conditions, which manifest themselves as illusions.
>
> (Shams and Kim, 2010: 280)

Synesthesia, in contrast, is robustly or persistently illusory. It involves experiences conjured from whole cloth.[13] Synesthesia is typically unprincipled. It does not result from more general perceptual strategies for dealing with the world that are realized in other multisensory contexts. It does not typically stem from broader regularities that help to overcome perceptual limitations, inaccuracies, or ambiguities. Unlike ordinary crossmodal biases and recalibrations that sometimes lead to illusion, synesthesia is not in this way intelligible as adaptive. It is accidentally beneficial. That is, the benefits it confers do not come from its implementing strategies that enhance perceptual reliability. Mnemonic, learning, and aesthetic enhancements, for instance, stem from associations or characteristics internal to experience rather than from improvements to perceptual resolution or accuracy.

To summarize, the sound-induced flash illusion and a battery of other cases show that the predisposition toward intermodal perceptual recalibration and reconciliation in typical human perceivers is strong. That effects such as crossmodal biasing and recalibration are so prevalent across multisensory contexts suggests that crossmodal illusions are neither aberrations nor mere quirks that stem from mere accidents or miscuing. Instead, they are intelligible responses to unusual or atypical circumstances.

[13] Macpherson (2007) suggests that the distinction between crossmodal illusions and synesthesia depends on the difference between illusion and hallucination. According to the standard philosophical understanding, illusion involves perceiving an object but misperceiving its features, and hallucination involves failing to perceive an object at all. On this conception, synesthesia is not necessarily hallucinatory. In many cases, synesthetes perceive an object but misperceive its features. For instance, a synesthete might see a grapheme but misattribute some color to it. Perhaps, however, this should be understood as involving an *attribute* or *property hallucination* rather than mere illusion. This would require developing and appealing to an independently motivated conception of an attribute or property hallucination. One way to characterize the distinction between property illusion and hallucination is to appeal to determinables and determinates. In property illusion, you perceive some determinable feature but misperceive its determinate value; in property hallucination, you fail to perceive the relevant determinable. Nevertheless, being hallucinatory does not appear to suffice for being a case of synesthesia. The sound-induced flash effect, a crossmodal illusion, may involve hallucinating at least one visually apparent event. Perhaps, however, it involves illusorily perceiving an event's numerosity. Given these obstacles, I won't rely on this way of drawing the distinction.

Table 2.1. Synesthesia vs. crossmodal illusions.

Synesthesia	*Crossmodal illusions*
uncommon	common
isolated	widespread
quirky	not quirky
generates	alters
suffices	doesn't suffice
inappropriate	appropriate
principled	unprincipled
accidentally beneficial	robustly beneficial
robustly illusory	accidentally illusory

In contrast with synesthesia, which is not as a rule the result of general perceptual strategies that enable typical human subjects to better perceive features in the world, crossmodal illusions stem from perceptual strategies that are readily intelligible as adaptive and advantageous. Crossmodal illusions result from intermodal processes that conform to multisensory principles or regularities that enhance the reliability of perception. In resolving conflicts, they demonstrate a perceptual concern for the common sources of stimulation to multiple sense modalities. The experimental results show that such multisensory organizing principles apply quite generally. They apply across various sets of sense modalities, and they concern a wide range of features. They constrain multisensory perception even under ordinary conditions when conflict and ambiguity are absent and no recalibration occurs. Crossmodal perceptual interactions thus reveal that multisensory processes are widespread and shape the organization and character of perceptual awareness in typical human subjects. Synesthesia generally does not. (See Table 2.1.)

2.5 Synesthesia and synesthesis

I began with two opposing perspectives on synesthesia. According to one, synesthesia is "the strangest thing." According to the other, synesthesia is pervasive. The considerations described here favor the first. Synesthesia differs in a number of diagnostic respects from common crossmodal interactions, including those that lead to illusion. It thus should be distinguished from those more typical crossmodal effects as an outlier.

Nonetheless, this discussion suggests a conciliatory position. Viewed in the right light, synesthesia is not an outlier of a wholly distinctive variety. It belongs to the extensive class of crossmodal phenomena. In particular, synesthesia is one among many effects in which stimulation to one sensory system has a relatively immediate impact upon experience that is typically associated with another sense modality.

This broader family of crossmodal effects includes crossmodal illusions, as well as accuracy-enhancing recalibrations, biasing, resolution of ambiguity, and cuing of attention. Synesthesia may even share certain inter-sensory mechanisms with typical crossmodal interactions. Crossmodal interactions among senses are surprising and may strike us as odd because they conflict with central aspects of historically prevalent commonsense, philosophical, and scientific conceptions, according to which the senses are explanatorily independent modes of awareness and domains for inquiry.

To be clear, however, synesthesia is not an utterly pervasive phenomenon. Instead, it involves an uncommon overproliferation of crossmodal influence. When operating in the usual manner, crossmodal interactions are straightforwardly intelligible as advantageous and as adaptive perceptual capacities. In synesthesia, cross-sensory effects occur in a manner that is untethered from the requisite regularities that generally hold between features experienced through differing senses. The resulting synesthetic experiences thus systematically fail to accurately reflect one's surroundings. As a result, synesthesia lacks an obvious world-revealing benefit or an enhancement to perceptual accuracy or reliability. Nevertheless, synesthesia may confer contingent benefits, such as learning, memory, aesthetic, and creative enhancements. For instance, Watson et al. (2012b,a, 2014) propose a novel account according to which synesthetic associations are remnants of complex childhood learning tasks in which they assisted. But such benefits are due primarily to qualitative features inherent in synesthetic experiences. Thus, on balance, I concur with the important *separatist* lesson of Deroy and Spence (2013), who distinguish synesthesia from crossmodal correspondences and thus argue that we are not all even weak synesthetes.

Of course, there *could* be far more typical crossmodal effects that share central characteristics with synesthesia and that are not best understood as crossmodal perceptual illusions. And such effects could be intelligible as perceptually adaptive. An experience of one sense might be enough to trigger an appropriate experience associated with another sense. For instance, seeing visible vocal gestures might suffice on an occasion to generate auditory imagery associated with the speech sounds that normally accompany those gestures.[14] Or audition could cause appropriate tactual experiences, as perhaps occurs when hearing fingernails or metal on slate. These could be relatively direct crossmodal effects. We can even imagine cases in which the induced phenomenology is sufficiently vivid and effectively externalized. We can imagine that the induced experience in fact is a *reliable* guide in most human subjects to audible or tactual features that are present but that otherwise would go unheard or unfelt. There could be such widespread, reliable crossmodal enhancements. And, in principle, creatures could evolve to make use of them.

[14] See, e.g., Calvert et al. (1997). For an example involving musical notation, see also Brodsky et al. (2003). For a useful, relevant review of auditory imagery, see Hubbard (2010).

According to my characterization, such synesthetic crossmodal enhancements would not count as synesthesia. Instead, I recommend that we go further and distinguish *synesthesia* from *synesthetic effects*. Any cross-sensory synesthetic effect is one in which stimulation to one sense modality suffices to cause or to generate an experience with phenomenal character that is associated with a perceptual experience typical of another sense modality. Synesthesia, however, is a condition in which this type of process occurs consistently and counternormatively, and which involves systematic illusion that is only ever accidentally veridical. Thus, there could be synesthetic effects without synesthesia. It remains highly speculative to claim that outside synesthesia there actually exist robust synesthetic effects that impact the phenomenal character of experience in a manner that is associated with the affected sensory modality. Induced imagery currently provides the most intriguing examples.

Given the contrast with typical crossmodal perceptual illusions (or even merely potential reliable synesthetic effects), synesthesia pales. Just as visual illusions illuminate the principles of vision and the structure of visual awareness, crossmodal illusions help us to elucidate intermodal organizing principles and the structure of multisensory awareness. Plain crossmodal perceptual illusions and recalibrations teach us more about the nature, character, and function of perceptual awareness than their more attention-grabbing relatives with the wild qualia.

References

Auvray, M. and Deroy, O. (2015). How do synaesthetes experience the world? In Matthen, M., editor, *Oxford Handbook of Philosophy of Perception*, pp. 640–58. Oxford University Press, New York.

Baron-Cohen, S., Burt, L., Smith-Laittan, F., Harrison, J., and Bolton, P. (1996). Synaesthesia: Prevalence and familiality. *Perception*, 25(9):1073–9.

Baron-Cohen, S. and Harrison, J. E. (1997). *Synaesthesia: Classic and Contemporary Readings*. Blackwell, Malden, MA.

Beauchamp, M. S. and Ro, T. (2008). Neural substrates of sound–touch synesthesia after a thalamic lesion. *The Journal of Neuroscience*, 28(50):13696–702.

Bertelson, P. (1999). Ventriloquism: A case of cross-modal perceptual grouping. In Aschersleben, G., Bachmann, T., and Müsseler, J., editors, *Cognitive Contributions to the Perception of Spatial and Temporal Events*, pp. 347–62. Elsevier, Amsterdam.

Botvinick, M. and Cohen, J. (1998). Rubber hands 'feel' touch that eyes see. *Nature*, 391:756.

Brodsky, W., Henik, A., Rubinstein, B., and Zorman, M. (2003). Auditory imagery from musical notation in expert musicians. *Perception & Psychophysics*, 65(4):602–12.

Brogaard, B. (2012). Color synesthesia. In Jameson, K. A., editor, *Encyclopedia of Color Science and Technology*, Cognition and Language. Springer, Dordrecht.

Calvert, G. A., Bullmore, E. T., Brammer, M. J., Campbell, R., Williams, S. C. R., McGuire, P. K., Woodruff, P. W. R., Iversen, S. D., and David, A. S. (1997). Activation of auditory cortex during silent lipreading. *Science*, 276(5312):593–6.

Cytowic, R. E. (2002). *Synesthesia: A Union of the Senses*. MIT Press, Cambridge, MA, 2nd edition.

Cytowic, R. E. and Eagleman, D. M. (2009). *Wednesday is Indigo Blue*. MIT Press, Cambridge, MA.

Deroy, O. and Spence, C. (2013). Why we are not all synesthetes (not even weakly so). *Psychonomic Bulletin & Review*, 20:1–22.

Eagleman, D. M., Kagan, A. D., Nelson, S. S., Sagaram, D., and Sarma, A. K. (2007). A standardized test battery for the study of synesthesia. *Journal of Neuroscience Methods*, 159:139–45.

Guest, S., Catmur, C., Lloyd, D., and Spence, C. (2002). Audiotactile interactions in roughness perception. *Experimental Brain Research*, 146:161–71.

Harrison, J. (2001). *Synaesthesia: The Strangest Thing*. Oxford University Press, New York.

Harrison, J. E. and Baron-Cohen, S. (1997). Synaesthesia: a review of psychological theories. In Baron-Cohen, S. and Harrison, J. E., editors, *Synaesthesia: Classic and Contemporary Readings*, pp. 109–22. Blackwell, Malden, MA.

Hay, J. C., Pick, H. L., and Ikeda, K. (1965). Visual capture produced by prism spectacles. *Psychonomic Science*, 2:215–16.

Hubbard, E. (2007). Neurophysiology of synesthesia. *Current Psychiatry Reports*, 9(3):193–9.

Hubbard, T. L. (2010). Auditory imagery: Emprical findings. *Psychological Bulletin*, 136(2):302–29.

Jousmäki, V. and Hari, R. (1998). Parchment-skin illusion: sound-biased touch. *Current Biology*, 8:R190.

Macpherson, F. (2007). Synaesthesia, functionalism and phenomenology. In Marraffa, M., de Caro, M., and Ferretti, F., editors, *Cartographies of the Mind: Philosophy and Psychology in Intersection*, volume 4 of *Studies in Brain and Mind*, pages 64–80. Springer, Dordrecht.

McGurk, H. and MacDonald, J. (1976). Hearing lips and seeing voices. *Nature*, 264:746–8.

Pick, H. L., Warren, D. H., and Hay, J. C. (1969). Sensory conflict in judgments of spatial direction. *Perception and Psychophysics*, 6:203–5.

Ramachandran, V. S. and Hubbard, E. M. (2001). Synaesthesia—a window into perception, thought, and language. *Journal of Consciousness Studies*, 8(12):3–34.

Ramachandran, V. S. and Hubbard, E. M. (2003a). Hearing colors, tasting shapes. *Scientific American*, 288(5):52–9.

Ramachandran, V. S. and Hubbard, E. M. (2003b). The phenomenology of synaesthesia. *Journal of Consciousness Studies*, 10(8):49–57.

Sekuler, R., Sekuler, A. B., and Lau, R. (1997). Sound alters visual motion perception. *Nature*, 385:308.

Shams, L., Kamitani, Y., and Shimojo, S. (2000). What you see is what you hear. *Nature*, 408:788.

Shams, L., Kamitani, Y., and Shimojo, S. (2002). Visual illusion induced by sound. *Cognitive Brain Research*, 14:147–52.

Shams, L. and Kim, R. (2010). Crossmodal influences on visual perception. *Physics of Life Reviews*, 7(3):269–84.

Shimojo, S. and Shams, L. (2001). Sensory modalities are not separate modalities: plasticity and interactions. *Current Opinion in Neurobiology*, 11:505–9.

Simner, J., Mulvenna, C., Sagiv, N., Tsakanikos, E., Witherby, S. A., Fraser, C., Scott, K., and Ward, J. (2006). Synaesthesia: The prevalence of atypical cross-modal experiences. *Perception*, 35(8):1024–33.

Smith, B. C. (2015). The chemical senses. In Matthen, M., editor, *Oxford Handbook of Philosophy of Perception*, pp. 314–52. Oxford University Press, Oxford.

Vroomen, J., Bertelson, P., and de Gelder, B. (2001). Auditory-visual spatial interactions: automatic versus intentional components. In de Gelder, B., de Haan, E., and Heywood, C., editors, *Out of Mind*, pp. 140–50. Oxford University Press, Oxford.

Vroomen, J. and de Gelder, B. (2000). Sound enhances visual perception: cross-modal effects of auditory organization on vision. *Journal of Experimental Psychology: Human Perception and Performance*, 26:1583–90.

Wager, A. (1999). The extra qualia problem: synaesthesia and representationism. *Philosophical Psychology*, 12(3):263–81.

Watson, M. R., Akins, K., Spiker, C., Crawford, L., and Enns, J. T. (2014). Synaesthesia and learning: a critical review and novel theory. *Frontiers in Human Neuroscience*, 8(98).

Watson, M. R., Akins, K. A., and Enns, J. T. (2012a). Second-order mappings in grapheme–color synesthesia. *Psychonomic Bulletin & Review*, 19(2):211–17.

Watson, M. R., Blair, M. R., Kozik, P., Akins, K. A., and Enns, J. T. (2012b). Grapheme–color synaesthesia benefits rule-based category learning. *Cognition*, 21(3):1533–40.

Witthoft, N. and Winawer, J. (2013). Learning, memory, and synesthesia. *Psychological Science*, 24(3):258–65.

Zampini, M. and Spence, C. (2004). The role of auditory cues in modulating the perceived crispness and staleness of potato chips. *Journal of Sensory Studies*, 19(5):347–63.

Zhou, W., Jiang, Y., He, S., and Chen, D. (2010). Olfaction modulates visual perception in binocular rivalry. *Current Biology*, 20(15):1356–8.

Zhou, W., Zhang, X., Chen, J., Wang, L., and Chen, D. (2012). Nostril-specific olfactory modulation of visual perception in binocular rivalry. *The Journal of Neuroscience*, 32(48):17225–9.

3

Synesthetic Perception as Continuous with Ordinary Perception, or

We're All Synesthetes Now

Jonathan Cohen[1]

> Rather than displaying merely some odd, fortuitous associations, these universal synesthetic experiences reflect important cognitive properties that in several respects are common to normal people as well as to synesthetes.
>
> (Marks, 1975: 303)

One of the central outstanding puzzles about synesthesia, and one that is at least partly to blame for the recent surge in attention given to the condition by philosophers and psychologists, is that of understanding the relationship between synesthetic perception and normal perception. Of course, the answer we give to this puzzle will depend on how we conceive of both synesthesia and normal perception. In this chapter I'll argue that, given what we know about both, the most plausible view is that synesthesia is not a fundamentally distinct, pathological outlier relative to normal perception; rather, it is best understood as continuous with capacities present in normal perception.

I'll argue for this conclusion in three ways. First, I'll argue that the feature at the very heart of our understanding of synesthesia—informational integration between psychological systems—is also ubiquitous in normal perception (§3.1). Second, I'll consider similarities and differences between synesthesia and informational integration in normal perception (§3.2). I'll review evidence to the effect that there are striking, detailed, and otherwise unexpected similarities between the two forms of informational integration (§3.2.1), and I'll argue that the evidence some have taken to

[1] Department of Philosophy, University of California, San Diego, 9500 Gilman Drive, La Jolla, CA 92093-0119, joncohen@aardvark.ucsd.edu.

reveal significant qualitative differences between informational integration in synesthetes and normal perceivers is far less decisive than it might first appear (§3.2.2). Finally, I'll show how an understanding of synesthesia as continuous with normal perceptual capacities correctly predicts the otherwise surprising result that synesthetes perform better than non-synesthetes in certain perceptual tasks that don't implicate synesthetic perception (§3.3). The upshot, I'll suggest, is that synesthetic perception is usefully viewed as much closer to non-synesthetic perception (a fortiori, less clearly pathological) than standard views allow.

3.1 Informational integration, synesthetic and otherwise

My first line of argument for construing synesthesia as continuous with normal perception rests on a piece of conceptual analysis: my claim is that the distinctive feature at the core of synesthesia is in fact present, ubiquitously, in normal perception. To make this case I'll first attempt to distill out a minimal essence of what is distinctive about synesthesia (§3.1.1); then I'll argue that that same feature shows up surprisingly often in normal perception, so long as the latter is seen aright (§3.1.2), and that this fact points us in the direction of thinking of synesthetic and normal perception as species of a common kind (§3.1.3).

3.1.1 Synesthesia

There is much about synesthesia that is understood poorly or not at all. Among other controversies, there is debate over the classification and definition of the condition (e.g., Cytowic, 2001; Hubbard, 2007; Macpherson, 2007), the diversity of its forms (Day, 2005),[2] its unity as a psychological kind (Ramachandran and Hubbard, 2001; Dixon et al., 2004; Simner, 2012),[3] and whether it is inherited or acquired (Armel and Ramachandran, 1999; Beauchamp and Ro, 2008; Harrison and Baron-Cohen, 1995; Cohen Kadosh et al., 2009; Asher et al., 2009). Similarly, there is controversy over whether the experience of an $A - B$ synesthete (one whose perceptual encounters with A cause an experience that is associated in normals with perception of B is like that of a normal subject but with an added, synesthetic layer of normal experience (as it were, a normal A-type experience conjoined with a normal B-type experience), or whether her synesthetic experience is simply alien/incomparable to the

[2] Sean Day lists "more than 65" types of synesthesia, individuated by inducer/concurrent pairs, at his website (http://www.daysyn.com/Types-of-Syn.html).

[3] Ramachandran and Hubbard (2001) distinguish between "lower" synesthetes, in whom the trigger is more closely linked to specific sensory features (e.g., in grapheme-color synesthesia, graphemes trigger the color reaction only when presented in particular fonts), and "higher" synesthetes, in whom the trigger seems less tied to particular perceived properties (thus, e.g., unusual fonts or Roman numerals will bring about the concurrent color representation). Dixon et al. (2004) mark a separate distinction between "projector" synesthetes, who experience their concurrents as located in space, and "associator" synesthetes, who do not.

experiential inventory of normals. There is controversy about the implications synesthesia has for the individuation of the senses (Keeley, 2013) and philosophical views such as functionalism (Gray et al., 1997, 2002; Macpherson, 2007), representationalism (Wager, 1999, 2001; Alter, 2006; Gray, 2001b; Rosenberg, 2004), and modularity (Baron-Cohen et al., 1993; Segal, 1997; Gray, 2001a).[4]

Despite all this controversy, there is at least one idea about synesthesia that seems uncontroversial: on more or less all accounts, synesthesia involves the presence of (abnormal) influence between systems that, in ordinary circumstances, represent distinct features. That is, what makes a grapheme-color synesthete's experience (more generally, an $A - B$ synesthete's experience) notable is that, in her, the system that in ordinary circumstances represents grapheme identity $(/A)$ activates or mediates representations in the system that, in, ordinary circumstances, represent color $(/B)$. Hence occurrences of A in such a subject (the "trigger"/"inducer") mediate representations of B (the "concurrent"). Moreover, notice that the link between the A system and the B system in synesthetic perception is not merely causal: it is not only that the activity of the A system initiates or triggers activity in the B system, but that the resulting particular state of (hence, information carried by) the B system counterfactually/informationally depends on the particular state of (hence, information carried by) the A system that does the triggering. Thus, in grapheme-color synesthesia, for example, it is not only that the activity of the grapheme-representation system causes activity in the color-representation system (though that is true). Crucially, and in addition, *which* color is synesthetically represented by the color system depends counterfactually/informationally on which grapheme is represented in the grapheme-representation system. Consequently, it makes sense to describe such cases by saying that the activity of the A system (unusually) draws on information represented in the A system—that there is here a kind of crosstalk, or informational integration between the A system and the B system.[5]

[4] For a useful overview of these and other controversies about synesthesia, see Auvray and Deroy (2013).

[5] Two remarks about the notion of informational integration at work are in order. (Thanks here to Matthew Fulkerson for discussion.)

First, the term 'informational integration' shouldn't be taken to imply that the states of the $(/A)$ and $(/B)$ systems between which there is an integration carry information about any single common distal feature type. Rather, the suggestion is that there is a causal interaction between two states that carry information, despite their carrying information about different feature types. (Thus, for example, in the case of grapheme-color synesthesia, the interaction obtains between a first state that carries information about distal grapheme form and a second state that carries information about distal color.)

Second, we shouldn't assume that the way the integration works is that there will always be a (non-synesthetically induced) B representation prior to the interaction, such that the integration consists in a modification of that prior B-representation in a way that depends on the A-representation. The point is only that, whether there is a B-representation prior to the synesthetic interaction or not, the resulting state of the B-representing system is counterfactually/informationally dependent on the information represented in the A-system. In this sense, the B system (unusually) draws on information represented in the A system, so there is no informational firewall between the two. (That said, there do appear to be cases where there is a prior B-representation. For example, a grapheme-color synesthete who synesthetically represents the grapheme 'L' as green will typically also non-synesthetically perceive the black color of the ink in which

Now, saying this much leaves a cornucopia of questions unanswered. Perhaps most significantly, it presupposes some method for individuating psychological systems and identifying them with ordinary content-types. It also leaves plenty of room for disagreement about the nature of the causal and informational connections between the systems, and just what systems (only perceptual systems? mid-level perceptual systems? cognitive systems?) will, when joined in the relevant way, count as synesthetically linked. And it leaves open all of the controversial issues gestured at in the beginning of this section. But this far-reaching agnosticism is just the point: the idea that synesthesia involves integration between normally unconnected psychological systems constitutes an island of consensus in a sea of controversy about the condition. And it has, I suggest, a good claim to the status of essential core of our understanding of what synesthesia amounts to.

This idea is present in the Greek etymological roots of the term: *syn-* (joining), *-aesthesis* (sensation). It is reflected in the standard characterization of the condition as a merging/mixing/union/unity of the senses,[6] and it shows up in some form in all of the proposed theoretical definitions and glosses. Thus, for example, Marks (1978: 8) defines synesthesia as "the transposition of sensory images or sensory attributes from one modality to another" (cf. Marks, 1975: 303). Harrison and Baron-Cohen (1997) "define synaesethesia as occurring when stimulation of one sensory modality automatically triggers a perception in a second modality, in the absence of any direct stimulation to this second modality" (3). Harrison (2001) describes the condition as "implying the experience of two or more sensations occurring together" (3). Cytowic (2001) offers the idea of a "sensory blending" (2). According to Ramachandran and Hubbard (2001), "Synaesthesia is a curious condition in which an otherwise normal person experiences sensations in one modality when a second modality is stimulated" (4). Similarly, Gray et al. (2002) write that "Synaesthesia is a condition in which, in otherwise normal individuals, stimulation in one sensory modality reliably elicits the report of a sensation in another" (5).[7] A more complicated expression of the idea comes out in Macpherson's definition:

Synaesthesia is a condition in which either:

(i) an experience in one sensory modality, or
(ii) an experience not in a sensory modality, such as an experience of emotion, or
(iii) an imagining or thought of what is so experienced, or

that grapheme is printed. (This point explains the possibility of Stroop-like interference between synesthetic and non-synesthetic representations—now a common diagnostic for synesthesia (Dixon et al., 2000; Mattingley et al., 2001; Mills et al., 1999) that, on its face, appears to be some kind of interesting computational combination between independently generated A and B representations.)

[6] Such phrases are used as titles or subtitles by, e.g., Marks (1978); Cytowic (2001); Ward (2008).

[7] This formulation puts more weight on the report of the concurrent, per se, than is probably wanted; surely the report is only instrumentally useful to the extent it serves as evidence of the real item of interest—the concurrent sensation itself. If so, an improved version would define synesthesia as a condition in which, in otherwise normal individuals, stimulation in a first sensory modality reliably elicits a sensation in another.

(iv) a mental state outlined in either (i)–(iii), together with recognition of what the mental state represents is either a sufficient automatic cause of, or has a common sufficient automatic cause (lying within the central nervous system of the subject) with, an experience or element of experience that is associated with some sensory modality and is distinct from (i).

This synaesthetic experience or element of experience can be associated with the same or a different sensory modality from that which may be ordinarily associated with the mental state in (i)–(iv). (Macpherson, 2007: 70)[8]

Without meaning to downplay or ignore the important and interesting differences between these competing definitions, I want to make the simple point that they are all, appropriately, agreeing on the central idea about synesthesia with which we started. Namely, they are agreeing (despite their differences) that the condition crucially involves the activation and informational mediation by a system that ordinarily represents a first type of information of a system that ordinarily represents a second type of information.

There is an obvious diagnosis of the convergence on this idea by so many different theoretical proposals: viz., that the idea genuinely captures what lies at the heart of our understanding of synesthesia. At any rate, I propose that we adopt this view, and carry out our comparison between synesthesia and normal perception by (at least in part) asking whether that core idea distinguishes synesthesia from normal perception. This will be the task of §3.1.2.

3.1.2 Normal perception

Needless to say, the view we take about the relationship between synesthetic and normal perception will depend not only on how we are thinking about synesthesia but also on our understanding of normal perception. This matters because there are ways of thinking of normal perception in currency that make the informational integration characteristic of synesthetic perception look more exceptional than I believe it is. I want to argue that, on the contrary, information integration is rife in normal perception. And this, I'll suggest, should give us an initial reason to take

[8] Note that Macpherson's definition (unlike the others quoted) does not restrict attention to associations between specifically sensory representations. Among other benefits, the absence of this restriction leaves Macpherson's definition in a better position than competitors to accommodate the "higher" synesthetes of Ramachandran and Hubbard (2001), in whose synesthetic experience the role of sensory or perceptual representation is at best incidental. This seems like an attractive feature of her proposal.

I am less sympathetic to another of the selling points Macpherson advertises: she points out that, by restricting attention to *sufficient* causes in clause (iv), her proposed definition respects her intuition that there is a difference in kind between synesthesia and cases of crossmodal illusion (e.g., the McGurk effect) in normal perception (cf. Macpherson, 2007: 70–1). Of course, it is one of the morals of the present chapter to question just this intuition (hence whether respecting it is a benefit of a proposed definition). However, whatever one thinks about the status of the disputed intuition at the end of the day, the point I'm making in the main text stands: Macpherson's definition, just like the simpler proposals considered above, makes central the idea that synesthesia involves abnormal causal influence between systems that, in ordinary circumstances, represent distinct features.

seriously the hypothesis that synesthetic perception is continuous with non-synesthetic perception.[9]

We can begin to address the issue of informational integration in normal perception by asking whether and to what extent the individual perceptual mechanisms extracting particular distal features in normal perception—e.g., shape, color, form, and motion (in vision); pitch, loudness, and timbre (in audition)—are mutually informationally encapsulated.[10]

One logically possible answer to this question—call it the *dedicated feature extraction view*—is that feature extractors in normal perception are, by and large, mutually informationally encapsulated. Thus, for example, this view would predict that the shape extractor (as it might be) carries out its computations in a way that is insensitive to, and independent of, the information extracted by the color extractor (as it might be), and vice versa.

Though the dedicated feature view is a logically possible answer to our question, I believe that that logically possible answer is incorrect as a matter of empirical fact, in that it ignores the extensive evidence of significant integration between separate extractors. In particular, I want to motivate an alternative *integrative view*, on which feature extractors are integrated in (inter alia) the informational sense discussed above. That is to say, first, that the operation of one extractor can have causal effects on the operation of another. More than this, it is to say that there is a kind of counterfactual/informational integration between feature extractors: the particular state taken on by a second extractor (hence, the information it carries about the world) depends counterfactually and informationally on the particular state taken on by a first (hence, the information it carries about the world).[11]

In §3.1.2.1, I will argue that, of these two competing pictures, the integrative conception offers us a more satisfying and empirically adequate way of thinking of perception. If I am right about this, then this will go some distance to showing

[9] The discussion in this subsection, and especially the presentation of evidence of informational integration in normal perception in §3.1.2.1, draws on material from Burnston and Cohen (2012).

[10] Clark (2000) argues persuasively that a picture of perception as a bundle of feature extractors is incomplete, and must be supplemented by mechanisms for binding extracted features to perceived objects. For present purposes I ignore this (serious) complication as well as all sorts of interesting and important questions about the relation between feature perception and object perception; for more on such themes, see Burnston and Cohen (2012).

[11] There is a further, distinct, sense in which separate extractors may reasonably be said to be integrated in normal perception. Namely, there is reason to think that separate extractors can be directed at the extraction of a common feature, such that they run independently and in parallel, but such that their output is then combined and reconciled at some later point. Thus, for example, it is plausible that visual representations of depth are computed from the output of several such independent extractors, each independently running its own characteristic algorithm over its own characteristic range of input (as it might be, one or more computing stereopsis from retinal disparity data, a cluster deriving depth information from pictorial cues, a further cluster computing depth information from familiar object size information, and so on—for evidence of this kind of integration and further discussion, see Burnston and Cohen, 2012). I'll put this further sense of integration aside in what follows.

that the forms of integration we found at the heart of synesthesia (§3.1.1) don't, after all, mark a significant qualitative distinction between synesthetic and normal perception.

3.1.2.1 INTEGRATION IN NORMAL PERCEPTION

There are, it would appear, many processes in normal perception that point to the kind of informational integration under discussion. For reasons of space I give only a few (sadly, mostly visuocentric) examples that I take to be illustrative of the general theme.

A first kind of evidence of informational interactions within a perceptual modality comes from Field et al. (2009), who show that rod photoreceptors, which ordinarily function under scotopic conditions, provide input to blue/yellow opponent pathways in the macaque retina. What is interesting and surprising about this finding is precisely that, even though rod photoreceptors and blue/yellow pathways are generally thought to extract quite different ranges of distal features (indeed, in what one might have thought were almost entirely non-overlapping conditions), the information represented by the blue/yellow pathway turns out to be systematically, counterfactually dependent on rod photoreceptor informational output.

Here is a related, and similarly low-level, albeit somewhat speculative, case concerning color vision. Broackes (2009) has suggested that human deuteranopes employ dynamic input from their intact S-cone receptors to extract color information that is ordinarily subserved in trichromats by the (non-dynamic) output of L-cones or M-cones. Again, if correct, this proposal speaks to the existence of informational integration at the photoreceptor level: the suggestion is that red/green extractors are not encapsulated from S-cone output, but instead that the state of the red/green system depends counterfactually/informationally on the state of the S-cones.

Moving above the photoreceptor level, there is increasing evidence that luminance/chromatic properties are used by the visual system to estimate shape, depth, texture, and more (see, for example, Mullen et al., 2000; Kingdom, 2003; den Ouden et al., 2005; Kingdom et al., 2006; Kingdom and Kasrai, 2006; Gheorghiu and Kingdom, 2007; Hansen and Gegenfurtner, 2009). If that is true, then it means that extractors for shape, depth, texture, and so on are not only causally triggered by, but also informationally/counterfactually dependent on the information carried by luminance and chromatic feature extractors. And the McCollough effect (McCollough, 1965) and similar illusions suggest that some of those dependencies may run in the other direction as well: these effects suggest that extractors of chromatic color information are causally triggered by, and informationally/counterfactually dependent on, the particular informational states of form, orientation, and motion extractors. Likewise, there is abundant evidence of interaction between visual representations of luminance and motion. Thus, researchers have shown that motion processing is impaired or qualitatively different at isoluminance—e.g., that motion is represented as slower at isoluminance, that the direction of motion is far more difficult to discriminate at isoluminance, and that isoluminant stimuli can induce a motion aftereffect on luminance stimuli (Anstis, 2003, 2004; Howe et al., 2006; Mullen and Baker, 1985; Thompson, 1982). Again, this means that extractors for visual motion are triggered by, and informationally/counterfactually depend on, the information carried by luminance extractors.

Nor are the sorts of perceptual interactions of interest limited to intramodal cases. Thus, to mention some well-known examples, the McGurk effect (in which subjects' visual perception of a mouth's motion affects their auditory perception of simultaneously heard speech sound (McGurk and MacDonald, 1976)) and the ventriloquist illusion (in which subjects perceive a ventriloquist's voice as originating from the location of the visually perceived dummy rather than that of the auditorily perceived ventriloquist (Pick et al., 1969; Vroomen and de Gelder, 2000, 2004)) give us reason for thinking that the state of at least some auditory feature extractors are causally, informationally, and counterfactually dependent on the state of at least some visual feature extractors. Similarly, the cutaneous rabbit illusion (Geldard and Sherrick, 1972) and cases of sensory substitution (e.g. Bach y Rita et al., 1969) are standardly taken to show that there is two-way informational/counterfactual dependence between the states of tactile and visual feature extractors.

All of these findings give us reason for doubting that the perceptual mechanisms for the extraction of distinct features in normal perception are mutually encapsulated in the way that the dedicated feature extraction view proposes. In turn, they motivate taking seriously the alternative, integrative picture as the correct view about normal perception.

3.1.2.2 MORALS

The instances of perceptual integration discussed above are, to all appearances, representative of the architecture of perception: informational integration (at many levels of organization) appears to be the rule rather than the exception in perceptual systems. Indeed, so overwhelming is the evidence in favor of integration that it can become hard to avoid seeing informational interaction in perceptual mechanisms once one begins to look.

On reflection, this is perhaps less surprising than one might have thought. First, given a fixed number of sensory receptors, and a large (if finite) number of perceptible features to which we are sensitive, it is more or less inevitable that feature extractors should share information at one level or another. Second, the very idea of perceptual computation, which is central to perception on nearly anyone's story, depends on sharing featural information. For, construed generally, perceptual computation means deriving values for new output features on the basis of features already extracted. Thus, when the perceptual system computes form from motion, or objecthood from edge locations, or illumination from higher-order scene statistics (for example), it is using prior featural information—representations of feature exemplifications that have already been extracted (possibly together with information about environmental regularities and channel conditions)—to extract novel featural information.[12] As such, the novel, extracted features depend systematically on the features used as input to the perceptual computation, which is just to say that the former cannot be informationally encapsulated from the latter.

Given these points, it is no surprise to learn of the many instances of informational integration in perception. If anything, the question is why the dedicated feature extraction view should have seemed plausible in the first place (to the extent it ever did).[13]

3.1.3 *Continuity and discontinuity*

In so far as the dedicated feature extraction view and the integrative view offer us quite different pictures of the degree of informational integration present in normal perception, they make available different views of the relation between synesthetic and normal perception.

From the vantage point of the dedicated feature extraction view, the informational integration characteristic of synesthesia amounts to a pathological form of crosstalk between distinct, normatively encapsulated feature extractors. As such, accepting that view of normal perception is tantamount to endorsing a discontinuity view about the relation between synesthetic and normal perception. On the other hand, because the integrative picture conceives crosstalk between distinct feature extractors as a routine part of normal perception, the occurrence of such crosstalk in synesthetic cases won't, by itself, mark the latter as pathological in the same way.

This is not to say that the integrative view of (normal) perception is unable to see any distinctions at all between normal and synesthetic perception. For one thing, even by the lights of the integrative view, the particular forms and degree of crosstalk characteristic of, say, grapheme-color synesthesia are statistically abnormal. For another, there's nothing to prevent the proponent of the integrative view from recognizing that synesthetic representations are unlike non-synesthetic perceptual representations in being typically erroneous: presumably, for example, the induced

[12] There are, to be sure, forms of radical enactivism and other anti-representational views of perception on which this sort of computation, defined over representations, plays a far less central role. However, I do not believe that these views can offer a descriptively adequate account of perception (for particularly persuasive arguments to this effect, see Gallistel, 2008; Burge, 2010), so will put them aside in what follows.

[13] This is perhaps the place to mention that there is no in principle conflict between the view that normal perception depends extensively on the sort of informational integration we have been discussing and the view that there is substantial modularity/cognitive impenetrability (in the sense of Fodor (1983)) in normal perception. First, the idea of integration between feature extractors leaves it open that the extractors might exhibit Fodor's hallmarks of modularity—they might be, for all I have said, domain-specific, mandatory, fast, informationally encapsulated from central cognition, fixed in their neural architecture, and so on. Second, nothing that has been said above requires that integrative processes should exhibit the "isotropic" or "Quinean" features Fodor (1983) takes to threaten modularity. For more extensive discussion, see Burnston and Cohen (2014).

synesthetic color representation occurring in a grapheme-color synesthete is (ordinarily) an erroneous representation of the color of the perceived grapheme.[14]

Such differences notwithstanding, the broad lesson stands: given the integrative view (but not given the dedicated feature extraction view), the integration present in synesthesia will look much more like an extension of integrative elements present in ordinary perception than an unprecedented, pathological case. To this extent, then, the integrative view of normal perception makes possible a continuity thesis about the relation between normal and synesthetic perception.

To see what such a continuity view amounts to, it may be helpful to compare the case of synesthesia against ordinary perceptual illusion, on the one hand, and tumor- or schizophrenia-induced hallucination, on the other. When I perceive the Müller-Lyer configuration, for example, I end up with a misrepresentation of the size of certain elements in the display. Plausibly, this occurs not because there is some radically discontinuous, pathological, and unusually error-prone mechanism for size representation at work in just these situations. Rather, the error comes about because the very same, highly reliable mechanisms for size and form perception that serve me well in ordinary contexts operate here as well, but misfire in predictable ways when extended to this configuration. Given all this, a continuity view about the relation between normal (veridical) perception and ordinary illusion seems appropriate. In contrast, perceptual (or apparently perceptual) hallucinations caused by certain tumors or schizophrenia are at least partly the result of mechanisms that *are* radically discontinuous, pathological, and unusually error-prone. As such, a continuity view about the relation between normal perception and such tumor- or schizophrenia-induced hallucinations is much less plausible. The continuity view about synesthesia is the view that the relation between synesthesia and normal perception is, in these senses, closer to that between ordinary perceptual illusion and normal perception than it is to that between tumor-/schizophrenia-induced hallucination and normal perception.

As we have seen, the evidence reviewed above supports the integrative view over the dedicated feature extraction view of normal perception. And since the former but not the latter position supports a continuity view concerning synesthesia, the evidence for the integrative view also supports construing normal and synesthetic perception as species of a common kind.

3.2 Synesthetic and non-synesthetic associations: compare and contrast

My second line of support for a continuity thesis about the relation between synesthetic and normal perception comes from consideration of similarities and

[14] Here I ignore complications connected with my own (somewhat idiosyncratic) account of errors of color representation (see Cohen, 2007, 2009). For the record, I don't believe that there is ultimately a clash between those views and what I say here.

differences between the two. After reviewing some of the evidence concerning such similarities (§3.2.1) and differences (§3.2.2), I'll turn briefly to the methodological question of just how we should think about the role of such similarities and differences in assessing the dispute between continuity and discontinuity views (§3.2.3).

3.2.1 *Similarities*

On the evidence, there appear to be interestingly deep similarities between cases of informational integration in synesthetic and non-synesthetic perception. Specifically, the evidence suggests that when non-synesthetes are asked to make deliberate, nonce (non-synesthetic) associations between domains linked in synesthetic subjects, they do so in ways that—to a surprising extent—mirror the automatic, non-deliberate, much more stable, synesthetically mediated associations made by their synesthetic counterparts.

3.2.1.1 GRAPHEME-COLOR INTRAMODAL MAPPING

We can begin by comparing grapheme-color associations made by synesthetes and normal controls.

What makes grapheme-color associations interesting as a test case for continuity between synesthetic and non-synesthetic perception is that, while grapheme-color synesthesia is by far the most common (Day, 2005) and (at least in the last twenty years) probably the most widely studied form of synesthesia, pairings between graphemes and colors do not play any significant role at all in the mental lives of non-synesthetes. Of course, non-synesthetes can deliberately construct (nonce) grapheme-color associations; but there is no prior reason to expect that the pairings they choose should be much like the pairings in grapheme-color synesthetes in any significant respect. As it turns out, however, grapheme-color synesthetes and normals display a surprising level of consistency (within and between groups) in pairing letters and colors (Simner et al., 2005). Thus, both within and between groups, 'a' tends to be associated with red, 'b' with blue, 'c' with yellow, and so on (cf. Baron-Cohen et al., 1993; Day, 2001, 2005; Rich et al., 2005).

To be fair, Simner et al. (2005) go on to report differences between synesthete and control performance on this task. Specifically, they report that the particular grapheme-color pairings in synesthetes (but not normal controls) are mediated by frequency: higher-frequency graphemes are paired with colors whose names are higher in lexical frequency.[15] They found that the pairings chosen by non-synesthetes were not mediated by these factors. Rather, they found that the pairings chosen by non-synesthetes were a function of the presentation order of materials and the

[15] Simner et al. (2005) note that a color term's lexical frequency correlates with its position in the Berlin and Kay hierarchy (Berlin and Kay, 1969; Lindsey and Brown, 2009), hence that synesthetes are also pairing high-frequency graphemes with colors whose lexical expression is more fundamental in the Berlin and Kay typology.

typicality of colors (as measured by standard category norm ranking (Battig and Montague, 1969)).

Thus, it seems that synesthetes and non-synesthetes converge, to a surprising extent, in their choices of specific grapheme-color pairings, though differences in the properties of these pairings suggest that there may be different mechanisms underpinning the observed convergence. Given this situation, whether we should view grapheme-color pairings in synesthetes as two manifestations of a single psychological capacity will depend on how we individuate capacities. But even on the two-capacities construal, the observed behavioral convergence suggests that synesthetic and non-synesthetic grapheme-color pairings are at least closely related.

Nonetheless, whether construed as two versions of one capacity or two separate capacities, there are clear senses in which synesthetes outperform non-synesthetes on grapheme-color pairings. Namely, synesthete pairings are more intrapersonally consistent over time, specific/fine-grained, and automatic than those of non-synesthetes. (It is unsurprising that synesthetes outperform non-synesthetes on these measures, which are often used as diagnostics for the condition (Baron-Cohen et al., 1987, 1993).)

3.2.1.2 SOUND-COLOR INTERMODAL MAPPING

Much of what I've said about intramodal associations between graphemes and colors holds true as well for intermodal associations between sounds and colors. Once again, the comparison of interest is between the synesthetically mediated pairings between sound and color and the sound-color pairings made by normal controls.[16]

There are a number of interesting shared trends in the sound-color pairings made by both synesthetes and non-synesthetes. First, synesthetes and normal controls exhibit significant within- and between-group convergence in associating higher pitches with lighter/brighter colors, and lower pitches with darker colors. This convergence holds both in cases where the sounds in question are vowel sounds in natural language (Wundt, 1874; Ortmann, 1933; Karwoski and Odbert, 1938; Wicker, 1968; Marks, 1974) and in cases where the sounds are produced by (non-vocal) musical instruments (Karwoski et al., 1942; Wicker, 1968; Marks, 1974, 1982, 1987; Hubbard, 1996; Melara, 1989; Ward et al., 2006).[17] Second, Ward et al. (2006) report that synesthetes and normal controls exhibit significant within- and between-group convergence in associating certain instrument timbres with particular chroma (cf. Mudge, 1920): in their (somewhat hyperbolic) words, "musical notes from the piano and strings are, literally, more colourful than pure tones" (7). Third, Bleuler

[16] Sound-color synesthesia—also called chromesthesia—is another common and (at least until recent years in which grapheme-color synesthesia may have pulled ahead) much-studied form of synesthesia.

[17] More specifically, the association is between frequency (of the second formant, in the case of vowel sounds; of the fundamental, in the case of non-linguistic sounds) and lightness/brightness. See Marks (1975) for an extensive review of the nineteenth and twentieth-century documentation of this convergence.

and Lehmann (1881), Voss (1929), and Marks (1975) report a further shared trend: synesthetes and normal controls exhibit significant within- and between-group convergence in associating softer/louder sounds with smaller/larger colored patches. Though size is not a dimension of color, this shows yet another systematic similarity in the way synesthetes and non-synesthetes associate auditory and visual features.

These results are interesting not simply in that they reveal that synesthetes and non-synesthetes can both match individual sounds to individual colors; rather, they are interesting because they show that synesthetes and non-synesthetes agree in the way they systematically map particular auditory dimensions onto particular visual dimensions. Because of the specificity of the agreement in synesthetic and non-synesthetic pairings that these findings reveal, they suggest that there may be a shared mechanism mediating the auditory-visual associations in synesthetes and non-synesthetes.

Be that as it may, there are, once again, clear respects in which synesthetes exhibit superior performance in matching sounds to colors. For, unsurprisingly, synesthetic sound-color pairings have both higher internal consistency and higher specificity in color selection relative to the sound-color pairings made by normals (Ward et al., 2006).

3.2.2 Differences

Notwithstanding the similarities noted in §3.2.1, there are certainly also interesting differences between the cases (also as already noted). Indeed, in a provocative recent paper, Deroy and Spence (2013) appeal to such differences to argue that the continuity view is untenable. In particular, and though they consider several other differences as well that they take to be less telling against the continuity view, Deroy and Spence urge that crossmodal associations in normal perception are unlike synesthetic associations in being (i) bidirectional rather than unidirectional, (ii) transitive rather than intransitive, (iii) relative rather than absolute, (iv) malleable rather than rigid, and (v) plausibly expressed in non-human animals and human infants.[18]

[18] Below I follow Deroy and Spence (2013) in restricting discussion to alleged disanalogies between synesthetic associations and crossmodal correspondences in normal perception, even though the latter constitute a proper subset of the informational integrations in normal perception discussed in §3.1.2.

Even within this range, I'll ignore for reasons of space several of the features they list but take not to be as clearly incompatible with the continuity view. (I agree with them that these other features are not serious obstacles to that view.)

Finally, I'll ignore Deroy's and Spence's more programmatic objections to the effect that running together perceptual integration in normal perception and synesthesia may exhibit a kind of bias, is likely to confuse investigators, or makes unconfirmed empirical predictions—all of which I find untroubling. After all, I would have thought it is problematic to exhibit such bias only if the view it favors is false (which is just what is at issue). Similarly, if the continuity view is true, then entertaining or adopting it will lead to desirable enlightenment, rather than undesirable confusion. Finally, if it is true that the view makes unconfirmed empirical predictions, I suggest that that fact should be counted among its epistemic features rather than bugs (by both its fans and foes).

Unfortunately, I want to argue that the evidence of difference these authors rely on in arguing against the continuity view is substantially less decisive than they suppose.

3.2.2.1 UNIDIRECTIONALITY AND TRANSITIVITY

Deroy and Spence (2013: 653–4) claim that (at least historically) researchers have taken synesthetic relations to be unidirectional/asymmetric (if an inducer *I* synesthetically elicits a concurrent *C*, then *C* will not in general serve as an inducer that synesthetically elicits *I* in the same subject), while they have taken crossmodal associations in normal perception to be bidirectional/symmetric (e.g., visual large size primes auditory low pitch iff auditory low pitch primes visual large size). Additionally, they conjecture that crossmodal associations in normal perception may be transitive, while there is no evidence indicating that the same is true of synesthetic associations (655).

However, though Deroy and Spence appear to treat these differences as central to their case against continuity, I think it is fair to say that the evidence they offer concerning unidirectionality and transitivity is, at best, mixed. On the side of unidirectionality, they themselves point out that a number of investigators have recently reported finding bidirectional synesthetic elicitations (Cohen Kadosh et al., 2007; Cohen Kadosh and Henik, 2006; Cohen Kadosh et al., 2008; Gebuis et al., 2009; Johnson et al., 2007; Knoch et al., 2005; Richer et al., 2011), but worry that the cases reported are so far limited in number and breadth. Of course, Deroy and Spence are surely right that it would be nicer to have a richer range of data on the question. However, I don't see why that should be counted as a reason to doubt the data points that we have so far, and that, on their face, seem to suggest that the criterion of unidirectionality does not pull synesthesia apart from crossmodal association in normal perception. Turning to transitivity, Deroy and Spence admit freely that the question of whether crossmodal associations in normal perception are transitive "has, to [their] knowledge, not been investigated in any detail yet," and that their case for it remains entirely speculative.

In short, the evidence Deroy and Spence present under this heading falls far short of a decisive demonstration of a significant difference between the two sorts of cases.

3.2.2.2 RELATIVITY/CONTEXT-SENSITIVITY

Deroy and Spence (2013: 655–6) hold that "the concurrent in the case of synesthesia ... seems to be dependent solely on the nature of the inducer, and not on the other objects along which that inducer happens to be presented," whereas "the evidence concerning crossmodal correspondences suggests that they are very often relative. It is, for example, the relative, not the absolute, size that matters in the case of size-pitch correspondences."

Now, Deroy and Spence admit that this difference is less clearcut than it would seem, since, for example, it appears that the concurrent elicited by a bistable grapheme in grapheme-color synesthesia depends on the presence of surrounding characters that can induce one disambiguation rather than another (Dixon et al., 2006; Rich and Mattingly, 2003). But they respond to this apparent counterevidence by redescribing the case in a way that does not involve contextually relative concurrent elicitation by a single, bistable grapheme inducer. On their alternative description, there is a single, bistable *shape*, which can then be resolved (with contextual cues) into one of two context-insensitive, unambiguous *graphemes*, each of which elicits a single concurrent. In other words, their suggestion is that the context-relativity occurs prior to the representation of graphemes, and that each grapheme synesthetically elicits a concurrent in a context-insensitive (/"absolute") way. In this way, they hope to hold on to their claim that synesthetic associations are context-insensitive ("absolute"), while crossmodal associations in normal perception are context-sensitive.

I find this attempt to explain away the putative counterexamples to their criterion unconvincing.

First, just as a matter of dialectical burden-pushing, it should be clear that the criterion at issue will fail in its intended purpose of distinguishing synesthetic from non-synesthetic correspondences unless Deroy's and Spence's interpretation of the evidence is mandatory, as opposed to merely available; and they have done nothing to show that it is.[19]

Second, note that the interpretation Deroy and Spence propose for the apparent effects of context on synesthetic grapheme-color associations can be applied just as well or poorly as a description of the apparent effects of context on crossmodal size-pitch correspondence (or any other apparently context-sensitive crossmodal association) in normal perception. Here, too, we might deny that there is one single size that can be contextually modified to elicit different crossmodally associated pitches. Rather, we could say that there are two different values of a parameter we might call 'proximal size' that is computationally prior to the representation of object size. And the thought would be that there is a single, ambiguous *proximal size*, which can then be resolved (with contextual cues) into one of many possible context-insensitive, unambiguous *(object) sizes*, each of which elicits a single crossmodally associated pitch. In other words, the suggestion is that the context-relativity occurs prior to the representation of object sizes, and that each object size crossmodally elicits an associated pitch in a context-insensitive (/"absolute") way.

In general, the lesson seems to be that it is no more or less possible to apply the contemplated strategy of redescription as a way of denying context-sensitivity in both the synesthetic and non-synesthetic cases. Pending further argument or evidence that

[19] A further worry: the proposed re-explanation depends on supposing that a single context-relative shape is ambiguous between distinct context-mediated graphemic resolutions. If this is to avoid simply pushing back a contextually mediated synesthetic link by one step, it had better turn out that we have good reasons for denying that what takes us from context-relative shape to a grapheme is a synesthetic correspondence.

would break this symmetry, it would appear that the proposed criterion of difference does not, after all, distinguish between the kinds of cases.

3.2.2.3 MALLEABILITY

Deroy and Spence further maintain that crossmodal and synesthetic correspondences are differentially malleable by training/experience. On the one hand, they point out that inducer-concurrent relations in adult synesthetes are stable over time and relatively invulnerable to modification by learning/experience. On the other hand, they review evidence suggesting that "a subset of crossmodal correspondences (i.e., semantic ones) can be learned very rapidly, in a matter of trials" by adults (Deroy and Spence, 2013: 657).

But, once again, the alleged distinction in malleability is less clear than this lets on. First, Deroy and Spence are right to restrict their claim about malleability to a proper subset of crossmodal cases, since there are plenty of crossmodal correspondences (e.g., parade cases such as the ventriloquist illusion mentioned in §3.1.2.1, or the motion-bounce illusion (Sekuler et al., 1997)) that appear to be (at least) significantly less malleable. This shows, minimally, that the criterion under discussion fails to divide cleanly between synesthetic and crossmodal correspondences. But, second, if the unity of the class of crossmodal illusions withstands variation in malleability, as it appears to, then it's hard to see how variation in malleability could be a kind-distinguishing boundary that would separate off synesthetic from crossmodal correspondences in the way that Deroy and Spence say it does.[20]

3.2.2.4 INFRAVERBAL EXPRESSION

Deroy and Spence also propose to distinguish between crossmodal and synesthetic correspondences on the grounds that the former, but not the latter, are expressed in non-human animals (652) and human neonates and infants (645). Unfortunately, and as Deroy and Spence recognize in places (e.g., 645), it is controversial whether the specific cases they cite as evidence of crossmodal correspondence in infraverbals are crossmodal or synesthetic in nature, so this evidence fails to draw the distinction for which they enlist it. Moreover, it should be noted that one of the two leading current accounts locates the ontogenesis of adult human synesthesia in inadequate synaptic pruning over the normal course of development (Maurer and Maurer, 1988; Maurer and Mondlach, 2005; Baron-Cohen, 1996). Though this view, too, is controversial, if correct, it would suggest that synesthesia is indeed expressed widely

[20] A further concern about application of the malleability criterion is that apparent differences in malleability may reflect hidden asymmetries in regularity and reinforcement. Thus, it may be that synesthetic correspondences are, in principle, no less malleable than crossmodal correspondences, but seem so only because they are reinforced much more consistently in the experience of synesthetes relative to the transient crossmodal coincidences (such as those between, say, colors and flavors) mentioned by Deroy and Spence (2013: 657).

in early development.[21] Once again, it is hard to see this criterion as representing a boundary between distinct qualitative kinds.

3.2.3 *Methodological interlude*

In this section I have compared cases of informational integration in synesthetic and normal perception, and have argued that the similarities are deeper, and the differences shallower, than it might seem. Without retracting any of what I have said, however, I want to emphasize that the comparative component of the case for continuity, as I understand it, does not rest in simply pointing to similarities between the cases, or in (absurdly) denying the existence of disanalogies between the cases (as I suppose it would if it were an identity view rather than a continuity view). It is undeniable that there are both similarities and differences. But this observation leaves open whether such similarities and differences as there are merit treating the two kinds of associations as falling into different taxonomic kinds (as we do when, for example, we decide that, on reflection, it serves our explanatory purposes to treat jadeite and nephrite as different kinds) or not (as we do when, for example, we decide that, on reflection, it serves our explanatory purposes to treat adult and childhood expressions of chicken pox as different forms of the same underlying condition, or to treat whales and orangutans as members of the common kind *mammalia*). Which taxonomic choice we make in a given case depends not merely on spotting bare similarities or differences, but (among other things) on the explanatory needs in place, and how alternative choices serve those needs.

In applying these lessons to the choice between continuity and discontinuity views about the relation between synesthesia and normal perception, we should bear in mind the wide variety of cases of informational integration in normal perception, involving many different mechanisms at many different levels of perceptual processing, as discussed in §3.1.2. Consideration of this range naturally invites the worry that Deroy and Spence (2013) distinguish between synesthetic and non-synesthetic integration on the basis of differences that are not obviously wider or more important than those that separate instances of non-synesthetic integration. That is, if Deroy's and Spence's differences are sufficient to warrant a discontinuity view about synesthesia and normal perceptual integration, it is not at all obvious that we should count as instances of a common kind such normal perceptual phenomena as, e.g., postreceptoral integration, dominance, suppression, crossmodal dependence, spatiotemporal integration, and feature binding—which are all plausibly at least as different from one another across a range of criteria as synesthetic integration is from crossmodal

[21] On the main alternative account, synesthesia arises from feedback disinhibition between primary sensory areas and higher cortical areas in the brain (Grossenbacher and Lovelace, 2001). It's worth noting that, though the feedback disinhibition story doesn't have to be told in a way that predicts the expression of synesthesia in early development, this account is also potentially conducive to the continuity view, assuming (not implausibly) that there is a similar form of feedback disinhibition at work in normal crossmodal integration.

association. My defense of the continuity view is grounded in the thought that it sometimes serves explanation to be able to see the commonalities at work here—while also acknowledging the differences. (Though I intend this lesson to apply generally, see §3.3 for one dramatic class of findings whose explanation seems to hang on being able to see such commonalities.) If this is right, it would seem that the continuity view represents an attractive explanatory framework for thinking about perception.

3.3 Synesthetic enhancement of crossmodal integration

The third line of support I want to offer for the continuity view comes from recent work by Brang et al. (2012) showing that synesthetic performance on integrative perceptual tasks is enhanced relative to normal controls.[22] This evidence adds to the case for continuity because it amounts to a surprising connection between synesthetic and non-synesthetic informational integration that cries out for explanation, and that is easily explained if the continuity view is correct, but not easily explained otherwise.

Brang et al. (2012) compare synesthetic and non-synthetic integration by exploiting two much-studied intermodal interactions between visual and auditory perception known to be present in normal/non-synesthetic subjects. The first is the so-called double-flash illusion, in which a single visual flash is perceived as two visual flashes when accompanied by two auditory beeps (Shams et al., 2000). The second is the intersensory facilitation of reaction time—the finding that reaction times in congruent multimodal (simultaneously presented auditory and visual) stimulus detection tasks are significantly lower than reaction times for detection carried out in either modality alone (Hershenson, 1962), and, indeed, relative to what would be expected from a statistical summation of two independent, unimodal target detection processes (Miller, 1982, 1986).

These tasks are interesting for the purpose of assessing the continuity thesis, since they are known instances of perceptual integration in non-synesthetic subjects, and therefore afford an opportunity to test how and whether the relevant sorts of integration are affected by the presence of synesthesia. Significantly, however, Brang et al. (2012) chose to run these experiments on grapheme-color synesthetes. Since none of the stimuli in either of their tasks involved graphemes, the grapheme-color synesthesia of their synesthetic subjects should not have been engaged directly on these particular tasks.[23]

As usual, given our purposes of assessing the continuity/discontinuity controversy, we are interested in the comparison between synesthetes and normal controls, as

[22] To be clear, I am using 'enhancement' merely to describe an increased effect size; the claim is not that synesthetic perception is in these respects more accurate or reliable than, an improvement upon, or adaptively/teleologically superior to perception in normal controls.

[23] Brang et al. (2012) add that "None of the synesthetes experienced a synesthetic percept for any of the auditory or visual targets used. By utilizing stimuli that caused no synesthetic experiences, we can be confident that group differences reflect generalized processing, as opposed to differences driven by synesthetic percepts" (632).

measured by their susceptibility to the double-flash illusion, on the one hand, and the intersensory facilitation of reaction time on a detection task, on the other. For, if the types of perceptual interaction one sees in normal perception are different in kind from what occurs in synesthesia, as per a discontinuity view, one would not expect that the presence of synesthesia would have any systematic effect on them. In contrast, if perceptual interaction in normal perception is continuous with—a weaker or less pervasive form of the same kind as—perceptual interaction in normal controls, one would expect that the presence of synesthesia would enhance such forms of perceptual interaction.

Brang et al. (2012) report results on both experiments that fall squarely into line with the predictions of the continuity view. Thus, in the double-flash experiment, they found that (grapheme-color) synesthetes were significantly less likely than normals to report veridically that there was only a single flash accompanied by two beeps (viz., synesthetes were significantly more susceptible to the crossmodal illusion). And in the intersensory facilitation experiments, they found that synesthetic subjects benefited significantly more (relative to their unimodal baselines) from a multimodal stimulus than did normal controls.

These results are particularly significant because they show not only that there are systematic similarities between synesthetic and non-synesthetic performance in associating elements within or across perceptual modalities (as do the cases discussed in §3.2.1), but that the effects are exaggerated in synesthetes even in domains where their synesthesia is unengaged. This fact is explicable on the hypothesis that the enhancement is due to an interaction between synesthesia and some shared associative mechanism operating in both populations. In contrast, if normal perception and synesthesia are fundamentally discontinuous, then one would not expect the form of crosstalk that underlies synesthesia to have any systematic effect on performance on tasks involving unrelated forms of perceptual integration (relative to the performance of normal controls).[24] It would appear, then, that the observed results are (at least partly) explicable on the continuity view, while it is very hard to imagine what a discontinuity-friendly explanation would look like. As such, these results strongly support the continuity view.

3.4 Conclusion

The initial question with which we began was how we should understand the relationship between synesthetic and non-synesthetic perception. The answer to this question that I've been advancing in the foregoing—the continuity view—is

[24] Indeed, we might even predict that performance on such tasks would be *degraded* in synesthetes (relative to the performance of normal controls), on the hypothesis that the (unrelated) perceptual integration occurring in the perceptual systems of synesthetic subjects may place additional load on capacities enlisted in the perceptual tasks we test.

that the two are less different, hence that synesthesia is less of a pathological outlier, than traditional views would allow.

To be sure, there are ways of thinking about normal perception, such as the dedicated feature extraction view, that exaggerate the difference between it and synesthesia. But it has been my contention that these ways of thinking about normal perception are unjustified. I claim that once we adopt a more adequate view of normal perception—one that recognizes informational integration occurring within and between modalities—it is much more difficult to construe the (admittedly more extensive) informational integration characteristic of synesthetic perception as fundamentally different in kind. Moreover, the view that synesthetic and non-synesthetic perception are species of a common kind is far easier to reconcile with the observed systematic similarities between synesthetic and non-synesthetic cross-domain associations. And while there are undeniably also differences between synesthetic and non-synesthetic informational integration, there is reason (given standard explanatory needs in perceptual science) to regard these differences as relatively shallow, quantitative variations between elements of a common kind, rather than fundamental, qualitative, and kind-demarcating. Finally, the continuity view predicts the otherwise surprising finding that integrative effects in perception are enhanced in synesthetes relative to normal controls (even when the tasks do not involve the specific triggers that generate synesthetic percepts in the synesthetes). To the extent that having an explanation of these findings is better than not having one, these considerations further support the continuity view.

Of course, in advocating continuity I don't mean to suggest that synesthetic and normal perception are in all, or all interesting, respects alike. Nor do I claim that there are no differences between informational integration in normal and synesthetic perception. Rather, the claim is that when we think about ordinary perception as displaying various kinds of integration that are less controversially present in synesthetic perception, this gives us an explanatorily richer way of thinking of the ordinary cases, and more fully reveals and explains what is shared by both types of perceivers.[25]

References

Alter, T. (2006). Does synaesthesia undermine representationalism? *Psyche,* **12**(5), 1–11.

Anstis, S. M. (2003). Moving objects appear to slow down at low contrasts. *Neural Networks,* **16**, 933–8.

[25] Thanks to David Brang, Daniel Burnston, Ophelia Deroy, John Dougherty, Matthew Fulkerson, Don MacLeod, Eliot Michaelson, Elizabeth Seckel, Chris Wüthrich, and two anonymous referees, and to audiences at the Varieties of Human Cortical Colour Vision conference in Vancouver and the Institut d'Etude de la Cognition, Ecole Normale Supérieure, for many useful suggestions that have improved this chapter considerably.

Anstis, S. M. (2004). Factors affecting footsteps: contrast can change the apparent speed, amplitude and direction of motion. *Vision Research*, **44**, 2171–8.

Armel, K. C. and Ramachandran, V. S. (1999). Acquired synesthesia in retinitis pigmentosa. *Neurocase*, **5**, 293–6.

Asher, J. E., Lamb, J. A., Brocklebank, D., Cazier, J.-B., Maestrini, E., Addis, L., Sen, M., Baron-Cohen, S., and Monaco, A. P. (2009). A whole-genome scan and fine-mapping linkage study of auditory-visual synesthesia reveals evidence of linkage to chromosomes 2q24, 5q33, 6p12, and 12p12. *The American Journal of Human Genetics*, **84**(2), 279–85.

Auvray, M. and Deroy, O. (2013). Synesthesia: phenomenal enrichment and its challenges. In M. Matthen, editor, *The Oxford Handbook of Philosophy of Perception*. Oxford University Press, Oxford.

Bach y Rita, P., Collins, C. C., Saunders, F., White, B., and Scadden, L. (1969). Vision substitution by tactile image projection. *Nature*, **221**, 963–4.

Baron-Cohen, S. (1996). Is there a normal phase of synaesthesia in development? *Psyche*, **2**(27).

Baron-Cohen, S., Harrison, J., Goldstein, L. H., and Wyke, M. (1993). Coloured speech perception: is synaesthesia what happens when modularity breaks down? *Perception*, **22**, 419–26.

Baron-Cohen, S., Wyke, M., and Binnie, C. (1987). Hearing words and seeing colours: an experimental investigation of synaesthesia. *Perception*, **16**, 761–7.

Battig, W. F. and Montague, W. E. (1969). Category norms for verbal items in 56 categories: a replication and extension of the Connecticut norms. *Journal of Experimental Psychology*, **80**, 1–46.

Beauchamp, M. S. and Ro, T. (2008). Neural substrates of sound-touch synesthesia after a thalamic lesion. *The Journal of Neuroscience*, **28**(50), 13696–702.

Berlin, B. and Kay, P. (1969). *Basic Color Terms: Their Universality and Evolution*. University of California Press, Berkeley.

Bleuler, E. and Lehmann, K. (1881). *Zwangsmäßige Lichtempfindungen durch Schall und verwandte Erscheinungen auf dem Gebiete der anderen Sinnesempfindungen*. Verlag, Leipzig.

Brang, D., Williams, L. E., and Ramachandran, V. S. (2012). Grapheme-color synesthetes show enhanced crossmodal processing between auditory and visual modalities. *Cortex*, **48**(5), 630–7.

Broackes, J. (2009). What do the colour-blind see? In J. Cohen and M. Matthen, editors, *Color Ontology and Color Science*. MIT Press, Cambridge, Massachusetts.

Burge, T. (2010). *Origins of Objectivity*. Oxford University Press, Oxford.

Burnston, D. and Cohen, J. (2012). Perception of features and perception of objects. *The Croatian Journal of Philosophy*, **36**, 283–314.

Burnston, D. and Cohen, J. (2014). Perceptual integration, modularity, and cognitive penetration. In A. Raftopoulos and J. Zeimbekis, editors, *Cognitive Influences on Perception: Implications for Philosophy of Mind, Epistemology, and Philosophy of Action*. Oxford University Press, Oxford.

Clark, A. (2000). *A Theory of Sentience*. Oxford University Press, New York.

Cohen, J. (2007). A relationalist's guide to error about color perception. *Nous*, **41**(2), 335–53.

Cohen, J. (2009). *The Red and The Real: An Essay on Color Ontology*. Oxford University Press, Oxford.

Cohen Kadosh, R., Cohen Kadosh, K., and Henik, A. (2007). The neuronal correlate of bidirectional synesthesia: a combined event-related potential and functional magnetic resonance imaging study. *Journal of Cognitive Neuroscience*, **19**(12), 2050–9.

Cohen Kadosh, R. and Henik, A. (2006). When a line is a number: color yields magnitude information in a digit-color synesthete. *Neuroscience*, **137**(1), 3–5.

Cohen Kadosh, R., Henik, A., and Walsh, V. (2009). Synaesthesia: learned or lost? *Developmental Science*, **12**(3), 484–91.

Cohen Kadosh, R., Tzelgov, J., and Henik, A. (2008). A synaesthetic walk on the mental number line: the size effect. *Cognition*, **106**(1), 548–57.

Cytowic, R. E. (2001). *Synesthesia: A Union of the Senses*. MIT Press, Cambridge, Massachusetts, 2nd edition.

Day, S. A. (2001). Trends in synesthetically colored graphemes and phonemes. *Iconicity in Language*. Available at http://www.daysyn.com/Day2004Trends.pdf.

Day, S. A. (2005). Some demographic and socio-cultural aspects of synesthesia. In L. C. Robertson and N. Sagiv, editors, *Synesthesia: Perspectives from Cognitive Neuroscience*, pp. 11–33. Oxford University Press, Oxford.

Deroy, O. and Spence, C. (2013). Why we are not all synesthetes (not even weakly so). *Psychonomic Bulletin & Review*, **20**, 643–64.

Dixon, M. J., Smilek, D., Cudahy, C., and Merikle, P. M. (2000). Five plus two equals yellow. *Nature*, **406**, 365.

Dixon, M. J., Smilek, D., Duffy, P. L., Zanna, M. P., and Merikle, P. M. (2006). The role of meaning in grapheme-colour synaesthesia. *Cortex*, **42**(2), 243–52.

Dixon, M. J., Smilek, D., and Merikle, P. M. (2004). Not all synaesthetes are created equal: projector versus associator synesthetes. *Cognitive, Affective and Behavioral Neuroscience*, **4**(3), 335–43.

Field, G. D., Greschner, M., Gauthier, J. L., Rangel, C., Shlens, J., Sher, A., Marshak, D. W., Litke, A. M., and Chichilnisky, E. J. (2009). High-sensitivity rod photoreceptor input to the blue-yellow color opponent pathway in macaque retina. *Nature Neuroscience*, **12**, 1159–64.

Fodor, J. A. (1983). *The Modularity of Mind*. MIT Press, Cambridge, Massachusetts.

Gallistel, C. R. (2008). Learning and representation. In R. Menzel, editor, *Learning Theory and Behavior*, volume 1 of *Learning and Memory: A Comprehensive Reference*, pp. 227–42. Elsevier, Oxford.

Gebuis, T., Nijboer, T. C. W., and Van der Smagt, M. J. (2009). Multiple dimensions in bi-directional synesthesia. *European Journal of Neuroscience*, **29**(8), 1703–10.

Geldard, F. A. and Sherrick, C. E. (1972). The cutaneous "rabbit": A perceptual illusion. *Science*, **178**(4057), 178–9.

Gheorghiu, E. and Kingdom, F. A. A. (2007). Chromatic tuning of contour-shape mechanisms revealed through the shape-frequency and shape-amplitude after-effects. *Vision Research*, **47**(14), 1935–49.

Gray, J., Williams, S., Nunn, J., and Baron-Cohen, S. (1997). Possible implications of synaesthesia for the hard question of consciousness. In S. Baron-Cohen, editor, *Synaesthesia: Classic and Contemporary Readings*. Blackwell, Oxford.

Gray, J. A., Chopping, S., Nunn, J., Parslow, D., Gregory, L., Williams, S., Brammer, M. J., and Baron-Cohen, S. (2002). Implications of synaesthesia for functionalism: theory and experiments. *Journal of Consciousness Studies*, **9**(12), 5–31.

Gray, R. (2001a). Cognitive modules, synaesthesia and the constitution of psychological natural kinds. *Philosophical Psychology*, **14**(1), 65–82.

Gray, R. (2001b). Synaesthesia and misrepresentation: a reply to Wager. *Philosophical Psychology*, **14**(3), 339–46.

Grossenbacher, P. G. and Lovelace, C. T. (2001). Mechanisms of synesthesia: cognitive and physiological constraints. *Trends in Cognitive Sciences*, **5**(1), 36–41.

Hansen, T. and Gegenfurtner, K. R. (2009). Independence of color and luminance edges in natural scenes. *Visual Neuroscience*, **26**(1), 35–49.

Harrison, J. (2001). *Synaesthesia: The Strangest Thing*. Oxford University Press, Oxford.

Harrison, J. and Baron-Cohen, S. (1995). Synaesthesia: reconciling the subjective with the objective. *Endeavour*, **19**(4), 157–60.

Harrison, J. E. and Baron-Cohen, S. (1997). Synaesthesia: an introduction. In S. Baron-Cohen and J. E. Harrison, editors, *Synaesthesia: Classic and Contemporary Readings*, pp. 3–16. Wiley-Blackwell, Oxford.

Hershenson, M. (1962). Reaction time as a measure of intersensory facilitation. *Journal of Experimental Psychology*, **63**(3), 289–93.

Howe, P. D. L., Thompson, P. G., Anstis, S. M., Sagreiya, H., and Livingstone, M. J. (2006). Explaining the footsteps, belly dancer, wenceslas, and kickback illusions. *Journal of Vision*, **6**, 1396–405.

Hubbard, E. M. (2007). Neurophysiology of synesthesia. *Current Psychiatry Reports*, **9**(3), 193–9.

Hubbard, T. L. (1996). Synesthesia-like mappings of lightness, pitch, and melodic interval. *The American Journal of Psychology*, **109**(2), 219–38.

Johnson, A., Jepma, M., and de Jong, R. (2007). Colours sometimes count: awareness and bidirectionality in grapheme-colour synaesthesia. *The Quarterly Journal of Experimental Psychology*, **60**(10), 1406–22.

Karwoski, T. F. and Odbert, H. S. (1938). *Color-Music*, volume 50 of *Psychological Monographs*, ed. by J. F. Dashiell. American Psychological Association.

Karwoski, T. F., Odbert, H. S., and Osgood, C. E. (1942). Studies in synesthetic thinking: II. The role of form in visual responses to music. *Journal of General Psychology*, **26**, 199–222.

Keeley, B. L. (2013). What exactly is a sense? In J. Simner and E. M. Hubbard, editors, *The Oxford Handbook of Synaesthesia*. Oxford University Press, Oxford.

Kingdom, F. A. A. (2003). Colour brings relief to human vision. *Nature Neuroscience*, **6**, 641–4.

Kingdom, F. A. A. and Kasrai, R. (2006). Colour unmasks dark targets in complex displays. *Vision Research*, **46**(6–7), 814–22.

Kingdom, F. A. A., Wong, K., Yoonessi, A., and Malkoc, G. (2006). Colour contrast influences perceived shape in combined shading and texture patterns. *Spatial Vision*, **192**(2–4), 147–59.

Knoch, D., Gianotti, L. R., Mohr, C., and Brugger, P. (2005). Synesthesia: when colors count. *Cognitive Brain Research*, **25**(1), 372–4.

Lindsey, D. T. and Brown, A. M. (2009). World color survey color naming reveals universal motifs and their within-language diversity. *Proceedings of the National Academy of Sciences of the USA*, **106**(47), 19785–90.

Macpherson, F. (2007). Synaesthesia, functionalism and phenomenology. In M. de Caro, F. Ferretti, and M. Marraffa, editors, *Cartographies of the Mind: Philosophy and Psychology in Intersection Series: Studies in Brain and Mind, Vol. 4*, pp. 65–80. Kleuwer.

Marks, L. E. (1974). On associations of light and sound: the mediation of brightness, pitch, and loudness. *The American Journal of Psychology*, **87**(1/2), 173–88.

Marks, L. E. (1975). On colored-hearing synesthesia: cross-modal translations of sensory dimensions. *Psychological Bulletin*, **82**(3), 303–31.

Marks, L. E. (1978). *The Unity of the Senses*. Academic Press, New York.

Marks, L. E. (1982). Bright sneezes and dark coughs, loud sunlight and soft moonlight. *Journal of Experimental Psychology: Human Perception and Performance*, **8**(2), 177–93.

Marks, L. E. (1987). On cross-modal similarity: auditory-visual interactions in speeded discrimination. *Journal of Experimental Psychology: Human Perception and Performance*, **13**(3), 384–94.

Mattingley, J. B., Rich, A. N., and Bradshaw, J. L. (2001). Unconscious priming eliminates automatic binding of colour and alphanumeric form in synaesthesia. *Nature*, **410**, 580–2.

Maurer, D. and Maurer, C. (1988). *The World of the Newborn*. Basic Books, New York.

Maurer, D. and Mondlach, C. J. (2005). Neonatal synaesthesia: A reevaluation. In L. C. Robertson and N. Sagiv, editors, *Synaesthesia: Perspectives from Cognitive Neuroscience*, pp. 193–213. Oxford University Press, New York.

McCollough, C. (1965). Adaptation of edge-detectors in the human visual system. *Science*, **149**, 1115–16.

McGurk, H. and MacDonald, J. (1976). Hearing lips and seeing voices. *Nature*, **264**(5588), 746–8.

Melara, R. D. (1989). Dimensional interaction between color and pitch. *Journal of Experimental Psychology: Human Perception and Performance*, **15**(1), 69–79.

Miller, J. (1982). Divided attention: evidence for coactivation with redundant signals. *Cognitive Psychology*, **14**(2), 247–79.

Miller, J. (1986). Timecourse of coactivation in bimodal divided attention. *Attention, Perception & Psychophysics*, **40**(5), 331–43.

Mills, C. B., Boteler, E. H., and Oliver, G. K. (1999). Digit synaesthesia: a case study using a stroop-type test. *Cognitive Neuropsychology*, **16**, 181–91.

Mudge, E. L. (1920). The common synaesthesia of music. *Journal of Applied Psychology*, **4**(4), 342–5.

Mullen, K. T. and Baker, Jr, C. L. (1985). A motion aftereffect from an isoluminant stimulus. *Vision Research*, **25**(5), 685–8.

Mullen, K. T., Beaudot, W. H., and Mcllhagga, W. H. (2000). Contour integration in color vision: a common process for the blue-yellow, red-green and luminance mechanisms? *Vision Research*, **40**(6), 639–55.

Ortmann, O. (1933). Theories of synesthesia in the light of a case of color hearing. *Human Biology*, **51**, 155–211.

den Ouden, H., van Ee, R., and de Haan, E. (2005). Colour helps to solve the binocular matching problem. *The Journal of Physiology*, **567**(2).

Pick, Jr, H. L., Warren, D. H., and Hay, J. C. (1969). Sensory conflict in judgements of spatial direction. *Attention, Perception, & Psychophysics*, **6**(4), 203–5.

Ramachandran, V. S. and Hubbard, E. M. (2001). Synaesthesia: a window into perception thought and language. *Journal of Consciousness Studies*, **8**(12), 3–34.

Rich, A. N., Bradshaw, J. L., and Mattingly, J. B. (2005). A systematic, large-scale study of synaesthesia: implications for the role of early experience in lexical-colour associations. *Cognition*, **98**(1), 53–84.

Rich, A. N. and Mattingly, J. B. (2003). The effects of stimulus competition and voluntary attention on colour-graphemic synaesthesia. *NueroReport*, **14**, 1793–8.

Richer, F., Beaufils, G.-A., and Poirier, S. (2011). Bidirectional lexical-gustatory synesthesia. *Consciousness and Cognition,* **20**(4), 1738–43.

Rosenberg, G. (2004). *A Place for Consciousness: Probing the Deep Structure of the Natural World.* Oxford University Press, New York.

Segal, G. (1997). Synaesthesia: Implications for the modularity of mind. In S. Baron-Cohen, editor, *Synaesthesia: Classic and Contemporary Readings,* pp. 211–24. Blackwell, Oxford.

Sekuler, R., Sekuler, A. B., and Lau, R. (1997). Sound alters visual motion perception. *Nature,* **385**, 308.

Shams, L., Kamitani, Y., and Shimojo, S. (2000). What you see is what you hear. *Nature,* **408**(6814), 788.

Simner, J. (2012). Defining synaesthesia. *British Journal of Psychology,* **103**, 1–15.

Simner, J., Ward, J., Lanz, M., Janasari, A., Noonan, K., Glover, L., and Oakley, D. A. (2005). Non-random associations of graphemes to colours in synaesthetic and non-synaesthetic populations. *Cognitive Neuropsychology,* **22**(8), 1069–85.

Thompson, P. (1982). Perceived rate of movement depends on contrast. *Vision Research,* **22**, 377–80.

Voss, W. (1929). Das farbenhoren bei erblindeten. *Archiv fur die Gesamte Psychologie,* **73**, 407–524.

Vroomen, J. and de Gelder, B. (2000). Sound enhances visual perception: crossmodal effects of auditory organization on vision. *Journal of Experimental Psychology: Human Perception and Performance,* **26**(5), 1583–90.

Vroomen, J. and de Gelder, B. (2004). Ventriloquism and the freezing phenomenon. In G. A. Calvert, C. Spence, and B. E. Stein, editors, *The Handbook of Multisensory Processes,* pp. 141–50. MIT Press, Cambridge, MA.

Wager, A. (1999). The extra qualia problem: synaesthesia and representationalism. *Philosophical Psychology,* **12**, 263–81.

Wager, A. (2001). Synaesthesia misrepresented. *Philosophical Psychology,* **14**(3), 347–51.

Ward, J. (2008). *The Frog Who Croaked Blue: Synesthesia and the Mixing of the Senses.* Routledge, London.

Ward, J., Huckstep, B., and Tsakanikos, E. (2006). Sound-colour synaesthesia: to what extent does it use cross-modal mechanisms common to us all? *Cortex,* **42**, 264–80.

Wicker, F. W. (1968). Mapping the intersensory regions of perceptual space. *The American Journal of Psychology,* **81**(2), 178–88.

Wundt, W. (1874). *GrundzUge der physiologischen Psychologie.* Engelmann, Leipzig.

4

Reporting Color Experience in Grapheme-Color Synesthesia

On the Relation Between Color Appearance, Categories, and Terms

Yasmina Jraissati

Synesthesia is a genuinely perceptual phenomenon. In the most commonly observed case of grapheme-color synesthesia, the synesthete genuinely experiences a specific color when perceiving a grapheme. Several empirical data confirm the perceptual genuineness of the synesthetic experience. Neuro-imagery studies have shown that the cortical areas usually activated in color perception are activated when a synesthetic color is experienced (Nunn et al., 2002; Brang et al., 2011). Behavioral data, using the Stroop effect, also speak in favor of the perceptual nature of synesthesia. The Stroop effect is observed in the case of incongruence between a color term and the color of the ink in which the color term is printed. Participants' naming of the color of the ink is hindered by the incongruence of the color term. Take, for example, the term "red" printed in blue ink, compared to a patch of blue ink, with the task being to name the color of the ink (blue) in both conditions. The participant in this case is slower at naming the color of the ink (blue) in which the term "red" is printed than at naming the color of the ink (blue) in which the patch is printed (for a review and variants of the Stroop effect, see MacLeod, 1991). When it comes to the use of the Stroop effect in synesthesia, the incongruence occurs between the color of the ink in which the letter is printed and the synesthetic color induced by the letter. Take, for example, a synesthete, S., who associates the letter A with the color red. It has been shown (see for example Dixon et al., 2004; Nikolić et al., 2007) that synesthetes are slower at naming the color of the ink in which the letter A is printed when there is an incongruence between the color of the ink (say blue) and the color induced by the letter A (in this case red). This effect is an argument in favor of the fact that synesthesia is a genuinely perceptual phenomenon.

The perceptual genuineness of the synesthetic phenomenon is also indicated by the highly specific verbal reports that synesthetes make of their synesthetic experience.

In his paper, Eagleman reports artist Carol Steen's description of the concurrent of the letter *i* as a "hard metallic texture"; as for *z*, it is "the color of ale with a bubbly texture", while the number *1* has "the soft texture of a flannel blanket" (Eagleman and Goodale, 2009: 2). Referring to Sean Day's email forum for synesthetes, Eagleman also reports the synesthetic perceptual experiences of Catherine Y. Catherine says: "*A*: a buttery yellow with a linen texture, *E*: a deep velvety blue, *I*: white and slick, *O*: clear, like lucite, and 3-dimensional, *U*: grey" (Eagleman and Goodale, 2009: 2).

Yet studies of grapheme-color synesthesia typically ignore the visual complexity of the concurrent, and focus on the reported color only, especially in terms of hue. So, for example, Catherine Y.'s *A* would be typically reported as associated with yellow, *E* with blue, and *I* with white. These reports would therefore systematically discard any non-typically chromatic information—namely the buttery-ness of the reported yellow, the linen texture associated with *A*, the velvety smoothness of *E*, and the slickness of *I*. For this reason, it is understandable that some synesthetes complain about the way they are asked to report their color experiences and find it far too reductive (Eagleman and Goodale, 2009: 1).

Not only is non-chromatic information generally ignored in grapheme-color synesthesia studies, but on some occasions, the chromatic information itself is also simplified. Historically, we owe to Day the introduction of basic color categories (Berlin and Kay, 1969) in the synesthesia literature (Day, 2005). Day was collecting data from synesthetes across the world by written correspondence, and could only rely on verbal reports. Also, given that the synesthetes he was in contact with were from different linguistic communities, Day felt the need to use a universal typology for comparability purposes. For these practical reasons, Day referred to the Berlin and Kay theory. However, given the highly specific experiences reported by synesthetes, one should wonder whether such a simplification is justified when it is not practically unavoidable, and whether it might not have important theoretical implications for our understanding of synesthesia. In this chapter, I would like to uncover such implications.

The discussion between Simner and Beeli, spanning over three papers between 2005 and 2008, is a particularly eloquent case, regarding how critical color reporting is in grapheme-color synesthesia. The discussion that opposes Simner to Beeli pertains to the nature of the mediation occurring between inducer and concurrent. Based on the fact that letters are learned, Simner wants to argue that what mediates the association of a grapheme inducer with a color concurrent is of a conceptual nature (Simner et al., 2005; Simner and Ward, 2008). Further, Simner wants to argue that the association is conceptually mediated to the extent that the way the concurrent is associated with the inducer is linked to the color *term*, not its appearance. More specifically, Simner et al. contend that the association is mediated by language. Beeli et al., on the other hand, would like to argue that although the inducer may be of a conceptual and linguistic nature, the reason why a given color is associated with a given grapheme has to do with the appearance of the color, and is independent of the color term (Beeli et al., 2007).

Thus, the way synesthetic colors are reported in this discussion is key. I would like to show that the methodological choice of using basic color terms to report synesthetic experience has important theoretical implications. More specifically: (1) using the Berlin and Kay typology to argue for a linguistic and conceptual mediation of the synesthetic association in fact weakens the argument and is potentially incoherent; (2) the way this typology is used obscures other possibly interesting accounts that the broader framework of the basic color terms theory may be able to provide.

In what follows, I first present the discussion opposing Simner to Beeli. Next, I analyze the introduction of the Berlin and Kay typology in this discussion, clarify the notion of basic color terms as well as its theoretical framework, and finally go over the implications that the use of this notion entails. In the last section of this chapter, I point to a possible alternative account of the data in light of the color categorization literature.

4.1 Factors underpinning the color-grapheme association: the discussion

In their 2005 study, Simner et al. (2005) ask two questions: (a) What is the root of the grapheme-color association in synesthesia? (b) Does the phenomenon reflect an exaggeration of mechanisms of association common to all? As we shall see below, Simner et al. take their results to show both that there are common trends across synesthetes, and common trends across synesthetes and non-synesthetes. Also, both populations (synesthete and non-synesthete) seem to be influenced by color vocabulary. Thus, to the question (a) of what drives the non-random associations, Simner et al. (2005) answer that it is the linguistic content of both the inducer and the concurrent. When it comes to the second question (b), Simner et al. (2005) champion the continuity hypothesis, according to which synesthetic and non-synesthetic associations have common underlying mechanisms.

Simner et al. (2005) compare color associations of seventy native English-speaking synesthetes with those of 217 English-speaking and fifty-eight German-speaking non-synesthete control participants. Participants were asked to note on a form which color first came to mind in association with one of the twenty-six letters of the English alphabet and 0 to 9 digits. A German-speaking non-synesthete control group of fifty-eight participants also took the test. Given that synesthesia is most reliably established through consistency in time (Eagleman et al., 2007, but see Simner, 2012), a further control group of thirty-five English-speaking participants took the test twice with a 1–3-week interval. Synesthetes were re-tested 2–6 months later.

Synesthetic color terms were processed in the following way. Responses were considered consistent if the same response was elicited twice for the same grapheme. If the same term was not used twice, two independent coders assessed whether the terms were equivalent. So, for example, "beige" and "light brown" were considered equivalent, and both were therefore taken to be instances of "brown". Thus, all color terms produced in association with graphemes were reduced to the set of eleven basic color terms of the Berlin and Kay typology, namely: "white", "black", "red", "yellow", "green", "blue", "brown", "grey", "purple", "pink", and "orange" (Berlin and Kay, 1969).[1]

One of Simner's first notable results is the observation of some common trends across synesthetes. As shown in the introduction, synesthetic color experiences are highly specific. If at least some of these associations were found across synesthetic individuals, this would be a reason to grant that there are some neurological mechanisms underpinning these associations. The next question is then naturally what, in the content of the inducer and in that of the concurrent, drives the association? It could be either the appearance or the conceptual content of both the inducer and the concurrent.

Simner et al.'s account of the linguistically mediated association is in fact two-fold: there are two ways by which language seems to mediate associations. First, according to the "color vocabulary account", a given letter is associated with the color term featuring that letter at its beginning. According to Simner et al., the color vocabulary account is common to both synesthetes and non-synesthetes. In support of this first view, synesthetes were found to associate the letter b with "blue", and English-speaking controls the letter p with "purple". The fact that synesthetes and non-synesthetes seem to follow the same rule of association of a grapheme with a color in these two cases is an argument in favor of the continuity hypothesis. If at least in some cases a similar pattern seems to govern the letter/digit-color associations across synesthete and non-synesthete populations, then it may indeed be the case that synesthesia is caused by an exaggeration of a mechanism that exists in all human perceivers. Furthermore, German-speaking non-synesthete controls associate purple with the letter "l", knowing that the German term for purple is "lila". This is taken to confirm that the association is linguistically mediated, given that it seems to be determined by language-particular color vocabulary.

According to the second "color term frequency" account of grapheme-color associations, the most frequent graphemes are associated with the most frequent color terms. The color term frequency account, however, is only observed in synesthetes. Indeed, in synesthetes, it seems that vocabulary influenced only some associations, as the effect observed with the grapheme "b" and the term "blue" is not dominant: "Hence synesthetes were less likely to be influenced by the stimulus letter in their choice of colours, compared to controls. The lower-by-items significance in our interaction suggests that vocabulary-influenced colours are more likely for some

[1] Following Berlin and Kay's suggestion, and to avoid confusion, in this chapter I use capital letters to refer to Berlin and Kay's universal categories, e.g. WHITE. Color terms in a given language are between quotes, e.g. "white" in English, while the color is referred to with a term in lowercase and no quotes, e.g. white.

letters than others" (Simner et al., 2005: 1081). It might be argued that the fact that there seems to be evidence that the color term frequency account holds for synesthetes but not for non-synesthetes is problematic for the continuity hypothesis. However, this is not in the scope of this chapter. What matters to us here is the fact that Simner et al. mainly support the second "color term frequency" account when it comes to synesthetic associations, and how they argue for it:

> Synaesthetes tend to pair high frequency graphemes with high frequency colour names, and are sensitive too, to the typology of Berlin and Kay (1969). This reflects the order in which colours are introduced into human languages, and may also indicate the order in which colour distinctions are acquired in language development. (Simner et al., 2005: 1082)

According to Simner et al., then, what seems to mostly drive synesthetic color-grapheme associations is the frequency both of the inducer and the concurrent—more frequent inducers are associated with more frequent concurrents.

In a different study of factors underpinning grapheme-color synesthesia, Beeli et al. (2007) recruited nineteen native German-speaking synesthetes. In this experiment, unlike in Simner et al.'s 2005 study, the fact that synesthetes experience very specific color shades is taken into consideration. Consequently, participants are not asked to write on a form the color terms that refer to their induced color experiences. Instead, each letter or digit is spoken aloud by the experimenter, and the participants are asked to select the induced synesthetic color on a monitor. They could choose from 16,777,216 colors, and when they experienced textured, structured, or combined colors, they were asked to report only one color, for ease of data processing purposes (but see Eagleman and Goodale, 2009).

Next, colors were analyzed in terms of their hue, saturation, and lightness values, the three dimensions of color featured by most known color spaces. The data suggest a significant difference among the colors associated with the digits, in both saturation and brightness. For letters, a significant difference is also found among the associated colors in both saturation and brightness. Although the analysis of these results reveals that the tendency to associate letters with saturation and brightness of color is less clear than for numbers, the authors report that there nevertheless is a positive correlation between letter frequency and saturation: the more frequently the letter is used, the more saturated is the experienced synesthetic color.

Given that language is acquired, "some aspects of grapheme-color synaesthesia must be acquired" (Beeli et al., 2007: 791), according to the authors. However, such associations may not be entirely explained on the basis of language, because variations can be observed across synesthetes belonging to the same linguistic community. If language could explain grapheme-color associations, then synesthetes belonging to the same linguistic community should associate the same colors with the same graphemes. However, this is not the case, as an important degree of idiosyncrasy is observed in the specific associated colors. Thus, the trends that Beeli et al. observe across synesthetes are not in the choice of the *colors* per se, but in their respective dimensions, namely saturation and brightness. Furthermore, given the fact that letter and digit frequency are what seem to drive color correspondences, the synesthetic associations can only be due to implicit learning, not conscious associations (as reported by Witthoft and Winawer, 2006). Indeed, one is not conscious of the frequency of the letters and digits in use.

One important detail in the processing of the data in Beeli et al. (2007) is the following manipulation. Responses were measured in terms of the hue, saturation, and brightness of the associated colors. However, the digits 0 and 1 (except for two or three subjects out of nineteen) elicited achromatic responses. In other words, colors associated with 0 and 1 are mostly black and white, and less often some shades of grey. Black and white are achromatic colors which consequently have no hue. Therefore, they have no saturation value either, as saturation is a dimension of the perceived chromatic quality. Given that they were looking for a correlation with saturation, Beeli et al. therefore eliminated 0 and 1 from the statistical analysis:

> These digits [0 and 1] are typically different from other digits in synaesthesia and are often perceived as white or black. Thus, the relation between digit frequency and saturation was negative when all digits were included in the analysis, but the correlation became slightly positive when 0 and 1 were excluded. (Beeli et al., 2007: 790)

Had Beeli et al. included 0 and 1, they would have obtained a negative correlation where it would seem that the most frequent digits are associated with the least saturated colors, namely black and white. However, this analysis would have obscured the association of digits 2 to 9 with most saturated colors. Only after excluding 0 and 1 were they able to find a positive correlation between digit frequency and color saturation.

In Simner and Ward's (2008) respond to Beeli et al. (2007), they claim that color naming can better account for synesthetic grapheme-color associations in Beeli et al.'s study. Simner and Ward (2008) argue for this claim by converting the synesthetic colors obtained by Beeli et al. (2007) using a color picker into "the 11 irreducible color terms from Berlin and Kay" (Simner and Ward, 2008: 412). Next, Simner and Ward rank the letters, digits, and color terms according to the frequency of their use in German. In English, the ranking of German color terms is as follows: "white", "black", "red", "green", "blue", "pink", "yellow", "grey", "brown", "purple", "orange". In line with their previous 2005 study, Simner and Ward's 2008 analysis of Beeli et al.'s 2007 data shows that higher-frequency graphemes tend to be associated with higher-frequency color terms.

Further, Simner and Ward claim that their account is superior to Beeli et al.'s. Indeed, for their saturation hypothesis to be verified, Beeli et al. had eliminated 0 and 1 from the statistical analysis as seen above. Simner and Ward claim that the ad hoc nature of this manipulation is simply a sign of the insufficiency of the saturation account of grapheme-color synesthesia. The color term frequency approach, on the other hand, accounts for the association of 0 and 1 with white and black on the basis of the fact that "white" and "black" are the most frequently used color terms, and 0 and 1 the most frequently used digits.

Acknowledging that there probably is an independent relationship between color naming and color space which would account for Beeli et al.'s results, Simner and Ward refer to Jameson and D'Andrade (1997) and Regier et al. (2007) to argue that the structure of our perceptual space determines universal tendencies in color categorization. Based on their own previous study and on Beeli et al.'s results, Simner and Ward finally suggest an additional constraint to the Regier et al. model: not only does the structure of the perceptual space determine categorization, but there also seems to be a relationship between color term frequency and color saturation, where the most frequent color terms are the *least* saturated.

4.2 The Berlin and Kay typology: implications and limitations

4.2.1 The introduction of Berlin and Kay's typology

A striking and important difference between Simner et al. (2005) and Beeli et al. (2007) lies in their methodologies. The choice of methodology clearly results from their respective theoretical standpoints, and reflects the hypothesized linguistic or color appearance mediation of the association bias. Simner and colleagues argue for the linguistic mediation of synesthetic associations, while Beeli et al. seem more open to the possibility of a color appearance mediation. Consequently, in Simner et al. (2005), synesthetic colors are reported verbally. The rationale behind this methodological choice seems to be that if the synesthetic association results from a linguistic mediation, then color-naming data are required to show it.

Beeli et al. (2007), on the other hand, ask participants to produce the experienced color on a screen instead, and are explicitly critical of the use of verbal reports of experienced synesthetic color. Synesthetes report very specific color experiences, and reducing such fine-grained distinctions to linguistic categories might not reliably reflect the synesthetic colors and obscure meaningful features of these colors' appearance.

The fact that synesthetes experience highly specific concurrent colors is also apparent in their verbal reports. Typically, as Simner et al. point out (Simner et al., 2005), synesthetes produce more color words than non-synesthetes in association with graphemes. More specifically, Simner et al. report forty-five words on average for synesthetes vs/26.5 for non-synesthetes in the color to grapheme association task. Also, synesthetes produce 495 color variants compared to fifty-eight for controls (e.g. for the 195 "green" responses produced by synesthetes, there were fifty-four different color descriptors, while for the 219 "green" responses produced by non-synesthetes, there were only five different descriptors; Simner et al., 2005). This difference in the richness of vocabulary is taken to confirm the genuineness of the synesthetic experience. For Beeli et al., the richness of the experience might also indicate that what drives the synesthetic association is color appearance, not color terms.

Not only do Simner and colleagues rely on verbal reports in their procedure, they more specifically use a predetermined set of color categories, the so-called eleven basic color terms and categories introduced in 1969 by Berlin and Kay (Berlin and Kay, 1969). Thus, after eliciting verbal reports from synesthetes, they reduce the original color expressions to the set of the eleven basic color categories. It is on the basis of this reduction that they next proceed to show that high-frequency letters and digits correlate with the most frequently used color terms. Furthermore, the thereby reduced synesthetic colors are taken to reflect the Berlin and Kay evolutionary sequence, or the order in which color categories are taken to emerge in language (Berlin and Kay, 1969).

As noted in the introduction to this chapter, the use of Berlin and Kay's typology in studies of synesthesia was initiated by Day for practical reasons (Day, 2005). However, Simner et al.'s introduction of the Berlin and Kay typology is problematic. If the synesthetic association is supposedly linguistically mediated, the grounds on which "light brown" and "beige" are equated, then reduced to "brown", are not clear (see Eagleman et al., 2007 for a similar remark). Indeed, the only relation between "beige", "light brown", and "brown" is perceptual similarity or appearance. However, arguing for the reduction of "beige" to "light brown" on the basis of perceptual similarity contradicts the hypothesis the experiment was designed to verify. If synesthetes associate graphemes with colors on the basis of color term frequency, then the reported color term (i.e. "beige") is what matters, not its alleged semantic equivalent, the content of which is perceptual (i.e. the color beige). Indeed, note that the color term frequency account crucially relies on the used *term*, not its referent. More drastically, on the color term frequency account, the appearance of the term's referent should be completely irrelevant to the grapheme-color association. Thus, if the appearance of the concurrent is irrelevant, what is common to "beige" and "light brown"?

In what follows, I will first clarify a few notions from the Berlin and Kay theory that are misused in the discussion that interests us here. I will then argue that the adoption of the Berlin and Kay typology is to some extent in contradiction to the claim Simner et al. put forward. At best, the use of the Berlin and Kay typology prevents Simner et al. from reaching the conclusion of a linguistic mediation of synesthetic associations unequivocally.

4.2.2 Regarding basic color terms

Berlin and Kay's basic color terms theory was first proposed in 1969 to argue against the Sapir-Whorf hypothesis of linguistic relativism (Berlin and Kay, 1969; Whorf, 1956). Linguistic relativism is the view according to which color categories vary across languages. They are determined by a given community's needs, and result from language use (Boas, 1938; Whorf, 1940; and see also Davidoff et al., 1999;

Davidoff, 2001). Berlin and Kay suggested, contra relativism, that there was a set of eleven basic color categories that was found across languages, universally. Further, these eleven basic color categories emerge in the lexicon following a constrained evolutionary sequence. These two claims are the core of the basic color terms theory (BCTT).

Several questions naturally follow these initial statements, the first pertaining to the nature of basic color categories. What are these categories, and how do we identify them? An operational definition involving eight linguistic and psychological criteria was offered. Mainly: basic color terms are monolexemic (e.g. "blue-green" is not basic), they are not hyponyms, meaning that their extension is not included in that of another basic term (e.g. "crimson" is a kind of "red", therefore "crimson" is not basic), they are abstract and refer to all sorts of objects (e.g. "blond" is not a basic color term), and they are psychologically salient (e.g. they come first to mind; they are used most frequently; members of a given linguistic community refer to the same colors with the same terms; Berlin and Kay, 1969). From this definition, and more specifically from the criterion of non-hyponymy, it may be deduced that basic color terms are "irreducible", as Simner et al. claim. But, to be precise, it is not that these are irreducible terms but rather that they are at a level of categorization called "basic" that matters most to the BCTT (Rosch, 1972; Rosch, 1973).

It should be noted that the notion of "basic color categories" is far from being consensually accepted. Its operational definition was widely criticized in the literature (Hickerson, 1971; Kuschel and Monberg, 1974; Crawford, 1982; Lucy, 1997; Lyons, 1999; Saunders and Van Brakel, 1997, to name only a few). Also, anthropologists and psychologists who use this notion in the field or in their laboratories in fact disregard most of the eight criteria, and mainly (or even only, in some cases) rely on the criterion of psychological saliency (Berlin and Berlin, 1975; MacLaury, 1991; Maffi, 1990; Stanlaw, 1997; for a more detailed analysis of the basic color terms' definition see Jraissati et al., 2012).

Clearly, this is slightly problematic for the notion of irreducibility retained by Simner et al., according to which basic color terms are the simplest possible color terms in a given lexicon (Simner and Ward, 2008; Simner et al., 2005). For if all terms that are psychologically salient are basic, then, for example, if a term such as "crimson" was frequently used by a group, consistently used in reference to the same colors, and elicited fast reaction times, then "crimson" would be basic according to this definitional criterion. Consequently, would Simner et al. concede that "crimson" is irreducible'? The point here is that Simner and colleagues refer to the irreducibility of the basic color terms as a determining feature, while the notion of irreducibility is irrelevant outside the framework adopted by the BCTT—more on this point in section 4.3.

4.2.3 Regarding the evolutionary sequence

Simner et al. (2005) also evoke the evolutionary sequence of the BCTT in support of their color term frequency account. Two remarks need to be made here. First, the sequence Simner et al. seem to refer to was offered in 1969, and suggested that basic color categories emerge in a specific order: WHITE, BLACK, RED, YELLOW, GREEN, BLUE, BROWN, GREY, PURPLE, PINK, and ORANGE. This sequence was, however, revised as soon as 1975 (Berlin and Berlin, 1975). It reached its current version in 1999 (Kay and Maffi, 1999). The reason why the sequence changed in 1975 is linked to the fact that Berlin and Kay's understanding of categories evolved in the meantime. In 1969, Berlin and Kay thought that categories were defined by their focal color, or prototype, and consisted of sets to which colors were either members or not. The assumption was then that each color category emerged individually in the lexicon, in a given order. As a consequence, the speaker of a stage 3 language referred mostly to the same color when he said "white" in his language, as a speaker of English, which is a stage 7 language.

However, in 1975, the authors realized that the category extension, disregarded in 1969, was at least as important as the focal point. Thus, it is not that the term "white" emerges before the terms "red", "yellow", etc. Rather, in a system where there are three categories, the three categories would be WHITE, BLACK, and RED. However, the category WHITE in such a stage 2 language encompasses all light colors, including yellow, pink, light blue, and light green; BLACK encompasses all dark colors including most of blue, green, and purple; RED includes red, and perhaps some orange and brown. Thus, when the fourth category GREEN emerges, it is a composite category, like the previous WHITE and BLACK, which includes both blue and green in its extension. This composite category is later differentiated into two separate categories, GREEN and BLUE. Accordingly, saying that categories for "black", "white", "red", "yellow", etc. emerge in this order in language is not exactly accurate, and a correlation with color associations in synesthesia cannot be straightforward. The terms WHITE, BLACK, etc. of the sequence are just labels used by the BCTT to refer to categories, the extension of which varies depending on the lexicon's development stage, and could therefore be different from what we would call "white" or "black" in English.

The second, most important, remark pertaining to the evolutionary sequence of the emergence of color terms put forward in Simner et al. (2005) is its connection to universalism—i.e. the thesis according to which color categories are universals that are found cross-culturally. Indeed, Berlin and Kay's claim that the color lexicon evolves following a given sequence is tightly linked to the universalistic dimension of the BCTT.

More specifically, the idea of an evolutionary sequence was introduced by the BCTT to argue that categorization of color is universal, and not arbitrarily determined by language. Given that different languages have different numbers of basic color categories, there is no way one can argue for the universality of categorization unless one posits a universal evolutionary sequence, which would lead a lexicon from one stage into another. Remember that the category WHITE, although universal, does not necessarily have the same extension across languages. The extension of

WHITE depends on the number of basic color categories encoded in a given language, and therefore on its evolutionary stage. Given that color categories are taken to partition the color space jointly, languages with different numbers of basic color categories partition the space differently. Based on these different partitionings, one could argue that categorization is culturally relative. The only way different color space partitionings can be reconciled with universalism is by arguing that these different languages are only different to the extent that they belong to different stages of the universal evolutionary sequence. They are all bound to partition the color space in similar ways. In this sense, the idea of lexicon evolution is key in arguing for universalism in categorization.

The evolutionary sequence thesis, however, is also tightly linked to the proposed account of color categories' universality. Indeed, as is explained in the following paragraph, the idea of an evolving color lexicon presupposes the perceptual determination of these categories in the BCTT framework (Kay and McDaniel, 1978).

Proponents of the BCTT suggested that the universality of color categorization could be explained on the basis of biological reductions as soon as 1969. Universality of categorization does not necessarily imply that categories are perceptually determined. It can be argued that color categories are universal for reasons that are not exclusively biological (Shepard, 1992; Yendrikhovskij, 2001; Belpaeme and Bleys, 2005). Nevertheless, proponents of the BCTT adopted a biological and perceptual account of universal categorization. In the late 1970s, Kay and MacDaniel proposed that the evolutionary sequence was determined by Hering's unique hues: white, black, red, green, blue, and yellow (Hering, 1964), taken as resulting from the activity of the opponent cells in the lateral geniculate nucleus, an area specific to color processing at the end of the optic nerve (De Valois et al., 1966). Consequently, composite categories are categories that would encompass several outputs of these biological primaries, until they are singled out as categories in their own right. So, for example, in a stage 1 language, the category BLACK is a composition of the Hering primaries Blue/Black/Green, while WHITE is a composition of primaries White/Yellow/Red. In a stage 2 language where RED emerges as a category along with WHITE and BLACK, the extension of the category WHITE is reduced to include only the Hering primaries White/Yellow, and so on.

However, the standard theory of color vision was revised (De Valois and De Valois, 1993; Abramov and Gordon, 1994), and Hering's unique hues are no longer seen as being the direct output of the responses of the opponent cells. Consequently, proponents of the universalist view have suggested alternative models of categorization that no longer rest on these primaries (Kay et al., 1997; Regier et al., 2007). According to this new model of categorization, universal color categories would result from the interaction of an endowed capacity to optimally categorize with the irregularity of the perceptual space (Jameson and D'Andrade, 1997; Regier et al., 2007).

The irregularity of the perceptual space refers to the fact that due to the structure of our visual input system, our sensitivity to different areas of the color spectrum varies. Our sensitivity thresholds in the blue-green area are higher than in the red-yellow-green area. Consequently, an objective distance between two colors in the blue-green area is not perceived like a distance of the same magnitude in the yellow-red-green area (MacAdam, 1942; Churchland, 2007). Thus, our perceptual space is not uniform. In some areas of the space, where our thresholds are low, we can discriminate colors more finely. Such areas are "perceptually salient", for Regier et al. (2007). As a result, Regier et al. argue that some colors, such as white, black, red, yellow, then green and blue, are more perceptually salient than others.

Given that our capacity to optimally categorize refers to the fact that we have a tendency to group together perceptual objects that are most similar to each other and most dissimilar from other objects, the irregularities of the perceptual space will cause us to optimally categorize it in a given way. Although this model no longer rests on the opponent process mechanisms, it nevertheless still implies that our categorization is determined by perceptual mechanisms.

4.2.4 Perceptually determined color categories vs/linguistically mediated synesthetic associations

What, then, does the reliance on basic color terms and categories imply for Simner and colleagues? On a liberal reading of Simner and colleagues, the use of the basic colors terms' typology does not imply an endorsement of the BCTT account of universal categorization. We have seen that it was possible for the universality of basic color terms to result from factors that are not perceptual and biological. It might therefore be argued that when Simner and colleagues refer to the Berlin and Kay typology, they only refer to the observation that some color terms are most frequently and widely used. There are, however, two difficulties with this view.

First, if Simner and colleagues take basic color terms to simply be those terms that are most frequently used across a linguistic community, knowing that frequency of use varies across time and communities, what justifies their adopting in the UK a typology resulting from a study that was made in the USA, some forty years prior? If what matters to Simner and colleagues is the most frequent color terms, then those terms should have been identified within the group of study.

But more critically, it is not the frequency of use of the basic color terms that interests Simner and colleagues, who have explicitly justified the use of basic color terms by their irreducibility. Indeed, their interest in basic color terms stems from their belief that basic color terms are "irreducible". If Simner and colleagues claim that there are such irreducible terms, the question of what makes these terms irreducible is inescapable, and invites considerations that are beyond the scope of what Simner and colleagues are willing to concede. Either what makes some color terms irreducible is due to language use, or it is not due to language use. If what determines irreducible categories is language use, the first objection above is raised again, and the reason why Simner and colleagues did not determine the set of irreducible terms for their sample of participants is obscure, knowing that language use varies across cultures and time. If, however, what determines irreducible categories is not language use, then color categories are necessarily independent of language. In other words, universal categories exist independently of how they are named. In that case, the reason why the term "red" is associated with *A* across synesthetes may not be due to vocabulary, but to the universal category RED, whatever factors caused its categorization. It is therefore not obvious that what drives this association is the frequency of the basic color *term* "red". As a result, even if Simner and colleagues do not endorse the perceptual account of universal color categorization, the reliance on these universal categories prevents the unequivocal conclusion of a linguistic mediation in synesthetic associations.

This being said, in their 2008 study, it seems that Simner and Ward not only use Berlin and Kay's typology, but also do endorse the perceptual account of color categorization, at least to some extent. Indeed, in their response to Beeli et al. (2007), Simner and Ward (2008) acknowledge that there must be an independent connection between the structure of the color space and color term frequency, thereby adopting the line of argumentation of Regier et al. (2007), to which they refer. More specifically, Simner and Ward offer that the reason why the most frequent letters are associated with the most saturated colors can be explained by a link between color term frequency and saturation.

Thus, on a stricter reading of the Simner and Ward study, the adoption of the BCTT typology also involves the endorsement of the BCTT's perceptual account of color categorization. Yet the BCTT's account of universal categorization is in plain contradiction to what Simner and Ward's study is meant to show. Indeed, the BCTT argues that color categories result from perceptual (and cognitive) hard-wired mechanisms that are independent of language. Simner and Ward want to argue for a linguistic mediation of synesthetic associations via language and color vocabulary. By referring to the BCTT, Simner and Ward use perceptually based color categories to argue for a linguistic mediation of synesthetic associations.

This contradiction becomes obvious in a passage referring to the work of Davidoff, where Simner et al. claim the following:

> Neuropsychological studies have investigated the ways in which perceptual systems such as the organisation of colour space may be influenced by linguistic knowledge. Our research on grapheme-colour synaesthesia makes contact with this debate by showing that the linguistic composition of colour terms (e.g., the word-initial letter) can have direct repercussions within the visual perceptual system. (Simner et al., 2005: 1083)

If Simner et al. propose that their data speak in favor of an influence of language on perception, it is because they take their study to show that synesthetes experience a given color in association with a given grapheme on the basis of color vocabulary. However, according to Davidoff, a proponent of linguistic relativism in color categorization, there is no predetermined set of color universals, no irreducible or basic color terms. While for universalists it may be said that a given color C is named "x" because it belongs to a pre-existing category x, for relativists a given color C belongs to category x because it is named "x". In other words, for relativism, the only factor determining color categorization is language (Davidoff, 2001). A given speech community agrees to refer to a certain group of colors that are contiguously connected in color space in a given manner. The use of a term in reference to a given group of colors stabilizes, and as a result the color lexicon is formed. The lexicon may change in time, but it does not *evolve* in a predetermined direction. Relativism rejects the idea that the common patterns found across speech communities could be accounted for on the basis of universal and perceptually determined categories.

Thus, to argue along with Davidoff that language-relative categories may have repercussions for visual sensation (Simner et al., 2005), Simner et al. first need to show that the colors associated with graphemes in synesthesia are not perceptually determined in the first place. Yet because it uses the Berlin and Kay typology and endorses the universalistic perceptual account of categorization to some extent (Simner and Ward, 2008), their study, as it stands, does not allow them to make such a claim. Either color terms used by synesthetes are shaped by their language use—in which case their verbal reports should not be reduced to the Berlin and Kay typology, and consequently Simner et al.'s (2005) study could be taken to show that color terms affect synesthetes' color experience—or color terms used by synesthetes are basic color categories that are universal, in which case it cannot be excluded that they are perceptually determined, and consequently Simner et al.'s study cannot be taken to show that language affects perceptual experience.

4.3 Contributions to the discussion

4.3.1 The tensions in Simner and Ward's response to Beeli et al.

So far, we have shown that the possibility of the synesthetic association being mediated by the color's appearance on the concurrent's side could not be excluded due to the nature of the experimental paradigm and the introduction of the basic color categories more specifically. Thus, as long as the possibility that a color appearance mediation could be taking place is not excluded, the strength of the argument in favor of the linguistic mediation approach is at best considerably weakened. In this final section, I would like to show how the BCTT framework may in fact offer a possible response to Simner and Ward's (2008) take on Beeli et al.'s (2007) results, thereby allowing for the possibility of color appearance playing a role in synesthetic associations after all.

We have seen in section 4.1 that Beeli et al. suggested that letter and digit frequency positively correlated with color saturation—the most frequent graphemes are associated with the most saturated colors. In response to this study, Simner and Ward (2008) argue:

(1) There is an independent correlation between saturation and color term frequency
(2) But while the saturation approach does not account for the association of 0 and 1 to white and black, the color term frequency account does.

Consequently:

(3) The results obtained by Beeli et al. on the basis of an ad hoc elimination of 0 and 1 are better accounted for by color term frequency
(4) There is indeed a correlation between saturation and color term frequency but it is opposite to what Beeli et al.'s data seem to suggest: least saturated colors are most frequently named.

Simner and Ward's suggestion (1) that saturation of colors predicts color categories is their only way of explaining away Beeli et al.'s results. This move is required for them to argue that the data presented by Beeli et al. on associations based on color saturation can be accounted for by color term frequency instead. Yet to show that the color term frequency model is superior to Beeli et al.'s saturation model, Simner and Ward also need to show that color term frequency can account for the association of 0 and 1 with white and black, an observation Beeli et al. could not account for on the basis of saturation. Thus, Simner and Ward argue (2) that given that 0 and 1 are the most frequent digits, and "white" and "black" the most frequent color terms, the color term frequency approach is better equipped to account for Beeli et al.'s data.

However, having acknowledged that there exists an independent correlation between saturation and color term frequency in (1), Simner and Ward need to reconcile claims (1) and (2). In other words, there should be no tension between color term frequency accounting for the association of 0 and 1 with "white" and "black", and color term frequency being predicted by color saturation. As a solution, Simner and Ward offer that (4) the least saturated colors are named most frequently. In support of their claim that the structure of the space determines color naming, Simner and Ward refer to the studies of Jameson and D'Andrade (1997) and Regier et al. (2007) and propose "an additional link between color names and color space.... We found a significant negative correlation between saturation and color-term frequency, indicating that colors with the highest linguistic frequency are those that are least saturated" (Simner and Ward, 2008: 413).

There is, however, a clear contradiction between claim (1) and the conclusion in (4). We have seen that (1) was necessary to explain away Beeli et al.'s results. If Beeli et al.'s results can be accounted for on the basis of the link between color space structure and color naming, then there should be a *positive* correlation between color term frequency and saturation (i.e. the most frequent graphemes are associated with the most saturated colors). However, conclusion (4) suggests that the correlation between color term frequency and saturation is *negative* (i.e. the most frequent graphemes are associated with the least saturated colors). To avoid this contradiction between (1) and (4), Simner and Ward would have to abandon either claim (1) or claim (4). Either high saturation does not determine color naming and color term frequency, in which case Simner and Ward can claim (4), but not (1); or high saturation does predict color naming and color term frequency, in which case Simner and Ward can claim (1), but not (4).

However, Simner and Ward cannot abandon either claim. Because of Beeli et al.'s results, there has to be (1) some connection between color space structure and color naming. On the other hand, if there is a connection between color space structure and color naming, such a connection should be predicted by color term frequency for this approach to be validated. Therefore, Simner and Ward's account requires (4) that low saturation determines color naming and color term frequency. Thus, there is a necessary tension in Simner and Ward's response to Beeli et al. In what follows, I would like to suggest a way to resolve it.

4.3.2 Saturation or color term frequency? How the basic color terms theory may offer an alternative account for the data

As mentioned in section 4.2, Regier et al.'s (2007) model, based on a proposition by Jameson and D'Andrade (1997), is an attempt to account for universal color categorization on perceptual and cognitive grounds. As Simner and Ward (2008) rightly note, the interaction of hue, saturation, and brightness, the three supposed dimensions of color, yields an irregular color space (see section 4.2). However, this irregularity of the space does not amount to an irregularity in saturation alone. Regier et al.'s claim is *not* that some areas of the space are most saturated, and therefore that these areas ground universal categories. As we have seen in section 4.2, their claim is that different areas of the space are differently *perceptually salient*, where perceptual saliency refers to our varying sensitivity thresholds across the space. We are not more or less sensitive to saturation, or to brightness or hue. Our sensitivity thresholds pertain to our color experience as a whole; that is, as resulting from the interaction of the three, or more, dimensions taken together. In Regier et al.'s perspective, white, black, red, yellow, green, and blue are the most perceptually salient colors. Consequently, if white and black are perceptually salient, then perhaps perceptual saliency can account for Beeli et al.'s results where saturation had failed, and the synesthetic associations can be explained on the basis of color appearance after all.

The notion of perceptual saliency could therefore shed new light on the Simner et al./Beeli et al. discussion. The notion of optimality could be of further interest. Indeed, beyond perceptual saliency, the BCTT adds optimality to its account of universal color categorization. It is because of our endowed capacity to optimally categorize that color categories appear in our lexicon following a certain order—most optimal categories being the first to be named. We form our categories based on how similar and dissimilar the colors of the space are, knowing that these similarity relations are precisely determined by different degrees of perceptual saliency. Thus, in a space with two color categories, the most optimal categories are WHITE and BLACK, because the colors white and black are most perceptually salient, and are most dissimilar from each other. The third category would be RED, because red is perceptually salient and most dissimilar from white and black, and so on. Apart from the perceptual saliency of white and black, then, the reason why they would be associated with the most frequent digits, one might argue, is that WHITE and BLACK are also the most optimal categories.

In this context, suggesting that the most frequent terms are the ones that are least saturated is a mere observation: it so happens that "white" and "black" are the most frequent terms, and they happen to be the least saturated. There is no causal relation between low saturation and color term frequency. There may, however, be one between perceptual saliency coupled with optimal categorization, and color term frequency.

Color term frequency was often studied in relation to the BCTT. The frequency of the first terms of the sequence (i.e. "black", "white", "red") was shown (Pollnac, 1975; Bolton, 1978), and it was also shown that the frequency of the color terms more or less followed their appearance in the lexicon (Corbett and Morgan, 1988; Corbett and Davies, 1997, although some terms also disappear, see Kristol, 1980): the older the terms, the more frequent their use. But more importantly, frequency of use is a criterion of basic color categories. Indeed, frequency of use is a measure of psychological saliency, and we have seen in section 4.2 that psychological saliency is the most reliable criterion for basic color term identification. In other words, basic color terms are frequently used *by definition*. Thus, in the BCTT's framework, there is an indirect connection between color term frequency and the mechanisms underlying color categorization. To the extent that color space structure and optimality are taken to determine color categorization and naming, and that the color categories are identified on the basis of frequency of use (among other measures of psychological saliency), then most salient and optimal categories are referred to with names that are most frequently used. From this perspective, the Beeli et al. type of color appearance approach to grapheme-color associations would account for the positive results of Simner et al.'s frequency of use approach; not the other way around.

4.3.3 Beyond synesthesia: the possible implications for color categorization

It is important to note, however, that the universalistic model of color categorization (Regier et al., 2007) presented here has its own limitations, and the point of this chapter is not to argue for the color appearance mediation of synesthetic associations, nor is it to minimize the importance of Simner et al.'s findings. My aim is to show that the way color experience is reported in empirical studies of grapheme-color synesthesia has important consequences. More specifically, Simner and colleagues' methodology in this discussion is questionable because of the problematic implications of their reliance on the Berlin and Kay typology.

This being said, I would like to make one last remark: Whether the associations in grapheme-color synesthesia are conceptually mediated has not been directly addressed in the Simner et al./Beeli et al. discussion. Indeed, Simner et al. argue for the conceptual mediation of synesthetic associations by showing that the associations are based on language. The presupposition therefore seems to be that if the mediation is conceptual, than it has to be linguistic. Consequently, if the association can be shown to rest on language, the conceptual mediation of synesthetic associations will have been established.

However, this presupposition rests on a confused notion of color categorization that conflates color categories and color lexicon. It is precisely the existence of perceptually, non-linguistically determined color categories that the BCTT purports to show. The discussion opposing universalism to relativism revolves around whether color categories are independent of language. The relation between concept, language, and color appearance has yet to be clarified. By showing that the linguistic, color term frequency account of synesthetic associations was not convincing, I have not excluded that the mediation may be conceptual. Indeed, note that introducing optimality in an account of synesthetic associations implies that what mediates synesthetic associations is not only of a perceptual but a conceptual nature as well. This would, however, not mean that the associations are determined by our color vocabulary. According to this categorization model, perceptual saliency and optimal categorization both result from hard-wired mechanisms that are independent of language.

Therefore, with regards to what mediates the synesthetic associations, the categorization literature would seem to suggest that there are three, not two possibilities to explore: (1) synesthetic associations are mediated by the appearance of the concurrent; (2) synesthetic associations are mediated by the appearance of the concurrent and non-linguistic cognitive constraints of optimality in categorization; (3) synesthetic associations are linguistically mediated.

Clearly, the possible role of the notion of optimality in synesthetic associations is for the moment not supported by any empirical data. Nevertheless, the notions of optimality and perceptual saliency, as defined here, are possibly relevant for research into synesthesia. Conversely, this also shows a specific way in which research into synesthesia could possibly contribute to the wider field of color categorization. Part of the discussion opposing universalists to relativists in the color categorization literature pertains to what determines color categories. Universalists argue for perceptual and cognitive non-linguistic factors, while relativists argue for language use. If it could be shown that synesthetic associations are driven by color category optimality, a notion that rests both on color appearance and cognitive efficiency, then one might be able to argue that the mediation is indeed conceptual to some extent, although language independent. As a consequence, the possibility that color categories may be determined by perceptual and cognitive mechanisms independently of language would have gained an additional support in synesthesia. Conversely, if it could be shown that synesthetic associations are driven by color vocabulary, independently of universal optimal categories, this could be an argument in favor of the role of language in categorization.

References

Abramov, I. & Gordon, J. (1994) Color appearance: on seeing red—or yellow, or green, or blue. *Annual Review of Psychology* 45, 451–85.

Beeli, G., Esslen, M., & Jancke, L. (2007) Frequency correlates in grapheme-color synaesthesia. *Psychological Science* 18, 788–92.

Belpaeme, T. & Bleys, J. (2005) Explaining universal color categories through a constrained acquisition process. *Adaptive Behavior* 13, 293–310.

Berlin, B. & Berlin, E. A. (1975) Aguaruna color categories. *American Ethnologist* 2, 61–87.

Berlin, B. & Kay, P. (1969) *Basic Color Terms: Their Universality and Evolution*. Stanford, CA: CSLI Publications.

Boas, F. (1938) *The Mind of Primitive Man*. New York: The Macmillan Company.

Bolton, R. (1978) Black, white, and red all over: the riddle of color term salience. *Ethnology* 17, 287–311.

Brang, D., Rouw, R., Ramachandran, V. S., & Coulson, S. (2011) Similarly shaped letters evoke similar colors in grapheme-color synesthesia. *Neuropsychologia* 49, 1355–8.

Churchland, P. (2007) On the reality (and diversity) of objective colors: how color-qualia space is a map of reflectance-profile space. *Philosophy of Science* 74, 119–49.

Corbett, G. & Davies, I. R. L. (1997) Establishing basic color terms: measures and techniques. In C. L. Hardin & L. Maffi (Eds) *Color Categories in Thought and Language*. Cambridge: Cambridge University Press, 197–223.

Corbett, G. & Morgan, G. (1988) Colour terms in Russian: reflections of typological constraints in a single language. *Journal of Linguistics* 24, 31–64.

Crawford, T. D. (1982) Defining 'basic color term'. *Anthropological Linguistics* 24, 338–43.

Davidoff, J. (2001) Language and perceptual categorization. *TICS* 5, 382–7.

Davidoff, J., Davies, I., & Roberson, D. (1999) Colour categories of a stone-age tribe. *Nature* 398, 203–4.

Day, S. (2005) Some demographic and socio-cultural aspects of synesthesia. In L. C. Robertson & N. Sagiv (Eds) *Synesthesia: Perspectives from Cognitive Neuroscience*. Oxford: Oxford University Press, 11–33.

De Valois, R., Abramov, I., & Jacobs, G. H. J. (1966) Analysis of response patterns of LGN cells. *Journal of the Optical Society of America* 56, 966–77.

De Valois, R. & De Valois, K. (1993) A multi-stage color model. *Vision Research* 36, 833–6.

Dixon, M., Smilek, D., & Merikle, M. (2004) Not all synaesthetes are created equal: projector versus associator synesthetes. *Cognitive, Affective, & Behavioral Neuroscience* 4(3), 335–43.

Eagleman, D. M. & Goodale, M. A. (2009) Why color synesthesia involves more than color. *TICS* 13, 288–92.

Eagleman, D. M., Kagan, A. D., Nelson, S. S., Sagaram, D., & Sarma, A. K. (2007) A standardized test battery for the study of synesthesia. *Journal of Neuroscience Methods* 159, 139–45.

Hering, E. (1964) *Outlines of a Theory of the Light Sense*. Cambridge, MA: Harvard University Press.

Hickerson, N. (1971) Review of basic color terms: their universality and evolution. *International Journal of American Linguistics* 37, 257–70.

Jameson, K. & D'Andrade, R. G. (1997) It's not really red, green, yellow, blue: an inquiry into perceptual color space. In C. L. Hardin & L. Maffi (Eds) *Color Categories in Thought and Language*. Cambridge: Cambridge University Press, 295–320.

Jraissati, Y., Wakui, E., Decock, L., & Douven, I. (2012) Constraints on colour category formation. *International Studies in the Philosophy of Science* 26(2), 171–96.

Kay, P., Berlin, B., Maffi, L., & Merrifield, W. (1997) Color naming across languages. In C. L. Hardin & L. Maffi (Eds) *Color Categories in Thought and Language*. Cambridge: Cambridge University Press, 21–56.

Kay, P. & Maffi, L. (1999) Color appearance and the emergence of basic color lexicons. *American Anthropologist* 101, 743–60.

Kay, P. & McDaniel, C. K. (1978) The linguistic significance of the meanings of basic color terms. *Language* 54, 610–46.

Kristol, A. M. (1980) Color systems in Southern Italy: a case of regression. *Language* 56, 137–45.

Kuschel, R. & Monberg, T. (1974) 'We don't talk much about colour here': a study of colour semantics on Bellona Island. *Man* 9, 213–42.

Lucy, J. (1997) The linguistics of 'color'. In C. L. Hardin & L. Maffi (Eds) *Color Categories in Thought and Language*. Cambridge: Cambridge University Press, 321–46.

Lyons, J. (1999) The vocabulary of color with particular reference to Ancient Greek and classical Latin. In A. Borg (Ed.) *The Language of Color in the Mediterranean*. Wiesbaden: Otto Harrasowitz.

MacAdam, D. L. (1942) Visual sensitivities to color differences in daylight. *Journal of the Optical Society of America* 32, 247.

MacLaury, R. (1991) Social and cognitive motivations of change: measuring variability in color semantics. *Language* 67, 34–62.

MacLeod, C. M. (1991) Half a century of research on the Stroop effect: an integrative review. *Psychological Bulletin* 109(2), 163.

Maffi, L. (1990) Somali color term evolution: grammatical and semantic evidence. *Anthropological Linguistics* 32, 316–34.

Nikolić, D., Lichti, P., & Singer, W. (2007) Color opponency in synaesthetic experiences. *Psychological Science* 18(6), 481–6.

Nunn, J. A., Gregory, L. J., Brammer, M., Williams, S. C., Parslow, D. M., Morgan, M. J., . . . & Gray, J. A. (2002) Functional magnetic resonance imaging of synesthesia: activation of V4/V8 by spoken words. Nature *Neuroscience* 5(4), 371–5.

Pollnac, R. (1975) Intra-cultural variability in the structure of the subjective color lexicon in Buganda. *American Ethnologist* 2, 89–109.

Regier, T., Kay, P., & Khetarpal, N. (2007) Color naming reflects optimal partitions of color space. *PNAS* 104, 1436–41.

Rosch, E. (1972) Probabilities, sampling, and ethnographic method: the case of Dani Colour Names. *Man* 7, 448–66.

Rosch, E. (1973) Natural categories. *Cognitive Psychology* 4, 328–50.

Saunders, B. & Van Brakel, J. (1997) Are there non-trivial constraints on colour categorization? *Behavioral and Brain Sciences* 20, 167–228.

Shepard, R. N. (1992) The perceptual organization of colors. In J. Barkow, L. Cosmides, & J. Tooby (Eds) *The Adapted Mind*. Oxford: Oxford University Press.

Simner, J. (2012) Defining synaesthesia. *The British Psychological Society* 103, 1–15.

Simner, J. & Ward, J. (2008) Commentary: synaesthesia, color terms, and color space. *Psychological Science* 19, 412–14.

Simner, J., Ward, J., Lanz, M., Jansari, A., Glover, L., & Oakley, D. A. (2005) Non-random associations of grapheme to colours in synaesthetic and non-synaesthetic populations. *Cognitive Neuropsychology* 22, 1069–85.

Stanlaw, J. (1997) Color categories in thought and language. In C. L. Hardin & L. Maffi (Eds) *Color Categories in Thought and Language*. Cambridge: Cambridge University Press, 240–60.

Whorf, B.-L. (1956) *Language, Thought and Reality: Selected Writings*. J. B. Caroll (Ed.). New York: John Wiley Sons.

Whorf, B.-L. (1940) Science and linguistics. *Technological Review* 42, 229–31, 247–8.

Witthoft, N. & Winawer, J. (2006) Synesthetic colors determined by having colored refrigerator magnets in childhood. *Cortex* 42, 175–83.

Yendrikhovskij, S. N. (2001) Computing color categories from statistics of natural images. *Journal of Imaging Science and Technology* 45, 409–17.

PART II

Challenges Raised by Synaesthesia

5

Synesthesia and Consciousness

Exploring the Connections

Myrto Mylopoulos and Tony Ro

5.1 Introduction

Synesthesia is a condition in which individuals have atypical associations between a triggering stimulus ("inducer") and a mental response to that stimulus ("concurrent"), usually taking the form of a sensory experience.[1] For example, in some forms of grapheme-color synesthesia, individuals experience highly specific atypical color sensations when presented with certain alphanumerical characters, in addition to their regular experiences of the characters. Synesthesia comes in a wide range of forms; it can occur within a single modality or cross-modally. It can also be present from early in life or acquired under special circumstances, such as after a brain lesion (Ro et al., 2007).

In recent years, researchers have been making great strides in understanding this fascinating condition. Most of the focus has been on isolating the defining characteristics of synesthesia (e.g., Auvray and Deroy, forthcoming) and establishing suitable paradigms and tests for assessing it (e.g., Ramachandran and Hubbard, 2001; Eagleman et al. 2007). But while there has been a recent surge of interest surrounding synesthesia, one important question remains relatively unexplored: what is the relationship between synesthesia and consciousness? (For a recent exception, see Sagiv and Frith, 2013.)

This question deserves attention for a number of reasons. For one, synesthetic experiences typically occur consciously, so whatever is true of such experiences should fit comfortably with what is true about consciousness more generally. If it is determined that synesthetic experiences arise under certain conditions, these conditions should be consistent with those under which conscious states more generally are thought to arise.

[1] We say "usually" here because there are some forms of synesthesia in which the concurrent does not appear to take the form of a sensory experience. For example, ordinal linguistic personality (OLP) synesthesia involves attributing personality types (e.g., lazy, rude) to ordinal units (e.g., days of the week, letters).

Synesthesia thus provides a useful test case for evaluating theories of consciousness and their predictions.[2] Indeed, as Sagiv and Frith (2013) point out, synesthesia is especially valuable as a test case in that it comes in a wide variety of forms, involving a range of sensory modalities. It therefore has the potential to shed further light on a broad spectrum of conscious experiences and their underlying nature.

Second, exploring the relationship between synesthesia and consciousness requires addressing some important questions about how this condition manifests itself. Chief among these is the question of whether synesthesia can occur unconsciously, and what exactly this means. This question has largely been ignored in the literature. When synesthesia is described, it is typically by reference to its conscious experiential qualities. Indeed, part of what makes the condition so striking is the uniqueness of its subjective character, which is present in conscious experiences of "tasting shape," "hearing color," and so on. This emphasis on the subjective aspect of the condition, however, makes it easy to overlook the possibility that synesthesia sometimes occurs without being conscious at all.[3] In what follows, we seek to remedy this omission from the literature by evaluating this possibility directly.

In this chapter, we will consider some central aspects of the relationship between synesthesia and consciousness. First, we examine what can be learned about this relationship on the basis of existing empirical work, clarifying key questions along the way. We argue that there is good reason to accept synesthesia as a phenomenon that can occur in the absence of consciousness, and challenge the prevailing view that precludes that possibility by definition alone. In the second section, we review four main theories of consciousness: higher-order theory, neuronal global workspace theory, biological first-order theory, and attentional theory. We then lay out in the third section their predictions for where the neural signatures of consciousness are found and evaluate these predictions using synesthesia as a test case. Given that the empirical literature from which we are drawing is still in its very early stages, with little consensus thus far, we note that much of what we say here will be tentative and exploratory rather than firm and conclusive. Still, we think it is worthwhile to take these initial steps in opening up a discussion on the relationship between synesthesia and consciousness to help pave the way for future research.

5.2 Does synesthesia occur unconsciously?

As mentioned, synesthesia is characterized in terms of an atypical association between an inducer—that is, a triggering stimulus, and a concurrent—that is, a mental response

[2] Synaesthesia has also served as a case study in debates on functionalism and representationalism, with theorists arguing that it provides a counterexample to certain versions of these views (see MacPherson, 2007; Gray et al., 2002).

[3] By "synesthetic response," we simply mean the concurrent, or synesthetic event, triggered by the inducer rather than any overt behavioral response.

to that stimulus that typically takes the form of a sensory experience. So when it comes to determining whether synesthesia can occur unconsciously, two central questions naturally arise. The first is whether conscious awareness of the inducer is required for the associated concurrent to be triggered. Certainly, the inducer must be perceptually registered by the individual on some level, but this is compatible with its being subliminally perceived, with no conscious awareness involved. The question is whether a synesthetic response could nonetheless occur under such circumstances.

This question must be kept separate from the further important question of whether concurrents themselves can occur unconsciously. Even posing this question is rather controversial, since many view concurrents as necessarily conscious, eschewing the possibility of unconscious concurrents on the grounds that *by definition* synesthetic experiences are conscious experiences. On this view, if a mental response is unconscious, then it is not a synesthetic response. We will push back against this unwarranted assumption by arguing that, on the contrary, there is some reason to think that synesthetic responses do sometimes occur unconsciously and, furthermore, that there is no reason to define synesthesia in such a way that rules this possibility out.

5.2.1 Is conscious awareness of the inducer required for an associated concurrent to be triggered?

Investigation of this question is still in its early phases, and the results that we do have at this point are mixed. So while it is not possible to arrive at a solid verdict at this stage, it is useful to review the extant findings and make clear what they do and do not imply.

One of the earliest studies to address the question at hand is that conducted by Mattingley, Rich, Yelland, and Bradshaw (2001). Their study employed a variant of the Stroop task that is commonly used to study synesthesia, especially of the grapheme-color variety. In this paradigm, synesthetes are presented with stimuli and asked to name the colors in which they appear, as in the typical Stroop task (Macleod, 1991; Stroop, 1935). The twist is that the stimuli presented to the synesthetes are those that the synesthetes have previously specified as inducers for their synesthesia. In congruent trials, the color of the stimulus matches that of the synesthetic response that it triggers. For example, if a synesthete associates the letter "A" with the color red, in a congruent trial, the letter "A" would be presented in red. In incongruent trials, the color of the stimulus does not match that of the synesthetic response that it triggers. So using the grapheme-color matching above, the stimulus might be, for example, a blue letter "A." On such a task, synesthetes have been shown to be significantly slower to name the color of the stimulus in incongruent trials versus congruent trials compared with controls (Dixon, Smilek, Cudahy, and Merikle, 2000; Lupiáñez and Callejas, 2006; Mattingley, Rich, Yelland, and Bradshaw, 2001), suggesting that there is some interference between the color of the concurrent and the processing of the stimulus color for synesthetes.

In the pair of experiments of interest for our purposes, Mattingley et al. (2001) presented synesthetes and controls with achromatic letter primes. They were then asked to name the color of a patch that was congruent, incongruent, or neutral, relative to the color of the synesthetic response induced by the primes. In the first experiment, synesthetes were presented with the primes for 500 ms, so that they were consciously aware of them. Here, the synesthetes were significantly faster in naming the color of the patch in the congruent condition versus the incongruent and neutral conditions. Controls showed no such advantages in the "congruent" condition, as the color and letter pairings were meaningless to these subjects.

In the second experiment, synesthetes and controls were presented with the primes at brief intervals of either 56 or 28 ms. The primes were masked so that the participants did not consciously perceive them. Again, the synesthetes were asked to name the color of a patch that was congruent, incongruent, or neutral relative to the color of the concurrent that the primes were expected to induce. In this case there was no effect of congruency on the reaction times of the synesthetes; they performed on par with controls, suggesting that there was no priming effect of the sort that would be expected if a concurrent were present. These results therefore indicate that unless the synesthete is consciously aware of the inducing stimulus, no concurrent is triggered.

One might worry here that the participants did not perceive the priming stimuli *at all*, let alone unconsciously. If so, then this experiment would not offer support for anything stronger than the uncontroversial claim that unless the inducer stimulus is *seen*, consciously or not, no concurrent is triggered. To confirm that some unconscious visual processing of the stimuli did occur, Mattingley et al. (2001) used a separate task, in which participants were presented with letter primes for the same brief duration of time as in the target task, i.e., 56 or 28 ms, and asked the subjects to name letters that were either congruent (e.g., an "A" followed by "a") or incongruent (e.g., an "A" followed by "b") with those primes. Both synesthetes and controls were slower to name incongruent versus congruent letters, suggesting that they were processed to some degree, albeit unconsciously. Mattingley et al. (2001) conclude that in their key experiment, synesthetes did indeed unconsciously perceive the inducing stimuli, and so they interpret their results as support for the view that synesthetic responses do not occur unless the individual is *consciously* aware of the inducer stimulus. One concern with this study, however, is that the cross-dimensional priming measure (i.e., a letter priming a color as opposed to a letter priming a letter) may not have been sensitive enough to detect the synesthesia from the unconscious inducers.

Furthermore, not all studies point to the same conclusion as the Mattingley et al. studies. Other work seems rather to suggest that an unconsciously processed inducer can indeed give rise to a synesthetic response. Smilek, Dixon, Cudahy, and Merikle (2001) briefly presented a grapheme-color synesthete, C, with single black digits against backgrounds that were either congruent or incongruent with the color of her synesthetic responses. C's task was to identify the digit. Smilek et al. found that she was "less accurate" at identifying the target digit when it was presented against a congruent background color than when it was presented against an incongruent background. This difference was not found for controls performing the same task.

This result suggests, on at least one interpretation, that C undergoes her synesthetic experiences *before* she is consciously aware of the inducer digits, since otherwise she would not have difficulty consciously identifying the relevant digit against a congruent background (see, e.g., Smilek et al., 2005: 87). The idea is that before she consciously perceives the inducer digit, she processes its features to a degree, such that her synesthetic response is triggered. In congruent conditions, this response then interferes with the conscious identification of the inducer digit, appearing as it does against the same-colored background.[4]

A subsequent study by Wagar et al. (2002) may also provide some evidence that C's synesthetic response occurs despite no conscious awareness of the inducer. C and controls performed a task in which a target digit was presented among a set of distractors followed by an object substitution mask. After the mask, participants had to identify the target digit by pressing a key. C was significantly more accurate than controls at successfully identifying the digit when it was an inducer that produced an associated concurrent for her. Wagar et al. (2002) conclude that C's synesthetic response prevented object substitution masking by reducing the similarity between the target and mask, and that this did not occur for controls.

If Wagar and colleagues are right about this, then C's perception of the target inducer during this task was fully conscious, due to the associated photism blocking the object substitution masking. But the main source of evidence for the failure of the object substitution masking is that C was able to accurately identify the target significantly more often than controls, and this result also supports an alternative interpretation of the results that the authors do not consider. It could be, instead, that the object substitution masking did indeed succeed, and that C was not consciously aware of the inducer, though the associated concurrent was triggered. C would then be able to infer the identity of the inducer on the basis of the concurrent. And if so, then this too would be a case in which conscious awareness of the inducer is not required for a concurrent to be triggered. Unfortunately, the authors did not elicit subjective reports from the participants about whether they consciously saw the target. A subsequent study could incorporate this measure.

[4] In the paper reporting the original results, Smilek et al. (2001) do not make this claim, but explain the results by appeal to a reentrant processing model (Di Lollo, Enns, and Rensink, 2000; Lamme and Roelfsema, 2000) on which the activation of the synesthetic color interferes with processing in V4 that normally results in the segregation of the digit and the background. They speculate that this is due to interference between feedforward processing taking place through V1, V2, and V4, and feedback processing of the synesthetic color traveling through anterior fusiform and posterior inferotemporal areas back to V4 (933). While this interference in processing may be enough to explain the slower reaction times, it does not rule out the possibility that C has her synesthetic response before becoming consciously aware of the target digit, since the same interference could also suppress the conscious awareness of the target.

Others also argue on the basis of different results that synesthetic responses do not require conscious awareness of the inducer. For instance, Ramachandran and Hubbard (2001) describe a study in which a grapheme-color synesthete was presented with individual graphemes in their peripheral vision and asked to identify them. Typically, this is not a challenging task; however, when the target graphemes are "flanked" by other graphemes—that is, when they are presented with graphemes directly adjacent to them on both sides—identification becomes more difficult (a phenomenon known as "crowding"). When performing this task and presented with a flanked target grapheme, one synesthete commented that, "I can't see that middle letter but it must be an 'O' because it looks blue" (8). On this basis, Ramachandran and Hubbard (2001) conclude that "the [synesthetic] colour is evoked at an early sensory—indeed preconscious—level rather than at a higher cognitive level" (8).

We need to be careful here to distinguish between two importantly different questions: (i) Does a synesthetic response require conscious awareness of the inducer? and (ii) Does a synesthetic response require conscious awareness of the *identity* of the inducer? One could, for example, be aware of a target stimulus without being aware that it is a "2" or the letter "A," being aware of it instead in terms of other features it possesses, e.g. as a symbol with some indiscernible shape. Though Ramachandran and Hubbard's (2001) study, and their subsequent one (Hubbard et al., 2005), may be evidence for a negative response to the second question, they are *not* evidence in favor of a negative response to the first question, as the authors themselves seem to be suggesting. This is because the synesthete was clearly consciously aware of the stimulus; she simply could not consciously determine its identity. This verdict arguably also applies to Smilek et al. (2001). The results do not preclude the possibility that C was in many cases consciously aware of some target stimulus being present against a background, just not its specific identity. So neither of these studies can be used as solid evidence against the claim that a synesthetic response requires conscious awareness of the inducing stimulus to occur. They do provide some initial evidence, however, against the claim that a synesthetic response requires conscious awareness of the *identity* of the inducing stimulus.[5] (See Table 5.1.)

5.2.2 Do synesthetic responses occur unconsciously?

As we noted, it may seem odd to question whether synesthesia can be experienced unconsciously. After all, this phenomenon is primarily identified, at least initially, by subjective reports of the unusual and robust conscious sensory experiences that it involves, and this has become a definitional feature of the condition for many

[5] Note that the finding that ambiguous symbols (e.g., a symbol that may be read as either an "A" or an "H") generate different synesthetic responses depending on what their identity is taken to be given the context (see Simner, 2007) does not counter this evidence, since it does not establish that the grapheme needs to be *consciously* identified in a certain way for the response to occur, and this is the claim we are interested in.

Table 5.1. A summary of the main findings on the question of whether conscious awareness of the inducer or its identity are required for a synesthetic response to occur.

Study	Conscious awareness of inducer required?	Conscious awareness of the identity of the inducer required?
Mattingley et al. (2001)	Suggests yes	—
Smilek et al. (2001)	Suggests no, on one interpretation of findings	Suggests no
Ramachandran and Hubbard (2001)	—	Suggests no
Wagar et al. (2002)	Suggests no, on one interpretation of findings	—

theorists. As Deroy and Spence (2013) indicate, "of all the controversies surrounding the very existence, or definition, of synaesthesia that have been documented over the last 130 years or so... none have questioned that the fundamental characteristic of synaesthesia is the elicitation of a conscious concurrent" (5).

But though this may be so, we suggest that the possibility of unconscious concurrents is being unjustifiably overlooked. We need to distinguish here between the claim that synesthesia *always* involves a conscious concurrent, and the claim that it at least sometimes, or even typically, does. While we have reason to accept the latter claim, we have no reason to accept the former. It is worth keeping in mind here that the features by which we identify a certain phenomenon for the purposes of theorizing may not always be exhibited by the target phenomenon under other conditions. So though we may initially take synesthetic concurrents to refer to conscious experiences as a way of framing the phenomenon in question, this need not be the last word on the nature of the phenomenon.

To draw a simple analogy, water is properly identified, under some conditions, as a liquid substance. But this is no reason to deny that a solid or gaseous substance with the same chemical composition as the liquid substance we refer to as "water" is also properly described as such. Rather, the scientist's overall theory of water should be able to predict and explain these various forms that water takes under different conditions, with a proper understanding of its underlying chemical properties, which remain constant across these conditions.

Likewise, the fact that synesthetic responses associated with the inducing stimulus often occur consciously is no reason by itself to deny that they sometimes occur unconsciously as well. And if we have evidence that, under some conditions, inducing stimuli lead to psychological states that yield behavioral outputs that are similar to those yielded by conscious synesthetic experiences, e.g. interference in a Stroop-like task, but in the absence of consciousness, we have good reason, by virtue of this similarity, to construe these as synesthetic responses.

To approach this issue from another angle, we can consider what is true of sensory states more generally. While we often characterize the nature of our sensory states in terms of how we consciously experience them, and this is again a primary way by which we identify such states for the purposes of theorizing, there is nonetheless ample evidence that these very same types of states sometimes occur unconsciously, as in subliminal perception. This phenomenon has been well established in experimental settings. Persuh and Ro (2012), for example, have shown that the brightness of a stimulus can be affected by its context even when that stimulus is not consciously perceived, suggesting that unconscious sensations of brightness occur. These states are aptly termed sensations, despite occurring unconsciously, because they play the same psychological role within an individual's mental economy as their conscious counterparts in that they enable the individual to respond discriminately to sensory properties of stimuli. Importantly, the fact that they are not conscious states cannot itself be appealed to as a reason for denying them the status of "genuine" sensations, since the very question at issue is whether such states sometimes occur unconsciously.

Since synesthesia typically involves the triggering of sensory states in response to inducer stimuli in a way that results in characteristic behaviors, we urge that it may be that these states, like sensory states more generally, also sometimes occur unconsciously. This possibility has yet to be properly explored in the literature, due perhaps to the widespread insistence, as mentioned, on defining synesthesia as involving a conscious concurrent. But this could be tested using standard priming paradigms. For example, if a synesthete associates the letter "A" with the color red, a testing condition could be designed in which awareness of the synesthetic red response to the letter "A" is suppressed by other distracting stimuli. The synesthete could then be tested on whether he or she nonetheless responds faster to subsequent red stimuli than to those appearing in other colors.[6]

Indeed, there is evidence that something similar to this sometimes happens in so-called implicit bidirectional synesthesia. It has been found that certain grapheme-color synesthetes show behavioral priming effects for graphemes that act as inducers for concurrents when presented with stimuli whose colors match those of the relevant concurrents (e.g., Cohen et al., 2005; Cohen Kadosh, Cohen Kadosh, and Henik, 2007; see also Deroy and Spence, 2013). To take our earlier example, if they associate the letter "A" with the color red, they might be faster than controls to identify the letter "A" presented after a red stimulus. In some of these cases, there is no report of an inducer-related perceptual experience, suggesting that an unconscious response, e.g., a representation of the number or letter, is driving this priming effect. And if an unconscious representation of an inducer can be triggered in

[6] This is similar to the paradigm used by Mattingley et al. (2001), but importantly, their study does not rule out the possibility of unconscious synesthetic responses; it just provides some evidence against the occurrence of unconscious (or conscious) synesthetic responses when one is not consciously aware of the inducing stimulus.

response to the presentation of a stimulus matching the associated concurrent in relevant ways, it is not a stretch to think that, perhaps under certain conditions, an unconscious representation of a concurrent could be triggered in response to the presentation of the associated inducer. This remains an important question for future research.

Having clarified and explored the question of whether synesthesia occurs unconsciously, we turn now to evaluating major theories of consciousness using synesthesia as a test case for their predictions concerning the neural correlates of consciousness. We start, first, by reviewing the theories that will guide the remainder of our discussion.

5.3 Theories of consciousness

Theories of consciousness all undertake to explain the difference between conscious and unconscious mental states. We will not be able to survey all existing theories of consciousness in our discussion here. Instead, we describe the main commitments of four popular theories to draw out key implications that can be evaluated using synesthesia as a test case. The four theories are higher-order theory, neuronal global workspace theory, biological first-order theory, and attentional theory.

Higher-order theories are motivated by the commonsense observation that if one is not aware of being in a mental state, then that mental state is not conscious. For example, suppose that one desires to quit one's job, but one is completely unaware of having this desire. In this case, it would significantly strain our commonsense convictions if we were to nonetheless view this desire as a conscious one. Conscious mental states are those that one is aware of being in.

How does one become aware of one's own mental states? It is typically held that this awareness is had by way of being in a suitable higher-order state; that is, a mental state that represents oneself as being in a particular mental state.[7] On this type of view, unconscious mental states are those that are not targeted by any higher-order state, and so those of which one is unaware. There is some disagreement among theorists, however, regarding what kind of higher-order state is necessary for consciousness. On a popular version of the view, the higher-order state in question is a suitable thought to the effect that one is currently in a particular mental state (Rosenthal, 2005). On another influential variant, the higher-order state is viewed instead as a perception-like state (Armstrong, 1981; Lycan, 1996), which in some way senses or monitors the mental states that one is in. Yet an additional type of higher-order account holds that the higher-order state in question is the output of a decision

[7] This is all that is meant by "higher-order" here. A state is higher-order, on this terminology, insofar as it is about another mental state, not insofar as it engages "higher" or more complex cognitive functions, though this may be true as well.

process that determines whether a particular mental state, at least when it is a sensory state, constitutes a reliable sensory signal (Lau, 2008).

While higher-order views have their appeal, some theorists resist them on the grounds that there *are* cases, they argue, in which one is in a conscious mental state, but one is not aware of being in that state. These cases, it is urged, suggest that the deliverances of commonsense, which suggest that for a mental state to be conscious, one must be aware of it, are simply misguided. They therefore deny that a mental state must be the target of a higher-order state to be conscious. Such theorists are known as first-order theorists.

A popular version of this approach, defended by Dretske (1995), holds simply that a mental state is conscious if one is aware of something or aware that something is the case in virtue of being in that state. For example, on Dretske's view, if I am aware of a tree in front of me in virtue of being in some perceptual state, then that perceptual state is a conscious state. It need not be the case that I am also aware of the state that makes me aware of the tree by way of a higher-order state.

A variant of the first-order approach, and the one on which we will focus here, is the biological first-order approach favored by, among others, Block (2005, 2009) and Lamme (2003, 2006; see also Fahrenfort and Lamme, 2012). On this view, having a certain biological basis, in particular involving lower-level regions of the brain, is necessary and sufficient for conscious experiences of various types. To illustrate, Block (2005) argues by appeal to empirical evidence that the neural basis of the conscious visual experience of motion is likely a certain type of activation in MT/V5, which is part of a recurrent feedback loop to V1, and then back again to MT/V5. He argues for this claim in part on the basis of evidence that activation in this region occurs during motion perception (Heeger et al., 1999), and bilateral damage to a region including MT/V5 results in the inability to perceive motion (Zeki et al., 1991). On this view, for every type of conscious experience, we can expect to identify a corresponding neural basis; consciousness is necessarily a biological phenomenon.

A close cousin of the biological first-order approach is the neuronal global workspace theory. This view also denies that higher-order representation is required for a mental state to be conscious. But, unlike the biological first-order view, the neuronal global workspace view requires that the contents of a mental state be "globally broadcast"; that is, made available to areas of the brain responsible for verbal report, planning, intentional action, and memory (Baars, 1997; Dehaene and Naccache, 2001; Dehaene and Changeux, 2011). So while the biological first-order view allows that one might, in some cases, have a conscious experience despite being unable to report on it, the global workspace theory entails that if a state is conscious, then it is available for verbal report.

Finally, there are those theories that reserve a key role for attention to play in giving rise to consciousness (e.g., Cohen, Cavanagh, Chun, and Nakayama, 2012). Such views are motivated in large part by empirical findings that seem to suggest that in the absence of attention, a stimulus is not able to reach consciousness. In the condition known as hemispatial neglect, for example, individuals deny having conscious visual experiences of the left side of their visual field (Driver and Mattingley, 1998; Rafal, 1994). There is evidence, however, that they nonetheless process visual stimuli presented to them on that side (e.g., Volpe, LeDoux, and Gazzaniga, 1979; Ro and Rafal, 1996; Marshall and Halligan, 1988; Doricchi and Galati, 2000). Attentional theorists argue that this disorder is a result of damage to brain regions associated with attentional processing, in this case the inferior parietal lobe or superior temporal gyrus (Karnath, Ferber, and Himmelbach, 2001; Mort et al., 2003; Corbetta and Shulman, 2002; Prinz, 2012). And they use this to motivate their claim that attention is required for conscious awareness.[8]

Each of the theories that we have briefly reviewed here makes a different set of empirical predictions on the basis of which they may be evaluated. In the next section, our strategy will be to make explicit their predictions specifically related to the neural correlates of consciousness and determine whether they are consistent with what is presently known about conscious synesthetic experiences.

5.4 What can we learn about the neural correlates of consciousness from synesthesia?

The theories of consciousness we have surveyed each have something different to say about where the neural correlates of consciousness are likely to be found (see Lau and Rosenthal, 2011). Following others, we characterize these as the minimal neural basis sufficient for a conscious state with a specific content (see Koch, 2004; Chalmers, 2002; Block, 2005). Synesthesia researchers have also been working to determine the neural correlates of conscious synesthetic experiences and have begun establishing a body of empirical data. Drawing upon these predictions and findings, the question we will focus on in this section is whether synesthesia provides any useful insights with respect to what theories of consciousness predict about the neural correlates of consciousness.

If one accepts the higher-order approach to consciousness, the neural correlates of consciousness are likely to be located wherever the neural correlates of the relevant higher-order states are found. Since the likely neural correlates of higher-order states are neural events in prefrontal and parietal regions, the higher-order view predicts that the neural correlates of conscious states are likely somewhere in these areas as well. The neuronal global workspace view makes this prediction also, since the "workspace" is constituted by neurons in these same brain areas with long-range

[8] We note that studies that show the ability of individuals to orient attention without any conscious awareness (Kentridge, Nijboer, and Heywood, 2008; Kentridge, Heywood, and Weiskrantz, 1999; McCormick, 1997) pose serious challenges for such attentional theories insofar as they also make the claim that attention is sufficient for conscious awareness.

axons that make globally available the information they encode, thus giving rise to consciousness (Dehaene and Changeux, 2011).

By contrast, the biological first-order view associates conscious awareness with activity in early sensory regions, and does not specify a direct role for frontal or parietal brain regions. With respect to conscious visual states, for example, this view specifies recurrent feedback activity to V1 as being critical for these states to be conscious. As evidence for the necessity of recurrent activation, Lamme (2006) cites work by Boyer, Harrison, and Ro (2005), who found that they could induce blindsight-like behavior in healthy subjects by applying a TMS pulse to V1 with a delay of 100 ms after the onset of a stimulus. The thought is that, while the timing of the TMS leaves the feedforward sweep from V1 to extrastriate areas and regions in the parietal and temporal cortex intact, the recurrent feedback to V1 is disrupted, and so no conscious visual state results.

Attentional theories, on the other hand, propose that attention-related regions of the brain, including the temporoparietal junction (Corbetta and Shulman, 2002; Friedrich, Egly, Rafal, and Beck, 1998), are the neural correlates of conscious states. On Prinz's (2012) view in particular, attention is understood as a process by which information is made available to working memory. Prinz identifies the neural correlates of attention with a circuit involving perceptual pathways in early sensory regions, attention centers in parietal cortex, and brain regions associated with working memory, in this case the lateral frontal cortex. According to this view, damage or disruptions to these attention-related regions produces deficits in attention to affected regions of space and objects, which in turn produce deficits in conscious awareness.

It is worth noting that the empirical predictions of each of these theories are echoed in the main neural models of synesthesia. These models take as their basic premise the claim that synesthesia is a matter of hyperassociation between brain regions. They then seek to establish the precise nature of these associations. On the long-range disinhibited feedback model, the hyperassociation, at least in forms of synesthesia involving concurrents that are visual in character, is thought to result from aberrant long-range feedback between, for example, parietal regions and visual cortex. Due to the involvement of the parietal cortex, this falls in line with the predictions of the higher-order, the global neuronal workspace, and attention-based views of consciousness. On the re-entrant processing model of synesthesia, however, the hyperassociation for visual forms of synesthesia results from more local aberrant re-entrant feedback, for example from the anterior inferior temporal region back to posterior inferotemporal regions and back to V4. This fits more comfortably with the predictions of the biological first-order view.

Recently, some have been putting pressure on the prediction of the biological first-order view that activation in V1 is required for conscious visual experience. While numerous potential counterexamples have been put forward from various psychological conditions and studies (see Lau and Brown, 2011), it has gone largely unnoticed that the results of some neuroimaging studies on individuals with auditory-visual synesthesia also seem to challenge this prediction. In this form of synesthesia, individuals experience color sensations in response to spoken words. An early PET study by Paulesu et al. (1995) looked at six synesthetes with auditory-visual synesthesia. The participants showed significantly higher activation than controls when hearing spoken words in, among other regions, the right prefrontal cortex and the parieto-occipital junction, in keeping with the predictions of the higher-order, neuronal global workspace, and attentional views of consciousness. However, they did *not* show significantly higher activation in early visual areas such as V1, V2, and V4. The absence of activation in V1 is particularly noteworthy, given its supposed role in supporting conscious visual experiences according to the first-order biological view. As Cytowic (2002) puts it,

> [w]hat is most remarkable about Paulesu's study is that the primary visual area does not activate during the stimulus task, thus demonstrating—for the first time—that it is possible to have a conscious visual experience without the participation of V1, the classic primary visual area. (156)

Another study with auditory-visual synesthetes, by Nunn et al. (2002), this time using fMRI, found converging results with Paulesu et al.'s (1995) study. They did not find activation in V1 or V2 while synesthetes were undergoing their visual concurrents, though they did find activation in color areas of the brain; that is, in V4/V8, as well as V4α. They also found activation in various areas of the brain involved with higher functions, such as the inferior parietal lobe and the inferior frontal lobe. While these results, and those from other studies with similar findings (e.g., Hong and Blake, 2008; Hubbard et al., 2005), are problematic for the biological first-order view that takes V1 to be the neural correlate of conscious visual experience, they could be accommodated by higher-order, neuronal global workspace, and attentional views of consciousness.

In particular, on at least some versions of the higher-order view, higher-order mental states alone determine subjective experience, so that even if no corresponding first-order mental state is present, one will have the conscious experience of being in whatever mental state one's higher-order awareness represents oneself as being in. For example, if one is in a higher-order state representing oneself as seeing red, then one will have the conscious experience of seeing red, even if no corresponding first-order state representing red exists. This captures the idea that consciousness is a matter of how our mental lives appear to us; in other words, what mental states we represent ourselves as being in, and arguably how things subjectively appear can diverge from how they actually are, even within consciousness. Applying this here, a tempting interpretation of at least some conscious synesthetic experiences is that they are a function of higher-order states alone, since the relevant activation in V1, which would presumably correlate with the relevant first-order visual state, is not present.[9]

[9] We are grateful to David Rosenthal for this suggestion.

Still, the findings just discussed do not constitute a straightforward strike against the first-order view. Muddying the waters here is that yet other studies *have* found increased V1 activation in the case of auditory-visual synesthetes. For example, Aleman et al. (2001) used fMRI to test another synesthete who reported experiencing color in response to auditory linguistic stimuli. In one task, the synesthete was presented with auditory words or tones of different frequencies. In a second task, she was presented with either a single auditory letter or tones of different frequencies. The authors reported finding small clusters of activation in V1 during both tasks despite the lack of any visual input (see also Neufeld et al., 2012). And Hubbard and Ramachandran (2005) showed that some synesthetes with grapheme-color synesthesia showed greater activation in neighboring color regions of the brain when achromatic letters were presented to them. In addition, a fairly recent finding that would also seem to support the biological first-order view is that relevant early sensory areas appear to be implicated in non-visual cases of synesthesia. Furthermore, in patient SR, who has acquired auditory-tactile synesthesia and experiences sensations of touch in response to sounds, there is a much higher degree of activation in the secondary somatosensory cortex in response to sounds that she reports feeling in comparison to sounds that she does not reporting feeling (Beauchamp and Ro, 2008).

There is further evidence from neuroimaging studies on synesthesia that is consistent with the predictions of the attentional, higher-order, and neuronal global workspace accounts of consciousness insofar as they predict the participation of parietal regions in conscious experiences. This area is frequently implicated in synesthetic experiences (e.g., Weiss et al., 2005). In one study, it was even found that applying TMS to the posterior parietal lobe during a color-naming task performed by grapheme-color synesthetes attenuates synesthetic interference on a Stroop-like priming task (Esterman et al., 2006; see also Muggleton et al., 2007). These TMS results suggest that attentional mechanisms in the parietal cortex are involved with the visual feature binding of the concurrent with the inducer.

Taken together, neuroscientific studies of synesthesia, at least at this stage, do not unequivocally provide evidence in favor of one theory of consciousness over another in terms of their predictions regarding the neural correlates of conscious experience. However, such studies using neuroscientific approaches are illuminating in that they reveal some of the mechanisms that may give rise to conscious experiences in synesthesia and also provide at least some initial clues as to the neural correlates of conscious perceptual experiences more generally.

5.5 Conclusion

In this chapter, we have started to address important questions regarding the relationship between synesthesia and consciousness. We have reviewed what little work has been done in this area and we have argued that there is reason to accept that synesthesia sometimes occurs unconsciously and reason to reject the view that rules this out by definition alone. We have also taken some initial steps in evaluating popular theories of consciousness using synesthesia as a test case. It is too early to draw any firm conclusions regarding the neural correlates of consciousness on the basis of synesthesia. However, further explorations of synesthesia and consciousness should not only better inform us of the relationships between these two interesting and complex psychological phenomena, but should also allow us to more thoroughly understand the underlying natures of synesthesia and consciousness in and of themselves.

References

Aleman, A., Rutten, G. J., Sitskoorn, M. M., Dautzenberg, G., & Ramsey, N. F. (2001). Activation of striate cortex in the absence of visual stimulation: an fMRI study of synesthesia. *Neuroreport, 12*(13), 2827–30.

Armstrong, D. (1981). What is consciousness? In D. M. Armstrong (Ed.), *The Nature of Mind.* Ithaca, NY: Cornell University Press.

Baars, B. J. (1997). *In the Theater of Consciousness: The Workspace of the Mind.* Oxford: Oxford University Press.

Beauchamp, M. S., & Ro, T. (2008). Neural substrates of sound–touch synesthesia after a thalamic lesion. *Journal of Neuroscience, 28*, 13696–702.

Block, N. (2005). Two neural correlates of consciousness. *TRENDS in Cognitive Sciences, 9*(2), 46–52.

Block, N. (2009). Comparing the major theories of consciousness. In M. Gazzaniga (Ed.), *The Cognitive Neurosciences IV.* Cambridge, MA: MIT Press.

Boyer, J. L., Harrison, S., & Ro, T. (2005). Unconscious processing of orientation and color without primary visual cortex. *Proceedings of the National Academy of Science U. S. A., 102*, 16875–9.

Chalmers, D. (2002). What is a neural correlate of consciousness? In T. Metzinger (Ed.), *Neural Correlates of Consciousness: Empirical and Conceptual Questions.* Cambridge: MIT Press.

Cohen, M. A., Cavanagh, P., Chun, M. M., & Nakayama, K. (2012). The attentional requirements of consciousness. *Trends in Cognitive Sciences, 16*, 411–17.

Cohen Kadosh, R., Cohen Kadosh, K., & Henik, A. (2007). The neuronal correlate of bidirectional: a combined event-related potential and functional magnetic resonance imaging study. synesthesia. *Journal of Cognitive Neuroscience, 19*(12), 2050–9.

Cohen Kadosh, R., Sagiv, N., Linden, D. E. J., Robertson, L. C., Elinger, G., & Henik, A. (2005). When blue is larger than red: colors influence numerical cognition in synesthesia. *Journal of Cognitive Neuroscience, 17*, 1766–73.

Corbetta, M., & Shulman, G. L. (2002). Control of goal-directed and stimulus driven attention in the brain. *Nature Reviews Neuroscience, 3*, 201–15.

Cytowic, R. E. (2002). *Synesthesia: A Union of the Senses* (2nd ed.). Cambridge, MA: MIT Press.

Dehaene, S., & Changeux, J-P. (2011). Experimental and theoretical approaches to conscious processing. *Neuron, 70*, 200–27.

Dehaene, S., & Naccache, L. (2001). Towards a cognitive neuroscience of consciousness: basic evidence and a workspace framework. *Cognition, 79*, 1–37.

Deroy, O., & Auvray. M. (forthcoming). Synesthesia. In M. Matthen (Ed.), *The Oxford Handbook of the Philosophy of Perception*. Oxford: Oxford University Press.

Deroy, O., & Spence, C. (2013). Training, hypnosis, and drugs: artificial synaesthesia, or artificial paradises?. *Frontiers in Psychology, 4*.

Di Lollo, V., Enns, J. T., & Rensink, R. A. (2000). Competition for consciousness among visual events: the psychophysics of reentrant visual pathways. *Journal of Experimental Psychology: General, 129*, 481–507.

Doricchi, F., & Galati, G. (2000). Implicit semantic evaluation of object symmetry and contralesional visual denial in a case of left unilateral neglect with damage of the dorsal paraventricular white matter. *Cortex, 36*, 337–50.

Dretske, F. I. (1995). *Naturalizing the Mind*. Cambridge: MIT Press.

Driver, J., & Mattingley, J. B. (1998). Parietal neglect and visual awareness. *Nature Neuroscience, 1*, 1, 17–22.

Dixon, M. J., Smilek, D., Cudahy, C., & Merikle, P. M. (2000). Five plus two equals yellow. *Nature, 406*, 365.

Eagleman, D. M., Kagan, A. D., Nelson, S. S., Sagaram, D., & Sarma, A. K. (2007). A standardized test battery for the study of synesthesia. *Journal of Neuroscience Methods, 159*, 139–45.

Edquist, J., Rich, A. N., Brinkman, C., & Mattingley, J. B. (2006). Do synaesthetic colours act as unique features in visual search. *Cortex, 42*, 222–31.

Esterman, M., Verstynen, T., Ivry, R. B., & Robertson, L. C. (2006). Coming unbound: disrupting automatic integration of synesthetic color and graphemes by transcranial magnetic stimulation of the right parietal lobe. *Journal of Cognitive Neuroscience, 18*(9), 1570–6.

Fahrenfort, J. J., & Lamme, V. A. F. (2012). A true science of consciousness explains phenomenology: comment on Cohen and Dennett. *Trends in Cognitive Sciences, 16*(3), 138–9.

Friedrich, F. J., Egly, R., Rafal, R. D., & Beck, D. (1998). Spatial attention deficits in humans: a comparison of superior parietal and temporal-parietal junction lesions. *Neuropsychology, 12*(2), 193–207.

Gheri, C., Chopping, S., & Morgan, M. J. (2008). Synaesthetic colours do not camouflage form in visual search. *Proceedings of the Royal Society of London B Biological Sciences, 275*, 841–6.

Gray, J. A., Chopping S., Nunn, J., Parslow, D., Gregory, L. Williams, S. C. R., Brammer, M. J., & Baron-Cohen, S. (2002). Implications of synaesthesia for functionalism: theory and experiments. *Journal of Consciousness Studies, 9*(12), 5–31.

Heeger, D., Boynton, G. M., Demb, J. B., Seidemann, E., & Newsome, W. T. (1999). Motion opponency in visual cortex. *Journal of Neuroscience, 19(16)*, 7162–74.

Hong, S. W., & Blake, R. (2008). Early visual mechanisms do not contribute to synesthetic color experience. *Vision Research, 48*, 1018–26.

Hubbard, E. M., Arman, A. C., Ramachandran, V. S., & Boynton, G. M. (2005). Individual differences among grapheme-color synesthetes: brain-behavior correlations. *Neuron, 45*(6), 975–85.

Hubbard, E. M., Manohar, S., & Ramachandran, V. S. (2006). Contrast affects the strength of synesthetic colors. *Cortex, 42*, 184–94.

Karnath, H. O., Ferber, S., & Himmelbach, M. (2001). Spatial awareness is a function of the temporal not the posterior parietal lobe. *Nature, 411*(6840), 950–3.

Kentridge, R., Heywood, C. A., & Weiskrantz, L. (1999). Attention without awareness in blindsight. *Proceedings of the Royal Society of London B, 266*, 1805–11.

Kentridge, R., Nijboer, T. C. W., & Heywood, C. A. (2008). Attended but unseen: Visual attention is not sufficient for visual awareness. *Neuropsychologia, 46*, 864–9.

Koch, C. (2004). *The Quest for Consciousness: A Neuroscientific Approach*. Englewood, CO: Roberts & Company Publishers.

Laeng, B., Svartdal, F., & Oelmann, H. (2004). Does color synesthesia pose a paradox for early-selection theories of attention. *Psychological Sciences, 15*, 277–81.

Lamme, V. A. F. (2003). Why visual attention and awareness are different. *Trends in Cognitive Science, 7*(1), 12–18.

Lamme, V. A. F. (2006). Zap! Magnetic tricks on conscious and unconscious vision, *TRENDS in Cognitive Sciences, 10*(5), 193–5.

Lamme, V. A. F., & Roelfsema, P. R. (2000). The distinct modes of vision offered by feedforward and recurrent processing. *Trends in Neuroscience, 23*(11), 571–9.

Lau, H. (2008). A higher order Bayesian decision theory of consciousness. *Progressive Brain Research, 168*, 35–48.

Lau, H., & Brown, R. (2011). The emperor's new phenomenology? The empirical case for conscious experiences without first-order representations. In A. Pautz and D. Stoljar (Eds.), *Themes from Block*. Cambridge: MIT Press.

Lau, H., & Rosenthal, D. (2011). Empirical support for higher-order theories of conscious awareness. *Trends in Cognitive Sciences, 15*(8), 365–73.

Lupiáñez, J., & Callejas, A. (2006). Automatic perception and synaesthesia: evidence from colour and photism naming in a stroop-negative priming task. *Cortex, 42*, 204–12.

Lycan, W. G. (1996). *Consciousness and Experience*. Cambridge: MIT Press.

MacLeod, C. M. (1991). Half a century of research on the stroop effect: an integrative review. *Psychological Bulletin, 109*(2), 163–203.

Macpherson, F. (2007). Synaesthesia, functionalism, and phenomenology. In M. de Caro, F. Ferretti, and M. Marraffa (Eds.), *Cartographies of the Mind: Philosophy and Psychology in Intersection Series: Studies in Mind and Brain* (pp. 65–80). Dordrecht: Springer.

Marshall, J. C., & Halligan, P. W. (1988). Blindsight and insight in visuo-spatial neglect. *Nature, 336*, 766–7.

Mattingley, J. B., Rich, A. N., Yelland, G., & Bradshaw, J. L. (2001). Unconscious priming eliminates automatic binding of colour and alphanumeric form in synaesthesia. *Nature, 410*, 580–2.

McCormick, P. A. (1997). Orienting attention without awareness. *Journal of Experimental Psychology: Human Perception and Performance, 23*(1), 168–80.

Mort, D. J., Malhotra, P., Mannan, S. K., Rordern, C., Pambakian, A., Kennard, C., & Husain, M. (2003). The anatomy of visual neglect. *Brain, 126*, 1986–97.

Muggleton, N., Tsakanikos, E., Walsh, V., & Ward, J. (2007). Disruption of synaesthesia following TMS of the right posterior parietal cortex. *Neuropsychologia, 45*, 1582–5.

Mylopoulos, M. I., & Ro, T. (2013). Synesthesia: a colorful word with a touching sound? *Frontiers in Psychology, 4*, 1–9.

Neufeld, J., Sinke, C., Dillo, W., Emrich, H. M., Szycik, G. R., Dima, D., Bleich, S., & Zedler, M. (2012). The neural correlates of coloured music: a functional MRI investigation of auditory-visual synaesthesia. *Neuropsychologia, 50*(1), 85–9.

Nijboer, T. C. W., Satris, G., & van der Stigchel, S. (2011). The influence of synesthesia on eye movements: no synesthetic pop-out in an oculomotor target selection task. *Consciousness and Cognition, 20*, 1193–200.

Nunn, J. A., Gregory, L. J., Brammer, M., Williams, S. C. R., Parslow, D. M., Morgan, M. J., Morris, R. G., Bullmore, E. T., Baron-Cohen, S., & Gray, J. A. (2002). Functional magnetic resonance imaging of synesthesia: activation of V4/V8 by spoken words. *Nature Neuroscience, 5*(4), 371–5.

Palmeri, T. J., Blake, R., Marois, R., Flanery, M. A., & Whetsell, W. Jr. (2002). The perceptual reality of synesthetic colors. *Proceedings of the National Academy of Sciences U.S.A., 99*, 4127–31.

Paulesu, E., Harrison, J., Baron-Cohen, S., Watson, J. D. G., Goldstein, L., Heather, J., Frackowiak, R. S. J., & Frith, C. D. (1995). The physiology of coloured hearing: a PET activation study of colour-word synaesthesia. *Brain, 118*, 661–76.

Persuh, M., & Ro, T. (2012). Context-dependent brightness priming occurs without visual awareness. *Consciousness and Cognition, 21*(1), 177–85.

Prinz, J. J. (2012). *The Conscious Brain: How Attention Engenders Experience*. New York: Oxford University Press.

Rafal, R. D. (1994). Neglect. *Current Opinion in Neurobiology, 4*(2), 231–6.

Ramachandran, V. S., & Hubbard, E. M. (2001). Psychophysical investigations into the neural basis of synaesthesia. *Proc R Soc Lond B Biol Sci, 268*(1470), 979–83.

Rees, G., Kreiman, G., & Koch, C. (2002) Neural correlates of consciousness in humans. *Nature Review Neuroscience, 3*, 261–70.

Ro, T., Farnè, A., Johnson, R. M., Wedeen, V., Chu, Z., Wang, Z. J., Hunter, J. V., & Beauchamp, M. S. (2007). Feeling sounds after a thalamic lesion. *Annals of Neurology, 62*, 433–41.

Ro, T., & Rafal, R. D. (1996). Perception of geometric illusions in hemispatial neglect. *Neuropsychologia, 34*, 973–8.

Rolls, E. T. (2004). A higher order syntactic thought (HOST) theory of consciousness. In R. J. Gennaro (Ed.), *Higher-Order Theories of Consciousness* (pp. 137–72). Amsterdam & Philadelphia: John Benjamins Publishers.

Rosenthal, D. M. (2005). *Consciousness and Mind*. New York: Oxford University Press.

Rosenthal, D. M. (2008). Consciousness and its function. *Neuropsychologia, 46*(3), 829–40.

Rothen, N., & Meier, B. (2009). Do synesthetes have a general advantage in visual search and episodic memory? A case for group studies. *PLoS ONE, 4*(4), 1–9.

Sagiv, N., & Frith, C. (2013). Synesthesia and consciousness. In J. Simner and E. M. Hubbard (Eds.), *Oxford Handbook of Synesthesia* (pp. 924–40). Oxford: Oxford University Press.

Sagiv, N., Heer, J., & Robertson, L. (2006). Does binding of synesthetic color to the evoking grapheme require attention? *Cortex, 42*, 232–42.

Simner, J. (2007). Beyond perception: synaesthesia as a psycholinguistic phenomenon. *Trends in Cognitive Sciences, 11*(1), 23–9.

Smilek, D., Dixon, M. J., Cudahy, C., & Merikle, P. M. (2001). Synaesthetic photisms influence visual perception. *Journal of Cognitive Neuroscience, 13*(7), 930–6.

Smilek, D., Dixon, M. J., & Merikle, P. M. (2005). Binding of graphemes and synaesthetic colors in color-graphemic synaesthesia. In L. Robertson and N. Sagiv (Eds.), *Synesthesia: Perspectives from Cognitive Neuroscience* (pp. 74–89). Oxford: Oxford University Press.

Stroop, J. R. (1935). Studies of interference in serial verbal reactions. *Journal of Experimental Psychology, 18*, 643–62.

Volpe, B. T., LeDoux, J. E., & Gazzaniga, M. S. (1979). Information processing of visual stimuli in an 'extinguished' field. *Nature, 282*, 722–4.

Wagar, B. M., Dixon, M. J., Smilek, D., & Cudahy, C. (2002) Colored photisms prevent object-substitution masking in digit-color synesthesia. *Brain and Cognition, 48*, 606–11.

Ward, J., Jonas, C., Dienes, Z., & Seth, A. (2010). Grapheme-colour synaesthesia improves detection of embedded shapes, but without pre-attentive 'pop-out' of synaesthetic colour. *Proceedings of the Biological Sciences, 277*, 1021–6.

Weiss, P. H., Zilles, K., & Fink, G. R. (2005). When visual perception causes feeling: enhanced cross-modal processing in grapheme-color synesthesia. *NeuroImage, 28*, 859–68.

Zeki, S., Watson, J. D., Lueck, C. J., Friston, K. J., Kennard, C., & Frackowiak, R. S. (1991). A direct demonstration of functional specialization in human visual cortex. *Journal of Neuroscience, 11*(3), 641–9.

6

Synesthetic Binding and the Reactivation Model of Memory

Berit Brogaard

6.1 Introduction

Synesthesia is an unusual way of perceiving the world, in which internal or external stimuli provoke atypical sensations or thoughts (Baron-Cohen and Harrison, 1997; Cytowic, 1989; Ramachandran and Hubbard, 2001a; Grossenbacher and Lovelace, 2001; Emrich et al., 2002; Rich and Mattingley, 2002; Hubbard and Ramachandran, 2005; Sperling et al., 2005; Ward et al., 2005; Hubbard, 1996). For example, seeing the number 3 printed in black ink may lead to a sensation of copper green, hearing the word 'kiss' may flood the mouth with the flavor of tomato soup, and hearing the key of C# minor may elicit a slowly expanding purple spiral. In grapheme-color synesthesia, one of the most common forms of synesthesia, perceiving or thinking about an achromatic grapheme (also known as the 'inducer') gives rise to the sensation or thought (also known as the 'concurrent') that the grapheme has a specific color with a highly specific hue, brightness, and saturation (Simner et al., 2006). The concurrent images are either projected onto the external world (projector synesthesia) or perceived in the mind's eye (associator synesthesia) (Dixon et al., 2004). In projector synesthesia, the projected concurrent may be seen as instantiated like non-synesthetic colors, as floating above its inducer or as an 'after-image' that floats close to the subject's eyes. In associator synesthesia, the concurrent image is seen internally, much like a visual image retrieved from memory or generated by imagination.

Most cases of synesthesia are developmental. Subjects report having had the condition for as long as they can remember, and the condition appears to run in families (Baron-Cohen et al., 1996). While most cases of synesthesia are developmental, acquired cases have also been reported, for example following stroke (Beauchamp and Ro, 2008), optic nerve chiasm (Afra et al., 2009), extensive use of a sensory substitution device (Ward and Meijer, 2010), post-hypnotic suggestion (Cohen-Kadosh et al., 2009), and traumatic brain injury (Brogaard et al., 2012).

Synesthesia also occurs during intoxication resulting from exposure to psychedelic drugs, such as psilocybin, LSD, mescaline, peyote cactus, and DMT (Sinke et al., 2012; Brogaard, 2013). Drug-induced synesthesia differs from the other forms in being transient and less inducer-specific. Subjective reports suggest that, under intoxication, the same concurrent images can have a wide variety of inducers that happen to be present in the subject's environment (see Brogaard, 2013, for a review).

Up until the twenty-first century, the key evidence suggesting that synesthesia is a special condition that is fundamentally distinct from ordinary memory associations came from introspective reports. The idea that introspective reports can serve as evidence has been heavily criticized by behaviorists for almost a century, and introspective reports are still regarded as highly unreliable by most philosophers and scientists (Schwitzgebel, 2008; Hurlburt and Schwitzgebel, 2007). The widespread skepticism of phenomena that could not be subjected to objective testing, which accompanied the twentieth-century behaviorist movement, resulted in a lack of scientific interest in synesthesia during most of that century. The two main developments triggering a spark in research interest in synesthesia was the recent considerable progress in the area of neuroimaging as well as the development of the Synesthesia Battery, an automated online battery of tests that allows for rigorous testing for a range of different types of synesthesia (www.synesthete.org; Eagleman et al., 2007). It has recently been found that color differences in CIELUV and CIELAB space may be a more reliable way of diagnosing synesthesia (Rothen et al., 2013). However, a synesthesia battery based on CIELUV and CIELAB space is not yet available online.

The Synesthesia Battery consists of two sections: a color identification task and a color retrieval task. In the first task, the subject is presented with an inducer and must choose the concurrent she experiences among numerous options. When the concurrent is a color, the subject must choose a specific hue, brightness, and saturation from a color palette representing over 17.6 million distinct choices. The subject repeats the exercise three times for each inducer, which in the case of grapheme-color synesthesia amounts to 108 trials for graphemes A–Z and 0–9. The software then calculates the geometric distance among the subject's answers in red, green, and blue (RGB) color space. If the geometric distance in RGB color space is less than 1, that is strong evidence that the subject is a synesthete for that grapheme. However, a recent study by Rothen et al. (2013) generated a considerably higher cut-off value of 1.43. In the second task, the subject is presented with randomly ordered inducers one at a time together with a possible concurrent. The subject must determine whether the inducer elicits the concurrent in question as quickly as possible. A score higher than 90 percent further validates the results of the first task.

The online software tests for the presence of two features commonly regarded as diagnostic of synesthesia (Eagleman et al., 2007; Baron-Cohen et al., 1987). One is the specificness of inducer-concurrent pairs. The other is the automatic (and hence fast) associations between inducers and concurrents. If re-administered, the Battery can also be used to measure the stability of synesthetic connections over time, a third feature commonly regarded as diagnostic of synesthesia.

A further factor playing a role in the increased scientific interest in synesthesia over the last few decades is the realization that synesthesia can be informative in ways similar to other conditions that result from brain abnormalities. By studying how brain abnormalities affect normal perception, cognition, and action, we can gain insight into how these processes work in neurotypical individuals. One well-known hypothesis that has been validated by studies of lesions is the two-visual-stream hypothesis (Goodale et al., 1991; Goodale and Milner, 1992; Milner and Goodale, 1995, 2008). Research on subjects with lesions to the ventral stream but with intact dorsal systems as well as subjects with lesions to the dorsal stream but with intact ventral streams has led to a better understanding of how vision for perception and vision for action work as independent pathways (Brogaard, 2011). Though most forms of synesthesia do not result from brain lesions, but are the result of early developmental deviations in regions of the brain involved in perception and cognition, researchers believe that synesthesia can help elucidate models of perception, cognition, and action in neurotypical individuals. A good model of perception or cognition should be able to explain synesthesia by showing which processes or pathways in these models lead to the aberrant blending of sensory experiences.

It is still widely debated which models we should expect to be the best explanatory models of synesthesia. Typical early-perceptual models suggest that synesthesia is the result of interaction between brain regions via feedforward mechanisms (Ramachandran and Hubbard, 2001a, 2001b; Hubbard et al., 2005a, 2005b). Typical late-perceptual and cognitive models suggest that synesthesia is the result of aberrant feedback mechanisms (Grossenbacher and Lovelace, 2001; Dixon et al., 2006). In the first type of model the phenomenon is explained by unusual bottom-up interaction, for example between adjacent color and form areas. In the second type, the phenomenon is explained by unusual signal feedback from higher brain regions.

Earlier research on grapheme-color synesthesia has suggested that the phenomenon arises as a result of feedforward perceptual processes. Results from visual search tasks have indicated that when synesthetic inducers are hidden among distractors, this can lead to a pop-out effect and faster or more accurate response times (Ramachandran and Hubbard, 2001a, 2001b; Edquist et al., 2005; Rothen and Meier, 2009). As features computed in the early visual system are believed to be processed prior to a selection process facilitated by selective attention, these pop-out effects provide evidence that grapheme-color binding is an early visual phenomenon (Treisman, 1982). The claim that grapheme-color binding is an early visual phenomenon remains the subject of controversy, however. The location of inducers relative to distractors appears to influence search efficiency, suggesting that selective attention may be needed for synesthetic colors to reach consciousness (Laeng et al., 2004). Moreover, in more recent studies no clear evidence for pop-out effects among synesthetes has been found (Ward et al., 2010).

There are other aspects of synesthesia that are difficult for the early-perceptual models to explain. Though there is some degree of idiosyncrasy in which concurrent experiences are elicited by inducers, synesthetic connections are not completely arbitrary (Simner et al., 2005). A range of unrelated factors contribute to the formation of patterns across the concurrents experienced by synesthetes, including normal tendencies to associate certain items (e.g., high pitch and lighter colors) (Mondloch and Maurer, 2004), the visual or spectral shape of the inducer (Brang and Ramachandran, 2011), the contextual frequency of the inducer (Simner et al., 2005; Beeli et al., 2007), and exposure to the inducer-concurrent connection during early learning processes (Blake et al., 2005; Hancock, 2006; Witthoft and Winawer, 2006, 2013). In a recent study, Witthoft and Winawer (2013) looked at the letter-color associations in eleven grapheme-color synesthetes whose letter-color connections were remarkably similar. On the basis of battery tests, subjective reports and market investigations, the researchers were able to provide strong evidence that the eleven subjects acquired their synesthesia while learning the alphabet using refrigerator magnets.

It is important to note that Witthoft and Winawer's results do not show that synesthesia is just a memory association, similar to the association between sadness and the color blue, that we are all prone to make (Deroy and Spence, 2013). There are significant differences between stereotypical ties between two concepts and synesthetic binding. Unlike stereotypical memory associations, synesthetic connections are automatic, immediate, highly specific, and stable over time. Synesthetic associations also tend to have a different phenomenology compared to other types of associations. Many grapheme-color synesthetes, for example, *see* letters and numerals printed in black as having a specific color. However, Witthoft and Winawer's results do suggest that semantic memory may be importantly involved in generating the atypical, tightly interwoven connections that characterize the phenomenon. This, in turn, provides evidence that grapheme-color synesthesia need not be an early-perceptual phenomenon but may be associated with neurological processes occurring late in the perceptual system. Even if semantic memory is implicated in synesthesia, however, there is little reason to think that synesthesia is best explained by models of cognition as opposed to models of perception. Recent research on memory has revealed that there is considerable overlap between neural correlates of retrieved or actively maintained memories and those of sensory perception (Kahn et al., 2004; Polyn et al., 2005; Danker and Anderson, 2010; Rissman and Wagner, 2012). Retrieved and actively maintained memories originate in reinstated cortical representations of perceptual and semantic features.

In what follows, I review the evidence for thinking that there may be an intimate link between some cases of synesthetic binding and semantic memory connections. In the subsequent section I briefly review some results of recent memory research and show how this research can shed light on the mechanisms underlying synesthesia. Finally, I argue that synesthesia qua reinstatement of activity in sensory brain regions may help inform models of multisensory perception.

6.2 Evidence for semantic memory associations in synesthesia

The main evidence motivating local cross-activation as the mechanism underlying synesthesia has come from studies demonstrating higher accuracy or quicker response times in visual search tasks as a result of inducer pop-out effects. Synesthetes must experience inducers as having synesthetic colors prior to explicitly identifying them in order for them to have a pop-out effect (Treisman, 1982). So the initial results of visual search tasks suggested that synesthetic experience was the result of a preattentive bottom-up binding of inducer and concurrent and hence was an early-perceptual phenomenon (Ramachandran and Hubbard, 2001a, 2001b; Hubbard et al., 2005c; Rich and Karstoft, 2013) (see Figure 6.1).

The pop-out effects in grapheme-color synesthesia, however, have been questioned. Cytowic and Eagleman (2009) argue that the observed pop-out effects may not be due to preattentive bottom-up binding. Instead, when synesthetes pay attention to a grapheme during a visual search, the post-attentive synesthetic color experience may enhance their memory of the location of identified graphemes. The combined effect of the post-attentive synesthetic experiences of color-inducing graphemes organized in a particular pattern may be felt as the pop-out of a shape. Other research has supported the hypothesis that scan efficiency plays a role in synesthetes' increased response time in visual search tasks. One study found that increasing the number of elements in a matrix gives rise to a corresponding increase in reaction time for synesthetes (Palmeri et al., 2002). If true color-based pop-out is occurring in synesthetes' searches, then the target color-inducing graphemes should capture attention at the same rate regardless of the number of achromatic distractors in an array. However, the observed increase in reaction time when there is a greater number of elements in a display matrix is indicative of a limitation on the speed by which graphemes may be processed after selective attention, supporting the hypothesis that synesthetic experience may only make visual searches more efficient.

Other studies indicate that synesthetes may not be more efficient than controls in visual search tasks (Edquist et al., 2006; Rothen and Meier, 2009; Gheri et al., 2008; Ward et al., 2010). Edquist et al. (2006), for example, conducted a study involving

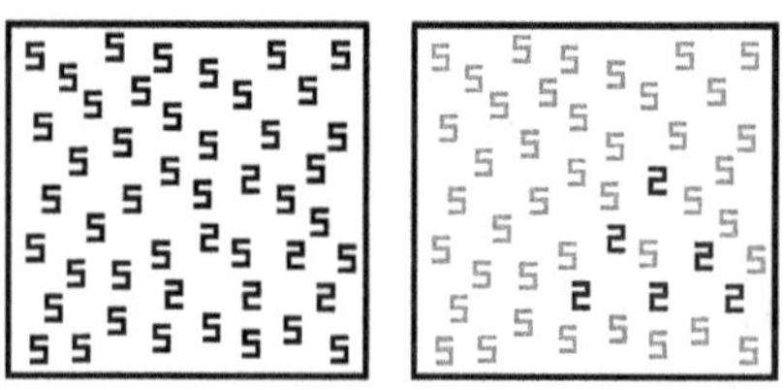

Figure 6.1. When normal subjects are presented with the figure on the left, it takes them several seconds to identify the hidden shape. Some grapheme-color synesthetes instantly see the triangular shape because they experience the 2s and the 5s as having different colors. See e.g. Rich and Karstoft (2013).

fourteen grapheme-color synesthetes and fourteen controls completing visual search tasks. The targets had a unique display color (e.g., red targets against a background of black distractors) in some trials. In other trials the targets were specifically chosen to induce colors in the synesthetes. Synesthetes and controls identified the targets equally efficiently when the target had a unique display color, but the two groups were equally inefficient when the target induced a synesthetic color. This study indicates that synesthetic experiences do not occur as a result of preattentive bottom-up perceptual mechanisms but, like higher-level perceptual phenomena, depend on selective attention. More recently, Ward et al. (2010) conducted a revised version of the Ramachandran and Hubbard (2001a, 2001b) and Hubbard and Ramachadran (2005) studies: in addition to the tasks included in the former studies, subjects were asked to report on their experiences of synesthetic colors after completing each task. Synesthetes scored higher than controls on visual search tasks, confirming the results of the former studies. However, the reported instances of synesthetic color experience did not correlate with the number of synesthetic inducers displayed to synesthetic participants, suggesting a disconnect between synesthetic phenomenology and task performance. The authors concluded that the better performance of synesthetes could not be due to cues provided by pre-attentively bound synesthetic color experience. Though there is still extensive debate about pop-out effects and search efficiency in grapheme-color synesthesia, the combined results of recent research indicate that the mechanisms underlying synesthesia need not merely involve local cross-activation.

Studies of cross-modal illusions also provide some evidence against the early-sensory models of synesthesia. Bargary et al. (2009) studied the effect of the McGurk illusion on synesthetic experience. The McGurk illusion occurs when one sound is played while a person is shown uttering a different sound. For example, the speaker is mouthing the word /ba-ba/ while the audio is dubbed as /ga-ga/. What you end up hearing is /da-da/. The researchers tested the reactions of nine word-color synesthetes to a version of the McGurk illusion. The auditory stimuli were recordings of words such as /bay/, /cup/, and /cap/. The visual inputs were recordings of a person mouthing words such as /gay/, /con/, and /can/. When the auditory and visual stimuli are played simultaneously, subjects will normally hear entirely different words, for example /day/, /cot/, and /cat/. The participants were presented with three videos: one in which the visuals were scrambled, so only the audio could be perceived, a second in which the sound was off, so only the visual could be perceived, and one where the audio and the visual were played simultaneously. After seeing the videos, the synesthetes clicked on a color in a large color array on a separate monitor. The researchers found that the synesthetes experienced significantly different colors depending on whether the McGurk illusion was present. For example, they would experience one color when hearing the word /bay/ in the scrambled video, a second color when seeing someone mouth the word /gay/ in the video with the sound off, and a third color when exposed to the combined output normally giving rise to a perception of the word /day/. As the McGurk effect results from integrating inputs from multiple senses, it is believed to occur relatively late in the perceptual process. Because the illusions affected the color experienced by the synesthetes, this provides some evidence that synesthetic experience is driven by late, multi-perceptual processing, rather than early, unisensory processing, although additive or interacting effects could not be ruled out on the basis of the study.

A different type of factor that counts against the early-perceptual models of synesthesia is the lack of complete idiosyncrasy in inducer-concurrent associations in grapheme-color synesthesia. There is greater agreement on letter-color associations among grapheme-color synesthetes than would be expected by chance (Rich and Mattingley, 2002; Simner et al., 2005). Letter shape, grapheme frequency, and color names can explain a good deal of these patterns. Brang and Ramachandran (2011) observed that graphemes that have similar shapes tend to elicit the same concurrents in grapheme-color synesthetes. Simner et al. (2005) found that frequently occurring letters tend to have common colors such as red, blue, and yellow, whereas less frequently occurring letters have more unusual colors such as purple or brown. They also found that letters more often give rise to a concurrent whose expression in English starts with that letter than expected by chance. Beeli et al. (2007) found inverse correlations between grapheme frequency and saturation and lightness in color space. Less frequent letters tend to be darker and less saturated than more frequent letters. While the shape-concurrent correlations observed by Brang and Ramachandran (2011) are consistent with the theory that grapheme-color binding occurs via interactions between color and shape areas in feedforward preattentive mechanisms, the findings showing correlations between letter frequency and color or colors and color names count against this possibility as a general explanatory mechanism.

Recent testing of patterns in grapheme-color binding suggests that synesthetic binding may be partially facilitated by semantic memory of graphemes and their colors. Witthoft and Winawer (2013) matched the data from eleven grapheme-color synesthetes who had completed the Synesthesia Battery. Ten of the eleven subjects reported having owned one of three sets of refrigerator magnets with the same color scheme sold by Fisher-Price between 1972 and 1989. The researchers found a remarkable similarity of letter-color associations among the synesthetes. The fewest matches among the synesthetes was fourteen letters. The probability of finding fourteen or more letter matches in twenty-six chances is less than one in 1 billion, which strongly supports the hypothesis that the subjects acquired their letter-color associations from the Fisher-Price toys. One possible alternative explanation is that the Fisher-Price associations are the same as generic grapheme-color associations that one is exposed to in daily life (e.g., A=red, B=blue), so the Fisher-Price associations did not directly shape the synesthetic associations, which were instead shaped by other environmental constraints that overlapped with the Fisher-Price associations. This possibility, however, seems unlikely, as the Fisher-Price associations do not appear to be particularly generic. Furthermore, if this were the case, then the synesthetic connections would still be the result of learned associations.

Witthoft and Winawer's results thus suggest that learning and memory may be involved in at least some instances of grapheme-color synesthesia.

While learning and memory may be implicated in synesthetic binding, attempts to train normal subjects to become synesthetes indicate that mere exposure to grapheme-color connections is not sufficient for inducing synesthesia. Several researchers have shown that training non-synesthetes can induce Stroop interference of the kind seen in synesthesia (Colizoli et al., 2012; Nunn et al., 2002; Meier and Rothen, 2009; Proulx, 2010). A Stroop effect is a reaction time interference in perceptual tasks (Stroop, 1935). The most common Stroop task demonstrates that neurotypical individuals take significantly longer to name the color in which a color word is printed if the color referred to by the word is incongruent with the printed color (MacLeod, 1991). The Stroop effect has also been found in grapheme-color synesthesia. Synesthetes can name the printed color of a grapheme much faster if the synesthetic color induced by the grapheme is congruent with the printed color (Mills et al., 1999; O'dgaard et al., 1999; Mattingley et al., 2001, 2006; Wollen and Ruggiero, 1983).

Although neurotypical controls trained to make semantic memory connections that mirror synesthetic connections are also subject to Stroop interference, this does not show that the trainees have acquired genuine synesthesia, as over-learned associations produce a Stroop effect. Neuroimaging also indicates a difference between synesthetes and trainees. Nunn et al. (2002) trained twenty-eight non-synesthetes to associate words and colors and measured brain activation using functional magnetic resonance imaging (fMRI). The non-synesthetes developed a condition similar to synesthesia but the trainees didn't have the same brain activation patterns as the synesthetes they were trained to mirror. This points to Stroop interference in the training cases as an indicator, not of synesthesia, but of semantic memory connections that are tightly interwoven and automatic. This, of course, does not *imply* that Stroop interference in cases of genuine synesthesia is also an indicator of semantic memory connections. First, the training studies typically do not produce congruency effects of a similar magnitude to those found in synesthesia. Second, projectors display larger congruency effects than associators (Dixon et al., 2004). So, there may well be different sources of congruency effects, and congruency effects may not reflect semantic associations in synesthetes. But the training studies show that congruency effects can be the result of semantic memory associations in synesthesia-like conditions. So, we do not necessarily need something beyond semantic memory connections to explain them. Together, the results of recent research indicate that synesthesia may not always be an early-perceptual phenomenon but could in some cases be a type of late, perceptual processing that involves semantic memory and reinstatement of activity in sensory areas.

6.3 The reactivation model of memory

Memory has traditionally been thought to be a result of higher cognitive functions. On an older conception of memory, short-term maintenance as well as the storage of semantic information and personal episodes involve the transfer of relevant stimulus representations to one or more dedicated storage regions in prefrontal/parietal cortices or hippocampus (Baddeley, 1992). Actively maintained or stored neural representations of stimuli were thought to be distinct from those encoded during sensory perception or proprioception. As synesthesia has a perceptual phenomenology and has been associated with neural activity in sensory areas of the brain (Nunn et al., 2002; Sperling et al., 2006; Paulesu et al., 1995; Elias et al., 2003), this older picture of memory makes it unlikely that semantic memory connections ever underlie genuine synesthesia.

Recent studies of memory, however, have found that the contents of our memories and the processes involved in the formation, storage, and retrieval of these memories are distributed across a wide range of neural assemblies in the brain that were active during encoding (e.g., Fuster, 2009; Eichenbaum and Cohen, 2001; Jonides et al., 2008, Martin and Chao, 2001; McClelland and Rogers, 2003; Schacter et al., 2007; Simons and Spiers, 2003; Danker and Anderson, 2010). Working memory maintains behaviorally relevant representations of stimuli that were just experienced or retrieved over short time intervals (Rissman and Wagner, 2012). According to a model of working memory that has been dubbed 'the sensory recruitment model' (Serences et al., 2009), working memory does not engage special working-memory neural ensembles but involves a maintenance of brain regions that were just activated. Neural regions in the prefrontal cortex execute this maintenance of activity via top-down modulatory control (D'Esposito, 2007; Postle, 2006; Fuster, 2009; Gazzaley et al., 2004). Top-down attentional processes also facilitate the generation and maintenance of mental images. Mental imagery activates many of the cortical regions associated with sensory perception (Kosslyn, 2005; Stokes et al., 2009, 2011). One of the main differences between sensory perception and stimulus maintenance turns on the lateralization of the activity. During initial stimulus processing from one eye, only contralateral visual areas are implicated. During the activity maintenance that is crucial to working memory, however, both hemispheres may be implicated. This strongly suggests that stimulus maintenance in short-term memory goes beyond the retinotopic representation of the stimulus.

There is also solid evidence that long-term storage of episodic memories involves the formation of neural networks in distributed neural assemblies that were originally activated during a given episode (Kahn et al., 2004; Polyn et al., 2005; Danker and Anderson, 2010; Rissman and Wagner, 2012). The brain regions associated with long-term memory are widely distributed, extending from sensory cortical areas to prefrontal cortex. Memory retrieval and recollection-based recognition involve a reactivation of these brain regions through coordination processes in the hippocampus. The process of retrieval begins with a reactivation of neural pathways associated with features of the event. These features are then contextualized by reinstating neural assemblies associated with contextual information. Which aspects of an event are retrieved will depend on attentional processes that can render one aspect of the event more relevant than others.

Reactivation of neural assemblies engaged during initial stimulus processing also occurs during familiarity-based recognition and recollection-based recognition involved in semantic memory (Brown and Aggleton, 2001; Gonsalves et al., 2005; Norman and O'Reilly, 2003; Yonelinas et al., 2005; Johnson et al., 2009; Chang et al., 2011). Whereas recollection-based recognition depends on pattern completion, familiarity-based recognition depends on pattern matching between retrieval cues and stored representations. Semantic memory of stimuli from discrete visual object categories, such as faces, houses, and chairs, may be more likely to be associated with specific cortical regions, viz., ventral temporal cortex (Aguirre et al., 1998; Epstein and Kanwisher, 1998; Kanwisher et al., 1997). But even memories of specific object categories are not highly modular. Most memory content is distributed across larger neural areas, and the brain regions encoding the contents of distinct memories may be overlapping (Haxby et al., 2001; Ishai et al., 1999, 2000). Memory of stimuli from discrete visual object categories, such as faces, houses, and chairs, is stored in a distributed pattern involving a weighing of features. The distributed activation pattern that reflects the mean feature weightings for stimuli from the category is also sometimes called a 'neural signature' (Rissman and Wagner, 2012; Haxby et al., 2001). Each category has its own neural signature insofar as exemplars within a category share more features with each other than they do with exemplars from different categories. So, even if the brain regions associated with memories of stimuli from, say, chairs and tables overlap, the memories of stimuli from the two object categories will have distinct neural signatures (Williams et al., 2007; Haushofer et al., 2008; Weber et al., 2009; Walther et al., 2009; Hsieh et al., 2010; Nyberg et al., 2000; Wheeler et al., 2000).

Together, the results of recent studies of memory strongly indicate that short-term memory maintenance as well as the retrieval of long-term episodic and semantic information involve a reinstatement of activity in brain regions initially activated during stimulus processing. Sensory perception and memory retrieval are thus not entirely distinct phenomena at the neurological level, even though there is a clear difference in phenomenology between the events of perceiving and remembering.

6.4 The memory model of synesthesia

The available evidence that suggests that semantic memory may play a role in synesthesia can be explained on the hypothesis that some forms of synesthetic experience are a kind of recollection-based recognition, which involves the hippocampus as an organizational unit. The hippocampus and its subregions are thought to be involved in relational information processing, including association between arbitrary stimuli (Eichenbaum and Cohen, 2001; Squire et al., 2004; Brown and Aggleton, 2001). Both the hippocampus and the inferior frontal gyrus (IFG) are critical for the retrieval of newly formed memories, whereas the hippocampus is believed to be less crucial for the retrieval of memories formed many years prior to current processing (Rissman and Wagner, 2012). If synesthesia is a kind of recollection-based recognition, then the hippocampus would be involved in encoding the inducer and the concurrent in a distributed neural network. The perception or thought of an inducer would trigger reinstated activity in the neural region that encoded the inducer via the IFG and the hippocampus. This would lead to the additional reinstantiation of activity in the associated neural region encoding the concurrent. For example, in the case of grapheme-color synesthesia, the hippocampus would bind together neural networks in visual form and color areas during the learning process. Once a strong association has been formed, exposure to achromatic grapheme-stimuli would trigger recognition of the grapheme *as* a particular grapheme (e.g., the numeral '3') and memory retrieval of synesthetic color (e.g., a particular shade of green). Retrieval of synesthetic color would involve reinstated neural activity in the color areas via the IFG and the hippocampus, yielding a synesthetic experience.

Although this scenario seems plausible in some cases of synesthesia, it cannot be the full explanation of how synesthesia develops and persists over time. There are no doubt ordinary memory associations that manifest the automaticity, specificity, and consistency commonly associated with synesthesia. For example, a particular smell may consistently lead to the automatic retrieval of a percept of a particular face. But even if ordinary memory associations sometimes manifest these characteristics, typical cases of synesthesia have a unique phenomenology and tend to involve a wide range of inducer-concurrent pairings. In grapheme-color synesthesia, for example, all numbers or letters tend to be associated with a specific color, and the experience is often distinctly perceptual in nature. Moreover, the hypothesis that memory associations may underlie synesthesia does not help us answer the questions of why only some people develop synesthesia and why only some synesthetes experience projections of concurrents. While specific episodes in a child's life, for example playing with refrigerator magnets, may contribute to the development of synesthesia, the inheritability of synesthesia makes it unlikely that specific episodes in early life are the only factor.

In all likelihood there are a multiplicity of factors involved in developing synesthesia. One may be increased sensitivity in neural regions that process the synesthetic concurrent. One type of research supporting this explanation has looked at the abilities of synesthetes to process stimuli that trigger their concurrent experiences without themselves triggering synesthesia. Yaro and Ward (2007) showed that in spite of the unidirectionality of grapheme-color synesthesia, grapheme-color synesthetes show superior perceptual discrimination of color compared to non-synesthetes. Banissy et al. (2009) looked at tactile and color discrimination in three groups of synesthetes with mirror-touch synesthesia and/or color synesthesia and a group of non-synesthetes. To test for discrimination, they subjected the participants to color and tactile discrimination tests using the Farnsworth–Munsell Colour Hue Test and the Gratings Orientation Test. They found that color synesthetes have enhanced color sensitivity, whereas synesthetes who experience touch have enhanced tactile sensitivity. A related kind of increased sensitivity was found in a recent study conducted by Terhune et al. (2011). The team looked at whether grapheme-color synesthesia involves increased cortical excitability in primary visual cortex. Using transcranial magnetic stimulation to stimulate primary visual cortex, a technique known to induce phosphenes spanning the visual field of normal subjects, they found that synesthetes experience phosphenes at a three-fold lower phosphene threshold compared to controls. They further showed that synesthetic experiences can be enhanced magnetically, indicating that the hyperexcitability of primary visual cortex in synesthetes helps strengthen neural activation in the primary visual cortex, thereby reaching the threshold of consciousness. The hypothesis that synesthetes may have increased neural sensitivity was corroborated more recently by findings of Arnold et al. (2012) and Terhune et al. (2013), both showing superior color processing (working memory in the latter) among synesthetes (see also Rothen et al., 2012). These results suggest that synesthetes have an increased sensitivity in neural regions that process the concurrent experiences.

Together with the reactivation model, these results indicate that whether a person develops synesthesia as a result of learning and memory and whether the synesthesia is of the projector or the associator type may depend on the degrees of hyperexcitability and reactivation of neurons in the primary visual cortex (or other sensory areas). Synesthetes may exhibit more hyperexcitability and reactivation of neural assemblies in visual areas than non-synesthetes, and projectors may exhibit more hyperexcitability and reactivation than associators. The increased color sensitivity found in synesthesia can also explain why synesthetic connections are not phenomenally on a par with ordinary memory retrieval.

The cognitive benefits of multisensory binding may be a further reason that some synesthetes develop memory associations that are more tightly interwoven and more perceptual than normal memory associations. Psychophysical studies of multisensory perception suggest that the integration of stimuli presented in different sensory modalities provides complementary information, leading to improved immediate performance (Doehrmann and Naumer, 2008). Laurienti et al. (2004), for example, found quicker response times for congruent audio and visual stimuli compared to unimodal stimulation but there was no improvement when the congruent stimuli were both visual. The response time for incongruent stimulations was significantly slower in both multisensory and intra-modal contexts. The integration of stimuli from different sensory modalities can also lead to enhanced memory performance over time. Murray et al. (2004) found that subjects had enhanced recognition abilities when shown repeated line drawings of common objects that were initially accompanied by semantically congruent sounds in comparison to an initial presentation of semantically incongruent sounds, sounds with no semantic content, or no sound.

On the basis of these considerations it is plausible to think that tightly interwoven, multisensory synesthetic connections prove to be particularly advantageous, both early on in learning processes involving the inducer and later on in memory retrievals involving inducer, concurrent, or both. While features associated in synesthetic binding may seem incongruent to normal individuals, synesthetes generally perceive the bound features as highly congruent. So, it is plausible that synesthetic binding could lead to improved immediate or long-term cognitive performance. This hypothesis has been validated by several recent studies (see Rothen et al., 2012 for a review). Smilek et al. (2002) presented a grapheme-color synesthete with a random selection of letters which were either randomly colored or colored in a manner consistent with their synesthesia and asked the subject to remember the letter selection. They subsequently tested the subject's recall of the letter selections and found that the selections that were consistent with the synesthesia were more accurately retrieved. Jarick et al. (2009) tested the experiences of a time-space synesthete L, who experiences the time of day and the months of the year as located in an imaginary space around her body in an order that depends on the particular perspective she takes in that space. Subject L and controls were exposed to a spatial cueing paradigm in which a visual month cue was presented to the subject followed by a square to the left or right. As subject L perceives some of the months to the left in her mental space and some to the right, the researchers predicted that the visual month cues would cause her to pay special attention to the left or right of the cue and would lead to a faster detection of squares in the regions she attends to compared to controls. These predictions were confirmed. Simner et al. (2009) further compared the performance of ten time-space synesthetes on eight memory tasks to controls. Tasks included tests of semantic and episodic retrieval of the dates of various events, non-verbal visual short-term memory, the manipulation and rotation of objects in three-dimensional space, and the recognition of 3D objects from 2D silhouettes. The synesthetes outperformed the non-synesthetes on all eight memory tasks.

The observation that synesthesia provides enhanced discriminatory abilities with respect to concurrent-related stimuli as well as superior performance on memory tasks points to enhanced cognition as a further factor in explaining why some people develop synesthetic connections. Though this factor is likely to play a greater role in explaining how the synesthesia gene has survived the obstacles of evolution (Brang and Ramachandran, 2011), it may also yield insight into the mystery of why particularly tightly interwoven memory associations are actually formed in people with the genetic disposition.

The hypothesis that semantic memory may underlie synesthetic binding is consistent with a type of feedback mechanism. However, memory mechanisms must be distinguished from standard cross-activation mechanisms and disinhibited feedback mechanisms. Enhanced anatomical connectivity near the fusiform gyrus confirming a feedforward mechanism has been reported for grapheme-color synesthesia (Rouw and Scholte, 2007; Jancke et al., 2009; Hanggi et al., 2011) and sound-color synesthesia (Zamm et al., 2013). Other evidence from psychophysical and neuroimaging studies favors a disinhibited feedback mechanism (Grossenbacher and Lovelace, 2001;

Dixon et al., 2006; Esterman et al., 2006; Neufeld et al., 2012). A recent imaging study of fourteen auditory-visual synesthetes, for example, found increased functional connectivity of the left inferior parietal cortex with the left primary auditory and right primary visual cortex (Neufeld et al., 2012), suggesting that synesthesia is the result of aberrant synesthetic binding in the parietal cortex and increased activation in sensory areas.

Although all models of synesthesia posit direct or indirect neural connections between sensory regions, the cross-activation and disinhibited feedback models predict that these connections are not mediated by the hippocampus or the IFG. Evidence of increased hippocampal activity in synesthetes at an early age would thus count in favor of a memory model of synesthesia. As the hippocampus may not be as critical for the retrieval of older memories, hippocampal activation may be less prominent in older synesthetes. Another piece of evidence that may point to a memory mechanism would be the persistence of synesthesia in individuals with a dysfunctional hippocampus, as a result of injury or disease. If the synesthesia persists in an unaltered form following hippocampal defects in younger individuals, that would be evidence against a memory mechanism. If injury or disease involving the hippocampus were to significantly alter or block the synesthesia, that would be evidence in favor of a memory mechanism, provided that other brain regions are not directly affected by the lesions.

6.5 Synesthesia as a model of multisensory perception

Though synesthesia is characterized as a blending of sensory or cognitive streams (perhaps within the same sensory modality), synesthesia is different from online interaction between different sensory modalities. Multisensory binding of incoming signals from different sensory channels occurs spontaneously when the spatial and temporal attributes of the signals match. For example, in the absence of evidence to the contrary, the brain assumes that simultaneous signals come from the same source (Stein and Meredith, 1993). This spontaneous, temporary binding of signals can be overridden if the semantic contents of the (largely) unimodal signals do not match relative to the individual's learning history, for example if you are viewing a cat but hearing the sound of a dog (Doehrmann and Naumer, 2008). Both high-level sensory integration and low-level, spontaneous integration consist in the binding of two incoming sensory stimuli. In synesthesia, a unimodal sensory or cognitive input triggers a concurrent experience, which makes synesthetic binding different from multisensory integration.

However, several authors have proposed that other forms of multisensory perception involving common mapping patterns are examples of synesthetic experience that is common to all of us (Bien et al., 2012; Martino and Marks, 2001). Bien et al. (2012) argue that the presence of a mental number line, a spatial distribution of small and large numerical values across horizontal mental space, could be considered a very common form of synesthesia. Mondloch and Maurer (2004) report on a study in which children consistently attribute a high-pitched tone to a small-sized or light-colored ball, which might be attributable to a synesthetic connection between high pitch and small size/light colors. Stevenson and Boakes (2004) point to the case of taste perception induced by odor as an example of widespread synesthesia. And Auvray and Spence (2008) consider, but ultimately reject, the idea that flavor perception (particularly sweetness enhancement) is a synesthetic experience induced by smell and taste (and perhaps by visual stimuli).

Regardless of how we decide on the categorical relationship between synesthesia and common mapping patterns across sensory modalities or pathways, the mechanisms underlying synesthesia and certain types of multisensory phenomena no doubt overlap considerably. As synesthesia offers the possibility of strict control of inducer and concurrent and it shares aspects of its mechanism with certain multisensory phenomena, synesthesia may be a good model in which to study these types of multisensory phenomena.

One less frequently discussed type of multisensory perception that may be anchored in mechanisms similar to those underlying synesthesia is auditory object recognition that proceeds via the interpretation of indexical sounds. Unlike symbolic sounds (e.g., words and narrative music), indexical sounds—when accurately interpreted—have meanings that are causally connected to the sound source, for example the sounds a dog makes when it is barking. The meaning of indexical sounds consists of low-level and high-level auditory features. Attributes such as pitch, spectral shape (pattern of amplitudes), temporal quality (continuous, oscillating, discrete serial units), transitions, on- and offset, and rhythm are examples of low-level auditory properties, whereas a dog barking, a ball bouncing, water dripping, your colleague passing by the office door, and the secretary getting ready to put on a fresh pot of coffee are examples of high-level auditory features.

Perceivers make use of memory associations between acoustic signals and the acoustic effects of the physical properties of objects on sound production to identify auditory objects from acoustic signals. Evidence from imaging studies suggests that retrieving information about the acoustic effects of the physical properties of objects on sound production involves reinstated neural activity in visual areas. Several studies have shown functional activation of visual areas by auditory stimulation in the blind (Buchel et al., 1998; Weeks et al., 2000; Arno et al., 2001; Roder et al., 2002; Gougoux et al., 2005; Burton and McLaren, 2006; Garg et al., 2007; Voss et al., 2008). Although auditory occipital activation has been absent in a vast number of neuroimaging studies of audition in sighted individuals, activation of visual areas has been observed in numerous brain imaging studies, including studies of music discrimination (Platel et al., 1997; Janata et al., 2002), word perception (Specht and Reul, 2003), sentence interpretation (Von Kriegstein et al., 2003), auditory sound discrimination (Eisenberg et al., 2005; Maeder et al., 2001), and auditory spatial attention (Wu et al., 2007). Cate et al. (2009) found that auditory occipital activation occurs only when auditory stimuli are attended to in the active discrimination of sounds. The magnitude of occipital activation does not depend on sound frequency or location but may reflect the meaning content of the sound. Because acoustic signals lead to visual representations in the perception of attended sounds, perception of attended sounds is thus multisensory, involving both the auditory and the occipital cortex. Although the phenomenologies of the conditions are very different, the cross-modal interactions in the perception of attended sounds are likely mechanistically akin to the cross-modal interactions found in some cases of synesthesia.

Another, related, multisensory phenomenon is language perception. The perception of language involves sound- or grapheme-imagery associations, either arbitrary associations or patterns unique to the individual. Language perception is thus associated with interactions between two sensory streams, e.g. the auditory and visual systems. Recent neuroimaging studies confirm the multisensory nature of language perception (for a review see Willems and Casasanto, 2011). Action-related sentences which describe actions with different effectors, such as *I grasp the knife*, *I bite an apple*, and *I kick the ball*, activate the premotor cortex in an effector-specific manner (Willems et al., 2010; Aziz-Zadeh et al., 2006; Tettamanti et al., 2005). Action-related nouns and verbs, such as *bookend*, *clock*, *door*, *cup*, and *hammer*, also activate premotor and inferior parietal areas, and the amount of action associated with an object word is reflected in the activation of the motor system during word reading (Rueschemeyer et al., 2010). Bookends, clocks, doors, cups, and hammers differ in how much action is needed to use the object effectively. Objects like hammers and cups that need active manipulation give rise to higher levels of activation than objects like bookends and clocks that can be used without actively manipulating them. Similar observations have been made for action verbs, such as *kick*, *jump*, and *run* (see Kemmerer and Gonzalez-Castillo, 2008 for discussion), and action sentences, such as *the wild horse crossed the barren field* (Saygin et al., 2010).

Language perception has also been linked to reinstated activity in perceptual areas. For example, object words followed by a word for a feature that typically belongs to the object are associated with reinstated activity in the neural region that would process the feature when it's perceived through a sensory modality (Simmons et al., 2007; Beauchamp and Martin, 2007). For example, if *cucumber* were followed by *green*, it would give rise to increased activation in extrastriate color areas compared to *blue*. Aziz-Zadeh et al. (2008) found that listening to sentences describing faces (e.g., *The girl has freckles on her cheeks*) or places (e.g., *The house has a futon near the fireplace*) reinstates activity in the fusiform face area and the parahippocampal place area.

These data indicating that perceptual and cortical motor systems can be selectively activated during auditory object recognition and language perception suggest that these types of perception may be multisensory in the same way as synesthetic experience involving semantic memory. All three phenomena are associated with the reinstatement of neural activity in separate cognitive or sensory pathways.

6.6 Conclusion

I have argued that a broad range of studies of developmental synesthesia indicate that the mechanism underlying the phenomenon may in some cases involve semantic memory associations. This idea may seem implausible if memory is thought of as a conceptual phenomenon entirely distinct from perception. Recent research on memory, however, suggests that the maintenance of working memory and the retrieval of semantic and episodic memory involve the reinstatement of neural processes in sensory (or other) areas originally activated in perceptual processes. The findings suggest that memory could have a perceptual phenomenology and neural activation profile very similar to those found in synesthesia. When the results from synesthesia research and studies of memory are put side by side, it becomes apparent that synesthetic connections may in some cases be a special case of common mapping patterns. The main difference between ordinary mapping patterns and synesthetic associations might consist simply in the tightness and stability of the association as well as the sensitivity of sensory neurons that process the concurrent. The suggestion that some cases of synesthesia are best understood as tightly interwoven semantic memory associations makes the phenomenon particularly suitable as a model of the types of multisensory perception that likewise consist in common mapping patterns.[1]

References

Afra P, Funke M, Matuso F (2009). Acquired auditory–visual synesthesia: a window to early cross-modal sensory interactions. *Psychol. Res. Behav. Manag.* 2: 31–7. doi: 10.2147/PRBM.S4481.

Aguirre GK, Zarahn E, D'Esposito M (1998). An area within human ventral cortex sensitive to "building" stimuli: evidence and implications. *Neuron* 21: 373–83.

Arno P, De Volder AG, Vanlierde A, Wanet-Defalque MC, Streel E, et al. (2001). Occipital activation by pattern recognition in the early blind using auditory substitution for vision. *Neuroimage* 13: 632–45.

Arnold DH, Wegener SV, Brown F, Mattingley JB (2012). Precision of synaesthetic colour matching resembles that for recollected colours rather than physical colours. *Journal of Experimental Psychology: Human Perception and Performance* 38: 1078–84.

Auvray, M, Spence C (2008). The multisensory perception of flavor. *Consciousness and Cognition* 17: 1016–31.

Aziz-Zadeh L, Fiebach CJ, Naranayan S, Feldman J, Dodge E, Ivry RB (2008). Modulation of the FFA and PPA by language related to faces and places. *Soc. Neurosci.* 3: 229–38.

Aziz-Zadeh L, Wilson SM, Rizzolatti G, Iacoboni M (2006). Congruent embodied representations for visually presented actions and linguistic phrases describing actions. *Curr. Biol.* 16: 1818–23.

Baddeley A (1992). Working memory. *Science* 255: 556–9.

[1] I am grateful to an anonymous reviewer for helpful comments on a previous version of this chapter.

Banissy MJ, Walsh V, Ward J (2009). Enhanced sensory perception in synaesthesia. *Experimental Brain Research* 196(4): 565–71.

Bargary G, Barnett KJ, Mitchell KJ, Newell FN (2009). Colored-speech synaesthesia is triggered by multisensory, not unisensory, perception. *Psychological Science* 20(5): 529–33.

Baron-Cohen S, Wyke M, Binnie C (1987). Hearing words and seeing colors: an experimental investigation of synesthesia. *Perception* 16: 761–7. doi: 10.1068/p160761.

Baron-Cohen S, Burt L, Smith-Laittan F, Harrison J, Bolton P (1996). Synaesthesia: prevalence and familiality. *Perception* 25: 1073–9.

Baron-Cohen S, Harrison J (eds) (1997). *Synaesthesia: Classic and Contemporary Readings*. Oxford: Blackwell.

Beauchamp MS, Martin A (2007). Grounding object concepts in perception and action: evidence from fMRI studies of tools. *Cortex* 43: 461–8.

Beauchamp MS, Ro T (2008). Neural substrates of sound-touch synesthesia after a thalamic lesion. *Journal of Neuroscience* 28: 13696–702.

Beeli G, Esslen M, Jancke L (2007). Frequency correlates in grapheme–color synaesthesia. *Psychol. Sci.* 18: 5.

Bertelson P (1999). Ventriloquism: a case of crossmodal perceptual grouping. In G Ashersleben, T Bachmann, J Müsseler (Eds.), *Cognitive Contributions to the Perception of Spatial and Temporal Events* (pp. 347–62). Amsterdam: Elsevier Science, B.V.

Bien N, ten Oever S, Goebel R, Sack AT (2012). The sound of size: crossmodal binding in pitch-size synesthesia: a combined TMS, EEG and psychophysics study. *Neuroimage* 2, 59(1): 663–72.

Blake R, Palmeri, TJ, Marois R, Kim C-Y (2005). On the perceptual reality of synesthetic color. In LC Robertson, N. Sagiv (Eds.), *Synesthesia: Perspectives from Cognitive Neuroscience* (pp. 47–73). New York: Oxford University Press.

Bor D, Billington J, Baron-Cohen S (2007). Savant memory for digits in a case of synaesthesia and Asperger syndrome is related to hyperactivity in the lateral prefrontal cortex. *Neurocase* 13: 311–19.

Brang D, Ramachandran VS (2011). Survival of the synesthesia gene: why do people hear colors and taste words? *PLoS Biol* 9(11): e1001205.

Brogaard B (2011). Conscious vision for action vs. unconscious vision for action. *Cognitive Science* 35: 1076–104.

Brogaard B (2013). Serotonergic hyperactivity as a potential factor in developmental, acquired and drug-induced synesthesia, serotonergic hyperactivity as a potential factor in developmental, acquired and drug-induced synesthesia. *Front. Hum. Neurosci.* 7: 657. doi: 10.3389/fnhum.2013.00657.

Brogaard B, Vanni S, Silvanto J (2012). Seeing mathematics: perceptual experience and brain activity in acquired synesthesia. *Neurocase*. doi: 10.1080/13554794.2012.701646.

Brown MW, Aggleton JP (2001). Recognition memory: what are the roles of the perirhinal cortex and hippocampus? *Nat. Rev. Neurosci.* 2: 51–61.

Buchel C, Price C, Frackowiak RS, Friston K (1998). Different activation patterns in the visual cortex of late and congenitally blind subjects. *Brain* 121 (Pt 3): 409–19.

Burton H, McLaren DG (2006). Visual cortex activation in late-onset, Braille naive blind individuals: an fMRI study during semantic and phonological tasks with heard words. *Neurosci. Lett.* 392: 38–42.

Cate AD, Herron TJ, Yund EW, Stecker GC, Rinne T, Kang X, Petkov CI, Disbrow EA, Woods DL (2009). Auditory attention activates peripheral visual cortex. *PLoS One* 4: e4645.

Chang K-MK, Mitchell T, Just MA (2011). Quantitative modeling of the neural representation of objects: how semantic feature norms can account for fMRI activation. *NeuroImage* 56: 716–27.

Colizoli O, Murre JM, Rouw R (2012). Pseudo-synesthesia through reading books with colored letters. *PloS One* 7(6).

Cohen Kadosh R, Henik A, Catena A, Walsh V, Fuentes LJ (2009). Induced cross-modal synaesthetic experiences without abnormal neuronal connections. *Psychological Science* 20(2): 258–65.

Cytowic RE (1989). *Synesthesia: A Union of the Senses.* New York: Springer Verlag.

Cytowic RE (1997). Synesthesia: phenomenology and neuropsychology. In S. Baron-Cohen (Ed.), *Synesthesia: Classic and Contemporary Readings* (pp. 17–39). Oxford: Blackwell.

Cytowic RE, Eagleman DM (2009). *Wednesday is Indigo Blue.* Cambridge: MIT Press.

D'Esposito M (2007). From cognitive to neural models of working memory. *Philos. Trans. R. Soc. Lond. B Biol. Sci.* 362: 761–72.

Danker JF, Anderson JR (2010). The ghosts of brain states past: remembering reactivates the brain regions engaged during encoding. *Psychol. Bull.* 136: 87–102.

Deroy O, Spence C (2013). Why we are not all synaesthetes (not even weakly so). *Psychonomic Bulletin & Review* 20(4): 643–64.

Dixon MJ, Smilek D, Merikle PM (2004). Not all synaesthetes are created equal: projector versus associator synaesthetes. *Cogn. Affect. Behav. Neurosci.* 4: 335–43.

Dixon MJ, Smilek D, Duffy PL, Zanna MP, Merikle PM (2006). The role of meaning in grapheme-colour synaesthesia. *Cortex* 42: 243–52.

Doehrmann O, Naumer MJ (2008). Semantics and the multisensory brain: how meaning modulates processes of audio-visual integration. *Brain Research* 1242: 136–50.

Eagleman DM, Kagan AD, Nelson SS, Sagaram D, Sarma AK (2007). A standardized test battery for the study of Synesthesia. *Journal of Neuroscience Methods* 159: 139–45.

Edquist J, Rich AN, Brinkman C, Mattingley JB (2006). Do synaesthetic colours act as unique features in visual search? *Cortex* 42: 222–31.

Eichenbaum H, Cohen NJ (2001). *From Conditioning to Conscious Recollection: Memory Systems of the Brain.* New York: Oxford University Press.

Eisenberg DP, London ED, Matochik JA, Derbyshire S, Cohen LJ, et al. (2005). Education-associated cortical glucose metabolism during sustained attention. *Neuroreport* 16: 1473–6.

Elias LJ, Saucier DM, Hardie C, Sarty GE (2003). Dissociating semantic and perceptual components of synaesthesia: behavioural and functional neuroanatomical investigations. *Brain Research, Cognitive Brain Research* 16: 232–7.

Emrich HM, Schneider U, Zelder M (2002). *Welche Farbe hat der Montag? Synästhesie: Das Leben mit verknüpften Sinnen.* Stuttgart: Hirzel-Verlag.

Epstein R, Kanwisher N (1998). A cortical representation of the local visual environment. *Nature* 392: 598–601.

Esterman M, Verstynen T, Ivry RB, Robertson LC (2006). Coming unbound: disrupting automatic integration of synesthetic color and graphemes by transcranial magnetic stimulation of the right parietal lobe. *J. Cogn. Neurosci.* 18: 1570–6.

Fuster JM (2009). Cortex and memory: emergence of a new paradigm. *J. Cogn. Neurosci.* 21: 2047–72.

Garg A, Schwartz D, Stevens AA (2007). Orienting auditory spatial attention engages frontal eye fields and medial occipital cortex in congenitally blind humans. *Neuropsychologia* 45: 2307–21.

Gazzaley A, Rissman J, D'Esposito M (2004). Functional connectivity during working memory maintenance. *Cogn. Affect. Behav. Neurosci.* 4: 580–99.

Gheri C, Chopping S, Morgan MJ (2008). Synaesthetic colours do not camouflage form in visual search. *Proceedings of the Royal Society B*, 275: 841–6.

Gonsalves BD, Kahn I, Curran T, Norman KA, Wagner AD (2005). Memory strength and repetition suppression: multimodal imaging of medial temporal cortical contributions to recognition. *Neuron* 47: 751–61.

Goodale MA, Milner AD (1992). Separate visual pathways for perception and action. *Trends in Neurosciences* 15: 20–5.

Goodale MA, Milner AD, Jakobson LS, Carey DP (1991). A neurological dissociation between perceiving objects and grasping them. *Nature* 349: 154–6.

Gougoux F, Zatorre RJ, Lassonde M, Voss P, Lepore F (2005). A functional neuroimaging study of sound localization: visual cortex activity predicts performance in early-blind individuals. *PLoS Biol* 3: e27.

Grossenbacher PG, Lovelace CT (2001). Mechanisms of synesthesia: cognitive and physiological constraints. *Trends Cogn. Sci.* 5: 36–41.

Hancock P (2006). Monozygotic twins' colour-number association: a case study. *Cortex* 42: 147–50. doi: 10.1016/S0010- 9452(08)70338-1.

Hanggi J, Wotruba D, Jäncke L (2011). Globally altered structural brain network topology in grapheme-color synesthesia. *J. Neurosci.* 31: 5816–28 doi: 10.1523/JNEUROSCI.0964-10.2011.

Haushofer J, Livingstone MS, Kanwisher N (2008). Multivariate patterns in object-selective cortex dissociate perceptual and physical shape similarity. *PLoS Biol.* 6: e187.

Haxby JV, Gobbini MI, Furey ML, Ishai A, Schouten JL, Pietrini P (2001). Distributed and overlapping representations of faces and objects in ventral temporal cortex. *Science* 293: 2425–30.

Hsieh P-J, Vul E, Kanwisher N (2010). Recognition alters the spatial pattern of fMRI activation in early retinotopic cortex. *J. Neurophysiol.* 103: 1501–7.

Hubbard TL (1996). Synesthesia-like mappings of lightness, pitch, and melodic interval. *Am. J. Psychol.* 109: 219–38.

Hubbard EM, Ramachandran VS (2005). Neurocognitive mechanisms of synesthesia. *Neuron* 48(3): 509–20.

Hubbard EM, Arman AC, Ramachandran VS, Boynton GM (2005a). Individual differences among grapheme-color synesthetes: brain-behavior correlations. *Neuron* 45: 975–85.

Hubbard EM, Piazza M, Pinel P, Dehaene S (2005b). Interactions between number and space in parietal cortex. *Nat. Rev. Neurosci.* 6: 435–48.

Hubbard EM, Manohar S, Ramachandran VS (2005c). Contrast affects the strength of synesthetic colors. *Cortex* 184–94.

Hurlburt R, Schwitzgebel, E (2007). *Describing Inner Experience? Proponent Meets Skeptic.* Cambridge, MA: MIT Press.

Ishai A, Ungerleider LG, Martin A, Haxby JV (2000). The representation of objects in the human occipital and temporal cortex. *J. Cogn. Neurosci.* 12(Suppl. 2): 35–51.

Ishai A, Ungerleider LG, Martin A, Schouten JL, Haxby JV (1999). Distributed representation of objects in the human ventral visual pathway. *Proc. Natl. Acad. Sci. USA* 96: 9379–84.

Janata P, Tillmann B, Bharucha JJ (2002). Listening to polyphonic music recruits domain-general attention and working memory circuits. *Cogn Affect Behav Neurosci* 2: 121–40.

Jancke L, Beel, G, Eulig C, Hanggi J (2009). The neuroanatomy of grapheme-color synesthesia. *Eur. J. Neurosci.* 29: 1287–93. doi: 10.1111/j.1460-9568.2009.06673.x.

Jarick M, Dixona MJ, Stewart MT, Maxwell EC, Smilek D (2009). A different outlook on time: visual and auditory month names elicit different mental vantage points for a time-space synaesthete. *Cortex* 45: 1217–28.

Johnson JD, McDuff SGR, Rugg MD, Norman KA (2009). Recollection, familiarity, and cortical reinstatement: a multivoxel pattern analysis. *Neuron* 63: 697–708.

Jonides J, Lewis RL, Nee DE, Lustig CA, Berman MG, Moore KS (2008). The mind and brain of short-term memory. *Annu. Rev. Psychol.* 59: 193–224.

Kahn I, Davachi L, Wagner AD (2004). Functional-neuroanatomic correlates of recollection: implications for models of recognition memory. *J. Neurosci.* 24: 4172–80.

Kanwisher N, McDermott J, Chun MM (1997). The fusiform face area: a module in human extrastriate cortex specialized for face perception. *J. Neurosci.* 17: 4302–11.

Kemmerer D, Gonzalez-Castillo J (2008). The two-level theory of verb meaning: an approach to integrating the semantics of action with the mirror neuron system. *Brain Lang.* 112: 54–76.

Kosslyn SM (2005). Mental images and the brain. *Cogn. Neuropsychol.* 22: 333–47.

Laeng B, Svartdal F, Oelmann H (2004). Does color synesthesia pose a paradox for early-selection theories of attention?. *Psychological Science* 15: 277–81.

Laurienti PJ, Kraft RA, Maldjian JA, Burdette JH, Wallace MT (2004). Semantic congruence is a critical factor in multisensory behavioral performance. *Exp. Brain Res.* 158: 405–14.

MacLeod CM (1991). Half a century of research on the Stroop effect: an integrative review. *Psychology Bulletin* 109: 163–203.

Maeder PP, Meuli RA, Adriani M, Bellmann A, Fornari E, Thiran J-P et al. (2001). Distinct pathways involved in sound recognition and localization: a human fMRI study. *Neuroimage* 14: 802–16. doi: 10.1006/nimg.2001.0888.

Martin A, Chao LL (2001). Semantic memory and the brain: structure and processes. *Curr. Opin. Neurobiol.* 11: 194–201.

Martino G, Marks LE (2001). Synesthesia: strong and weak. *Curr. Dir. Psychol. Sci.* 10: 61.

Mattingley JB, Rich AN, Yelland G, Bradshaw JL (2001). Unconscious priming eliminates automatic binding of colour and alphanumeric form in synaesthesia. *Nature* 410: 580–2. doi: 10.1038/35069062.

Mattingley JB, Payne J, Rich AN (2006). Attentional load attenuates synaesthetic priming effects in grapheme-colour synaesthesia. *Cortex* 42: 213–21.

Mattingley JB, Rich AN (2004). Behavioural and brain correlates of multisensory experience in synaesthesia. In G Calvert, C Spence, B Stein (Eds.), *Handbook of Multisensory Integration.* Cambridge, MA: MIT Press.

McClelland JL, Rogers TT (2003). The parallel distributed processing approach to semantic cognition. *Nat. Rev. Neurosci.* 4: 310–22.

Meier B, Rothen N (2009). Training grapheme-colour associations produces a synaesthetic Stroop effect, but not a conditioned synaesthetic response. *Neuropsychologia* 47(4): 1208–11.

Mills CB, Boteler EH, Oliver GK (1999). Digit synaesthesia: a case study using a Stroop-type test. *Cognitive Neuropsychology* 16: 181–91.

Milner AD, Goodale MA (2008). Two visual systems reviewed. *Neuropsychologia* 46: 774–85.

Milner D, Goodale MA (1995). *The Visual Brain in Action*. Oxford: Oxford University Press.

Mondloch CJ, Maurer D (2004). Do small white balls squeak? Pitch-object correspondences in young children. *Cogn. Affect. Behav. Neurosci.* 4: 133–6.

Murray MM, Michel CM, Grave de Peralta R, Ortigue S, Brunet D, Gonzalez Andino S, Schnider A (2004). Rapid discrimination of visual and multisensory memories revealed by electrical neuroimaging. *NeuroImage* 21: 125–35.

Neufeld J, Sinke C, Zedler M, Dillo W, Emrich HM, Bleich S, et al. (2012). Disinhibited feedback as a cause of synesthesia: evidence from a functional connectivity study on auditory-visual synesthetes. *Neuropsychologia* 50: 1471–7.

Norman KA, O'Reilly RC (2003). Modeling hippocampal and neocortical contributions to recognition memory: a complementary-learning-systems approach. *Psychol. Rev.* 110: 611–46.

Nunn JA, Gregory LJ, Brammer M, Williams SCR, Parslow DM, et al. (2002). Functional magnetic resonance imaging of synesthesia: activation of V4/V8 by spoken words. *Nature Neuroscience* 5: 371–5.

Nyberg L, Habib R, McIntosh AR, Tulving E (2000). Reactivation of encoding-related brain activity during memory retrieval. *Proc. Natl. Acad. Sci. USA* 97: 11120–4.

O'dgaard EC, Flowers JH, Bradman HL (1999). An investigation of the cognitive and perceptual dynamics of a colour-digit synaesthete. *Perception* 28: 651–64.

Palmeri TJ, Blake R, et al. (2002). The perceptual reality of synesthetic colors. *Proceedings of the National Academy of Sciences USA* 99: 4127–31.

Paulesu E, Harrison J, Baron-Cohen S, Watson JD, Goldstein L, Heather J, Frackowiak RS, Frith CD (1995). The physiology of coloured hearing: a PET activation study of colour-word synaesthesia. *Brain* 118: 661–76.

Platel H, Price C, Baron JC, Wise R, Lambert J, et al. (1997). The structural components of music perception: A functional anatomical study. *Brain* 120 (Pt 2): 229–43.

Polyn SM, Natu VS, Cohen JD, Norman KA (2005). Category-specific cortical activity precedes retrieval during memory search. *Science* 310: 1963–6.

Postle BR (2006). Working memory as an emergent property of the mind and brain. *Neuroscience* 139: 23–38.

Proulx MJ (2010). Synthetic synaesthesia and sensory substitution. *Consciousness and Cognition* 19(1): 501–3.

Ramachandran VS, Hubbard EM (2001a). Psychophysical investigations into the neural basis of synaesthesia. *Proceedings of the Royal Society B: Biological Sciences* 268: 979–83.

Ramachandran VS, Hubbard EM (2001b). Synaesthesia: a window into perception, thought and language. *Journal of Consciousness Studies* 8: 3–34.

Ramachandran VS, Hubbard EM (2003). The phenomenology of synaesthesia. *Journal of Consciousness Studies* 10: 49–57.

Rich AN, Karstoft KI (2013). Exploring the benefit of synaesthetic colours: testing for "pop-out" in individuals with grapheme-colour synaesthesia. *Cognitive Neuropsychology* doi: 10.1080/02643294.2013.805686.

Rich AN, Mattingley JB (2002). Anomalous perception in synaesthesia: A cognitive neuroscience perspective. *Nature Reviews Neuroscience* 3: 43–52.

Rissman J, Wagner AD (2012). Distributed representations in memory: insights from functional brain imaging. *Annual Review of Psychology* 63: 101–28.

Roder B, Stock O, Bien S, Neville H, Rosler F (2002). Speech processing activates visual cortex in congenitally blind humans. *Eur J Neurosci* 16: 930–6.

Rothen N, Meier B (2009). Do synesthetes have a general advantage in visual search and episodic memory? A case for group studies. *PLoS ONE* 4: 1–9.

Rothen N, Meier B, Ward J (2012). Enhanced memory ability: insights from synaesthesia. *Neurosci Biobehav Rev.* 36(8): 1952–63.

Rothen N, Seth AK, Witzel C, Ward J (2013). Diagnosing synaesthesia with online colour pickers: maximising sensitivity and specificity. *J. Neurosci. Methods* 215(1): 156–60.

Rouw R, Scholte HS (2007). Increased structural connectivity in grapheme-color synesthesia. *Nat. Neurosci.* 10: 792–7. doi: 10.1038/nn1906.

Rueschemeyer SA, van Rooij D, Lindemann O, Willems RM, Bekkering H (2010). The function of words: distinct neural correlates for words denoting differently manipulable objects. *J. Cogn. Neurosci.* 22: 1844–51.

Saygin AP, McCullough S, Alac M, Emmorey K (2010). Modulation of BOLD response in motion-sensitive lateral temporal cortex by real and fictive motion sentences. *J. Cogn. Neurosci.* 22: 2480–90.

Schacter DL, Addis DR, Buckner RL (2007). Remembering the past to imagine the future: the prospective brain. *Nat. Rev. Neurosci.* 8: 657–61.

Schwitzgebel E (2008). The unreliability of naive introspection. *Philosophical Review* 117: 245–73.

Serences JT, Ester EF, Vogel EK, Awh E (2009). Stimulus-specific delay activity in human primary visual cortex. *Psychol Sci.* 20(2): 207–14.

Simmons WK, Ramjee V, Beauchamp MS, McRae K, Martin A, Barsalou LW (2007). A common neural substrate for perceiving and knowing about color. *Neuropsychologia* 45: 2802–10.

Simner J, Mayo N, Spiller MJ (2009). A foundation for savantism? Visuo-spatial synaesthetes present with cognitive benefits. *Cortex* 45: 1246–60.

Simner J, Mulvenna C, Sagiv N, Tsakanikos E, Witherby SA, et al. (2006). Synaesthesia: the prevalence of atypical cross-modal experiences. *Perception* 35: 1024–33.

Simner J, Ward J, Lanz M, Jansari A, Noonan K, Glover L, et al. (2005). Non-random associations of graphemes to colours in synaesthetic and non-synaesthetic populations. *Cognitive Neuropsychology* 22(8): 1069.

Simons JS, Spiers HJ (2003). Prefrontal and medial temporal lobe interactions in long-term memory. *Nat. Rev. Neurosci.* 4: 637–48.

Sinke C, Halpern JH, Zedler M, Neufeld J, Emrich HM, Passie T (2012). Genuine and drug-induced synesthesia: a comparison. *Consciousness and Cognition* 21(3): 1419–34.

Smilek D, Dixon MJ, Cudahy C, Merikle PM (2002). Synesthetic color experiences influence memory. *Psychological Science* 13(6): 548–52.

Specht K, Reul J (2003). Functional segregation of the temporal lobes into highly differentiated subsystems for auditory perception: an auditory rapid event-related fMRI-task. *Neuroimage* 20: 1944–54.

Sperling JM, Prvulovic D, Linden DEJ, Singer W, Stirn, A (2005). Neuronal correlates of colour-graphemic synesthesia: a fMRI study. *Cortex* 42(2): 295–303.

Squire LR, Stark CE, Clark RE (2004). The medial temporal lobe. *Annu. Rev. Neurosci.* 21: 279–306.

Stein BE, Meredith MA (1993). *The Merging of the Senses.* Cambridge, MA: MIT Press.

Stevenson RJ, Boakes RA (2004). Sweet and sour smells: the acquisition of taste-like qualities by odours. In G Calvert, C Spence, BE Stein (Eds.), *Handbook of Multisensory Processes.* Cambridge, MA: MIT Press.

Stokes M, Saraiva A, Rohenkohl G, Nobre AC (2011). Imagery for shapes activates position-invariant representations in human visual cortex. *NeuroImage* 56: 1540–5.

Stokes M, Thompson R, Cusack R, Duncan J (2009). Top-down activation of shape-specific population codes in visual cortex during mental imagery. *J. Neurosci.* 29: 1565–72.

Stroop JR (1935). Studies of interference in serial verbal reactions. *Journal of Experimental Psychology* 18(6): 643–62.

Terhune DB, Tai S, Cowey A, Popescu T, Kadosh RC (2011). Enhanced cortical excitability in grapheme-color synesthesia and its modulation. *Current Biology* 21(23).

Terhune, DB, Wudarczyk OA, Kochuparampil P, Cohen Kadosh R (2013). Enhanced dimension-specific visual working memory in grapheme–color synesthesia. *Cognition* 129 (1): 123–37.

Tettamanti M, Buccino G, Saccuman MC, Gallese V, Danna M, Scifo P, Fazio F, Rizzolatti G, Cappa SF, Perani D (2005). Listening to action-related sentences activates fronto-parietal motor circuits. *J. Cogn. Neurosci.* 17: 273–81.

Treisman A (1982). Perceptual grouping and attention in visual search for features and for objects. *Journal of Experimental Psychology: Human Perception and Performance* 8(2): 194–214.

Von Kriegstein K, Eger E, Kleinschmidt A, Giraud AL (2003). Modulation of neural responses to speech by directing attention to voices or verbal content. *Brain Res Cogn Brain Res* 17: 48–55.

Voss P, Gougoux F, Zatorre RJ, Lassonde M, Lepore F (2008). Differential occipital responses in early- and late-blind individuals during a sound-source discrimination task. *Neuroimage* 40: 746–58.

Walther DB, Caddigan E, Fei-Fei L, Beck DM (2009). Natural scene categories revealed in distributed patterns of activity in the human brain. *J. Neurosci.* 29: 10573–81.

Ward J (2013). Synesthesia. *Annual Reviews of Psychology* 64: 49–75.

Ward J, Huckstep B, Tsakanikos E (2005). Sound-colour synaesthesia: to what extent does it use cross-modal mechanisms common to us all? *Cortex* 42(2): 264–80.

Ward J, Jonas C, Dienes Z, Seth A (2010). Grapheme-colour synaesthesia improves detection of embedded shapes, but without pre-attentive "pop-out" of synaesthetic colour. *Proceedings of the Royal Society B* 277: 1021–6.

Ward J, Meijer P (2010). Visual experiences in the blind induced by an auditory sensory substitution device. *Consciousness and Cognition* 19(1): 492–500.

Weber M, Thompson-Schill SL, Osherson D, Haxby J, Parsons L (2009). Predicting judged similarity of natural categories from their neural representations. *Neuropsychologia* 47: 859–68.

Weeks R, Horwitz B, Aziz-Sultan A, Tian B, Wessinger CM, et al. (2000). A positron emission tomographic study of auditory localization in the congenitally blind. *J. Neurosci.* 20: 2664–72.

Wheeler ME, Petersen SE, Buckner RL (2000). Memory's echo: vivid remembering reactivates sensory-specific cortex. *Proc. Natl. Acad. Sci. USA* 97: 11125–9.

Willems RM, Daniel Casasanto D (2011). Flexibility in embodied language understanding. *Front Psychol.* 2: 116.

Willems RM, Hagoort P, Casasanto D (2010). Body-specific representations of action verbs: neural evidence from right- and left-handers. *Psychol. Sci.* 21: 67–74.

Williams MA, Dang S, Kanwisher NG (2007). Only some spatial patterns of fMRI response are read out in task performance. *Nat. Neurosci.* 10: 685–6.

Witthoft N, Winawer J (2006). Synesthetic colors determined by having colored refrigerator magnets in childhood. *Cortex* 42: 175–83.

Witthoft N, Winawer J (2013). Learning, memory, and synesthesia. *Psychological Science* Jan 10; doi: 10.1177/0956797612452573.

Wollen KA, Ruggiero FT (1983). Colored-letter synesthesia. *Journal of Mental Imagery* 7: 83–6.

Wu CT, Weissman DH, Roberts KC, Woldorff MG (2007). The neural circuitry underlying the executive control of auditory spatial attention. *Brain Res.* 1134: 187–98.

Yaro C, Ward J (2007). Searching for shereshevskii: what is superior about the memory of synaesthetes? *Q. J. Exp. Psychol. (Hove)* 60: 681–95. doi: 10.1080/17470210600785208.

Yonelinas AP, Otten LJ, Shaw KN, Rugg MD (2005). Separating the brain regions involved in recollection and familiarity in recognition memory. *J. Neurosci.* 25: 3002–8.

Zamm A, Schlaug G, Eagleman DM, Loui P (2013). Pathways to seeing music: enhanced structural connectivity in colored-music synesthesia. *Neuroimage* 74: 359–66. doi: 10.1016/j.neuroimage.2013.02.024.

7

Merleau-Ponty and the Problem of Synaesthesia

André J. Abath

7.1 Introduction

There has recently been a renewal of interest in Merleau-Ponty's *Phenomenology of Perception*.[1] His general account of perceptual experience in terms of a bodily engagement with the world now seems appealing to many. Despite this renewed interest, however, his discussions of specific perceptual phenomena are still often ignored. Such is the case of his account of synaesthesia. According to Merleau-Ponty, we are all synaesthetes, at least potentially so. He writes:

> Synaesthetic perception is the rule, and we are unaware of it only because scientific knowledge shifts the centre of gravity of experience, so that we have unlearned how to see, hear, and generally speaking, feel, in order to deduce, from our bodily organization and the world as the physicist conceives it, what we are to see, hear and feel. (2002: 266)

Given the fact that synaesthesia is most often taken as being a rare phenomenon, this is a surprising claim. One could thus suppose that Merleau-Ponty's discussion is of no interest today. It would be a shame if we were to do so, however, for in his treatment of the phenomenon—although it is indeed mistaken in certain aspects—he happens to identify a form of sensory union which has been overlooked by contemporary accounts, or so I will try to show.[2]

This is how I will proceed. In section 7.2, I will present Merleau-Ponty's treatment of the problem of synaesthesia—as he calls it—and the account he offers as a solution to it. In section 7.3, I will show that his account is unsuccessful in dealing with what I call synaesthesia proper. In section 7.4, after showing that his account is also

[1] I am very grateful to Ophelia Deroy for her excellent comments on an earlier draft of this chapter.

[2] I will not discuss here Merleau-Ponty's treatment of synaesthesia in his unfinished book *The Visible and the Invisible* (1968), in which the phenomenon is addressed in relation to an ontological effort. For discussion, see Dillon (1988: 160–4).

unsuccessful in dealing with two other forms of sensory union—crossmodal correspondences and crossmodal mental imagery—I discuss the hitherto overlooked form of sensory union that emerges from it, which I will call *sensorimotor crossmodality*.

7.2 Merleau-Ponty's solution to the problem of synaesthesia

Let me start by making a distinction—important for our purposes—between what I will call synaesthesia proper and other cases of sensory union. By 'synaesthesia proper' I refer, using the words of Cytowic, to the "the rare capacity to hear colors, taste shapes, or experience other equally startling sensory blendings whose quality seems difficult for most of us to imagine" (1997: 18). The rarity of synaesthesia proper is contrasted by the everydayness of other cases of sensory union: people tend to match higher pitches with lighter colours and take certain colours as being warmer than others (Marks, 1975; Martino and Marks, 2001); people also tend to match a speech sound such as 'bouba' with round shapes, and a speech sound such as 'kiki' with jagged ones.[3] The number of examples here is enormous.[4] *Prima facie*, what these cases have in common with cases of synaesthesia proper is that they all involve a form of sensory union. But while in the latter cases we have "a tendency for a sensory feature, or attribute, in one modality— perceived or imagined—to be matched with a sensory feature in another modality" (Spence and Deroy, 2013: 644) (a tendency to match a given sound with a given shape, for instance), in synaesthesia proper we have a perception in a given modality triggering a *vivid experience* in a different modality, without a corresponding stimulus—the perception of a C sharp triggering the experience of bright blue, for instance; or, better put, the perception of a C sharp as being bright blue.

There is disagreement in the literature regarding whether we should treat all these cases as being synaesthesia, but distinguish between strong and weak forms (Martino and Marks, 2001), or take the phenomenon of synaesthesia as being restricted to what I am calling synaesthesia proper, and take the other cases of sensory union we have considered as being a different phenomenon, one of crossmodal correspondences (Gilbert, Martin, and Kemp, 1996; Spence, 2011; Deroy and Spence, 2013).[5] We need not directly engage this debate here. I will maintain a distinction between synaesthesia proper and crossmodal correspondences for explanatory purposes.

Now, what immediately catches our attention in Merleau-Ponty's discussion of the phenomenon of synaesthesia is how swiftly he moves from a typical case of

[3] This is the so-called buba/kiki effect. See Ramachandran and Hubbard (2001).

[4] See Spence (2011) for a detailed discussion of such cases.

[5] The terms here vary. Others talk, for instance, of *natural crossmodal mappings* (Evans and Treisman, 2010) or *crossmodal associations* (Crisinel and Spence, 2011).

synaesthesia proper to cases which, at a first glance, seem quite distinct. In synaesthesia, he writes, "*the subject does not say only that he has the sensation both of a sound and a colour: it is the sound itself that he sees where colours are formed*" (2002: 266, author's italics). This is a correct description of a case of synaesthesia proper—at least one which is in tune with subjects' reports. Almost immediately Merleau-Ponty goes on to list a number of other examples that count as synaesthesia for him. These cases, however, look (at first glance) quite different from the one considered at the beginning of his discussion:

> One sees the hardness and brittleness of glass, and when, with a tinkling sound, it breaks, this sound is conveyed by the visible glass. One sees the springiness of steel, the ductility of red-hot steel, the hardness of a plane blade, the softness of shavings.... In the jerk of the twig from which a bird has just flown, we read its flexibility or elasticity, and it is thus that a branch of an apple-tree or a birch are immediately distinguishable. One sees the weight of a block of cast iron which sinks in the sand, the fluidity of water and the viscosity of syrup. In the same way, I hear the hardness and unevenness of cobbles in the rattle of a carriage, and we speak appropriately of a 'soft', 'dull' or 'sharp' sound. (2002: 266–7)

These cases, for Merleau-Ponty, are ones in which we have an "an opening on to the structure of the thing" (Ibid: 266). Consider the first example, of one somehow seeing the hardness and brittleness of glass. What Merleau-Ponty has in mind here is that, in being visually (and only visually) presented with a piece of glass, one can somehow experience its hardness and brittleness—properties normally given by the sense of touch. These properties, moreover, are an indication of the inner (molecular) structure of the thing. And so is the case of several other properties of materials: springiness, ductility, softness, flexibility, elasticity. These are all properties normally presented as we manipulate objects, with or without the use of an instrument. Merleau-Ponty's point is that we can somehow experience them by only seeing the objects. Similarly, the viscosity or fluidity of a liquid is normally presented as we touch it or taste it, but we would somehow be able to experience these properties as we see the liquids. And finally, by only hearing a carriage moving over the cobbles outside we would be able to somehow experience their unevenness and hardness, properties normally presented by touch or vision (the latter for the case of unevenness).[6]

Now, in giving us an opening to the structure of the thing, these cases are quite unlike ones of synaesthesia proper, in which the relation between the inducer—the triggering stimulus, such as the hearing of a sound—and the concurrent—the experience triggered by perception, such as the experience of a colour in hearing a

[6] Curiously, Merleau-Ponty includes here a classic example of crossmodal correspondence, one between sounds and non-auditory properties, such as softness, dullness, and sharpness. This case is unlike the ones we have been describing in that it does not necessarily involve an opening on to the structure of the thing: soft sounds, for instance, are not necessarily emitted by soft objects. I thank Ophelia Deroy for pointing this out to me.

sound—seems arbitrary (Deroy and Spence, 2013). In no way a sound appearing red, for instance, is revealing of its structure.[7, 8]

If that is so, why would Merleau-Ponty be taking cases of synaesthesia proper and the ones just discussed as constituting a single phenomenon, captured under the label 'synaesthesia'? In part, he takes all these cases as being ones of sensory union. So he could be meaning exactly that by 'synaesthesia'. What he goes on to say, however, is far more interesting than merely describing different forms of sensory union and taking them, for this very reason, to constitute a single phenomenon.

Merleau-Ponty takes synaesthesia, in its more including sense—covering all the cases he mentions—as being a problem in need of a solution. In line with the general strategy of the *Phenomenology of Perception*, what he seeks is not an explanation in terms of brain physiology—what he frequently calls an explanation of "objective thought" (2002: 266)—but a phenomenological account of the phenomenon. The account itself is expressed in few and somehow mysterious words:

> The problem of forms of synaesthetic experience begins to look like being solved if the experience of quality is that of a certain mode of movement or of a form of conduct. When I say that I see a sound, I mean that I echo the vibration of the sound with my whole sensory being, and particularly with that sector of myself which is susceptible to colours. Movement, understood not as objective movement and transference in space, but as a project towards movement or 'potential movement' forms the basis for the unity of the senses. (1962: 272)

So, according to Merleau-Ponty, we need to bring into play potential movements of the subject, or projects towards movement, to give a phenomenological account of the problem of synaesthesia. But what does that mean?

Let me begin by discussing what it does *not* mean. It might be tempting to read Merleau-Ponty here as talking about acts of imagination. To engage in a project towards movement or potentially move would be to *imagine* oneself moving towards objects and interacting with them.[9] If one is so tempted, it is for good reason. When considering the cases described by him in which we have an access to the structure of the thing via union of the senses, there is a way of accounting for them in terms of acts imagination. Take the case of one seeing a piece of glass and somehow experiencing its hardness and brittleness. Is this a plausible case? Is this an experience of a

[7] I discuss the issue of arbitrariness in more detail below.

[8] These cases also seem different from typical cases of crossmodal correspondence, for instance the one in which subjects have a tendency to match higher pitches with lighter colours. It is not the case that, in being presented with higher pitches, we somehow experience lighter colours, but only that we have a tendency to match these sensory features. Moreover, matching higher pitches with lighter colours is not revealing of the structure of these sounds. I discuss the distinction between the cases presented by Merleau-Ponty and crossmodal correspondences in more detail below.

[9] We need not assume that to imagine oneself moving towards objects is a matter of entertaining sensory-like images, or picturing oneself in movement. It might be a case of propositional imagining: imagining *that* oneself is moving towards a certain object. For a discussion of propositional imagining, see Yablo (1993).

type we are familiar with, or one which we can somehow relate to? It seems to me that the following fictional case does not sound foreign to our ears:

While window shopping for antiquities, John's attention is caught by a set of 19th century Victorian glasses. They are far too expensive, so he does not dare asking to touch them. But, in his mind, he is carefully touching them right now. As he gets lost in his imaginings, he can *almost* feel the contours of their decoration, their hardness and brittleness.

We can all probably make sense of this case. It is one in which, by imagining himself touching the glasses, John somehow experiences their hardness and brittleness. His experience of these properties is certainly not like the one he would have if he were to actually touch the glasses. It does not feel to him like he is touching the glasses and being sensorily presented with their hardness and brittleness. What John has, instead, is a *quasi-sensory experience* of touching the glasses and of their hardness and brittleness. This is captured in everyday language by saying that he can *almost* touch the glasses and feel their hardness and brittleness.

It would be interesting if Merleau-Ponty had put his finger on this phenomenon, but I don't think that is the case, and for a simple reason: in the *Phenomenology of Perception* Merleau-Ponty discusses imagination only in passing,[10] mostly following Sartre. It plays no major role in the work.[11] It thus seems very unlikely that he would bring imagination into play in such a crucial moment of his discussion and not make it explicit, choosing instead to talk of "projects towards movement" and "potential movements". There are, however, aspects of this reading that seem correct as an interpretation of Merleau-Ponty's words, but that can be introduced without any talk of imagination, and under a framework which is in tune with some of the central ideas presented in the *Phenomenology of Perception*.

There is a famous passage in the work where Merleau-Ponty introduces the idea that, in perceptual experience, objects with which we happen to be familiar might be presented to us as "poles of action". He writes of a subject in the psychiatric literature, named Schneider:[12]

the subject, when put in front of his scissors, needle and familiar tasks, does not need to look for his hands or his fingers, because they are not objects to be discovered in objective space: bones, muscles and nerves, but potentialities already mobilized by the perception of scissors or needle, the central end of those 'intentional threads' which link him to the objects given. It is never our objective body that we move, but our phenomenal body, and there is no mystery in

[10] See, for instance, Merleau-Ponty (2002: 377).

[11] Galen A. Johnson (1993: 29–30) writes that, in the *Phenomenology of Perception*, "Merleau-Ponty takes Sartre's account [of imagination] as definitive, and given his own interests in the modalities of perception, employs Sartre's account as evidence for assigning an impoverished and reduced importance to imagination in comparison with perception". As also stressed by Johnson, Merleau-Ponty would get to rethink the issue of imagination in later works. See, for instance, his *Indirect Language and the Voices of Silence* (1964).

[12] Although Merleau-Ponty wishes to show that Schneider is unlike a normal subject in several aspects, the capacities here described are ones that Schneider and a normal subject share.

that, since our body, as the potentiality of this or that part of the world, surges towards objects to be grasped and perceives them.... The bench, scissors, pieces of leather offer themselves to the subject as poles of action. (2002: 121–2)

This is one of the central ideas in the *Phenomenology of Perception*, and one that is directed linked to Merleau-Ponty's account of synaesthesia. The example given here is clear enough: in perceptual experience, the subject might be presented not only with objects themselves, but objects as offering opportunities for action. The subject—who happens to be involved in the familiar task of manufacturing wallets—is presented to the bench, scissors, and pieces of leather as offering themselves for sitting, cutting up, and being cut, respectively. Similarly, when climbing up a rock, some of its faults appear to me as offering an opportunity for holding; others, an opportunity for placing my feet.[13, 14]

Now, what is also important to Merleau-Ponty is to stress that to be presented in perceptual experience to objects as offering opportunities for certain actions is to have our body mobilized for these very actions.[15] Thus, in perceiving a fault in a rock as offering an opportunity for holding, my body prepares itself for this very action. Similarly, in perceiving a track as offering itself for running through it, the athlete's body prepares itself for this very action. It is here that we find a place to talk of 'potential movements', or 'projects towards movement'. In being mobilized for action, or in preparation for action, our bodies are in a state of potential movement, or are involved in a project towards movement.

Notice that, in perceiving a fault in a rock as offering me an opportunity for holding, I may imagine myself acting according to opportunity: I may imagine myself moving and holding it. The point, however, is that I can have my body in preparation for action even if no act of imagination takes place. In fact, my body might be in such a preparation even if no reflexive thought takes place. Perceiving objects as offering

[13] The idea presented here is of course similar to the one introduced by Gibson (1977) under the label "affordance". For distinctions in detail between Merleau-Ponty and Gibson in this respect, see Dreyfus (2005) and Romdehn-Romluc (2012).

[14] Romdehn-Romluc (2013) raises the important issue that perceiving objects as offering opportunities might pull the subject to action in different degrees depending on background states, such as desires and emotions. Someone who profoundly wishes to conquer a certain rock will be strongly pulled to action as, nearing the top, he perceives a fault as offering the opportunity for holding. Similarly, a cup of water in front of me will strongly pull me to action if I perceive it as offering the opportunity for grasping and drinking from it when thirsty. If not thirsty, however, perceiving the cup as offering me this very opportunity will not pull me as strongly to action. In fact, if not thirsty, the cup may not be perceived as offering itself for grasping and drinking from it at all. This is another important point: whether an object appears as offering certain opportunities for action to a subject is in itself dependent on background states of the subject. Neither of these points receives much attention from Merleau-Ponty, since he is mostly concerned to discuss cases in which the subject is involved in a familiar task, and so objects strongly pull him to actions that will lead to a successful performance in the task.

[15] It should be stressed, however, that whether the subject's body is so affected by the perception of objects as offering opportunities for action will depend on how strongly the subject is pulled to these actions, which is itself dependent on background states of the subject, as we have seen. The cases that follow are ones in which subjects are strongly pulled to action.

opportunities for actions is sufficient for us to have our bodies in preparation to take up these opportunities, or to be in a state of potential movement.

We are now in a position to understand Merleau-Ponty's so-called solution (or beginning of a solution) to the problem of synaesthesia. Let us approach it by redescribing the case of John:

> While window shopping for antiquities, John's attention is caught by a set of 19th century Victorian glasses. As he inspects them with his eyes, they appear to pull his body for action: for grasping, and for delicately running his fingers through their decoration. Now John's body is in tension: he is about to move and touch the glasses. He can *almost* feel the contours of their decoration, their hardness and brittleness. They are far too expensive, however, and so John does not dare touching them. He walks away.

Unlike the previous description, John does not imagine himself touching the glasses. Instead, he perceives the glasses as offering themselves for certain bodily interactions. His body is then in preparation to take up these opportunities. It is in a state of potential movement, or involved in a project towards movement. So far, so good. What is important for our purposes, however, is another aspect of the experience being described here: in having his body in preparation for certain bodily interactions with the glasses, John somehow experiences their hardness and brittleness.

Once again, we are talking of quasi-sensory experiences. It does not feel to John like he is touching the glasses and being sensorily presented with their hardness and brittleness. His experience has a quasi-sensory aspect: he can *almost* feel their hardness and brittleness. And this is so even if he does not imagine himself touching the glasses. It suffices for the having of a quasi-tactile experience that, in being visually presented with the glasses, he is also presented with certain opportunities for bodily interactions; perceiving the glasses as offering these opportunities, in turn, involves having his body in preparation for these very interactions.

So, according to my reading of Merleau-Ponty, his account of synaesthesia—or his solution to the problem of synaesthesia—in its more including sense can be summed up as follows: in being presented with an object in a given sensory modality as offering opportunities for actions towards it, one's whole body can be engaged in the experience in being in preparation for taking up these opportunities. In having one's body so prepared, one can have quasi-sensory experiences related to another sensory modality, without a corresponding stimulus. In the case we have been considering, in being visually presented with objects as offering opportunities for certain bodily interactions with them, John's body is prepared to take up these opportunities, leading him to have a quasi-tactile experience.

For this to be a plausible story, there should be a systematic relation between the actions one is prepared to perform and the experiences one will end up having in the absence of a stimulus. For instance, if one is prepared to touch a glass, the experience one will end up having in the absence of a corresponding stimulus should have a tactile quality.

Also, I take it that the story is plausible only if having the body in preparation for action towards an object might lead us to somehow, quasi-sensorily, experience properties we expect the object to have, but that are sensorily hidden from us at a given moment, and not any old property. Thus, in being prepared to touch the Victorian glasses, John can somehow, quasi-sensorily, experience properties he expects glasses—or even Victorian glasses—to have, but not any old property.[16]

7.3 Merleau-Ponty's account and synaesthesia proper

Now, it seems clear that Merleau-Ponty wishes for his account to cover both cases of synaesthesia proper and the cases we have been discussing, ones in which subjects have an opening to the structure of the thing via union of the senses. In fact, if successful in doing so, it would give us a reason to consider these as constituting a single phenomenon. But is the account successful in this respect? In this section, I argue that it is not. The account fails when it comes to dealing with synaesthesia proper.

My discussion will focus on two aspects of synaesthesia proper: perceptual reality, from the subject's point of view, and arbitrariness. Let us start with perceptual reality. The relevant point for our purposes is well put by Deroy and Spence (2013: 651): "Most current definitions of synesthesia stress…that the concurrents are 'perceptually real' and, contrary to the case with mental images, subjectively indistinguishable from real percepts". As the literature on hallucination taught us, there are delicate issues surrounding the notions of subjective indistinguishability and perceptual reality.[17] For our purposes, however, it suffices to say that, in synaesthesia proper, to experience a property such as red in the absence of a corresponding stimulus—the concurrent—is phenomenologically just like experiencing the real thing. A synaesthetic perception of a letter as being green, when in fact it is black, is, for the synaesthete, phenomenologically just like the perception of a green letter. Thus, a common report of synaesthetic experience is for subjects to say that they *see* colours in letters or sounds. The use of 'see' should be taken as indicating the perceptual reality of the experience, in the sense relevant here: from the subject's point of view, to experience a concurrent in synaesthesia proper is phenomenologically just like experiencing the real thing.[18]

In the examples presented in the previous section, I talked of quasi-sensory experiences: of a subject *almost* feeling the hardness and brittleness of glass. The *quasi*-sensory aspect of these experiences is to be contrasted with the *sensory* aspect of synaesthesia proper: from the subject's point of view, it is not as if she could almost

16 I discuss this point in more detail below.

17 For discussion, see Fish (2008).

18 In one such report (available at http://www.experienceproject.com/stories/Have-Synesthesia/1090318), the subject writes: "My synesthesia allows me to see sounds, so to speak…I also see numbers and letters in colors. The letter R, for example, is a deep mahogany color and the number 2 is sunflower yellow."

see sunflower yellow when being presented with the number 2; instead, seeing the number 2 is just like seeing an instance of sunflower yellow.

Now, it seems phenomenologically correct to say that potential movements towards an object might lead to quasi-sensory experiences. It seems phenomenologically correct to say, for instance, that having the body in preparation for moving towards an apple and for eating it might lead to a quasi-sensory experience of its taste. I take it that we are familiar with such experiences. However, it does not seem phenomenologically correct to say that having the body in preparation for eating an apple might lead to a *sensory* experience of its taste; that is, to an experience like the one we would have if we were to actually eat the apple, or, to put it differently, to a perceptually real experience.[19] Similarly, it seems correct to say that, in seeing a set of Victorian glasses, John, being prepared to move and touch them, might somehow experience their hardness and brittleness, in the sense that he might have a quasi-sensory experience of these properties; as we have described, he might almost feel their hardness and brittleness. But it just seems phenomenologically incorrect to say that John, in being prepared to move and touch the glasses, could have an experience of these properties like the one he would have if he were to actually touch them: a perceptually real experience. In general terms, it does not seem phenomenologically correct to say that having the body in preparation for action towards an object might lead to a perceptually real experience of a property in the absence of a corresponding stimulus.

Curiously, in discussing having a body in preparation for action or for receiving certain stimuli, Merleau-Ponty explicitly links this to quasi-sensations. He gives the example of himself reading the word 'warm', and writes: "For the warmth which I feel when I read the word 'warm' is not an actual warmth. It is simply my body which prepares itself for heat and which, so to speak, roughs out its outline" (2002: 275). Similarly, if someone mentions to him a part of his body, he experiences "in the corresponding part a quasi-sensation of contact which is merely the emergence of that part of my body into the total body image" (Ibid). I think this is exactly right: to have the body in preparation for action (or for receiving a stimulus) might lead to quasi-sensory experiences or quasi-sensations of this sort. But it does not lead to perceptually real experiences like the ones observed in synaesthesia proper. This is a first reason for us to question the adequacy of Merleau-Ponty's account in dealing with synaesthesia proper.

Let us now turn to another hallmark of synaesthesia proper: arbitrariness. Deroy and Spence (2013: 647) write that, in synaesthesia proper, "there is no obvious

[19] I should stress that the idea is not that a quasi-sensory experience of an apple's taste cannot be vivid. In fact, given certain background states of the subject—such as her hunger and fondness for apples—the experience might be quite vivid. However, for one thing, vividness comes in degrees. The quasi-sensory experience might be vivid but less so than the experience one has in actually eating the apple. Be that as it may, my point is that, in having her body in preparation to eat an apple, it does not feel to her like she is eating the apple and tasting it. Instead, it feels like she can almost eat it and taste it.

(i.e., immediately explainable) relationship between the inducer and the concurrent; the mapping appears, in some sense, arbitrary (or surprising) to most". There need not be, from the subject's point of view, any obvious relationship between the number 2 and sunflower yellow, for instance. The subject might perceive the number 2 in sunflower yellow even if she hasn't been exposed to a number of occurrences of the number 2 in sunflower yellow. That is, in synaesthesia proper one need not—and typically does not—capture a regularity in one's environment, and so the phenomena cannot be explained in terms of exposure. It is this apparently arbitrary aspect of the experiences that makes synaesthesia proper surprising.

Merleau-Ponty's account, however, is ill suited to deal with arbitrariness. In having our bodies prepared for interaction with objects, we might somehow, quasi-sensorily, experience properties in the absence of corresponding stimuli. However, the properties we happen to experience are far from arbitrary. What we happen to experience reflects what we expect from objects, given prior bodily interactions. Thus John, in somehow experiencing the hardness and brittleness of the Victorian glasses by seeing them, is experiencing properties that glasses—or even Victorian glasses—revealed to him in prior tactile interactions. Similarly, in somehow experiencing the taste of an apple by seeing it, I am experiencing a property revealed to me by apples—or apples of this very sort—in prior gustatory interactions. Prior bodily interactions are one of the sources of expectations—testimony is another one[20]—regarding the properties of objects, and the properties we end up experiencing are guided by these expectations.

I take it that, if Merleau-Ponty's account is to retain its initial phenomenological plausibility, it must stick to the idea that having the body in preparation for action towards an object might lead us to somehow, quasi-sensorily, experience properties we expect the object to have, but that are sensorily hidden from us at the moment. This was, in fact, the whole point of Merleau-Ponty's discussion of us having an opening to the structure of the thing via a form of sensory union. By only seeing objects as offering opportunities for action may we somehow experience properties that they have but that happen to be hidden from us in visual experience; moreover, these properties might be indicative of their inner (molecular structure). We happen to experience these properties because they are the ones we expect the objects before us to have.

This is, I think, quite plausible. But insofar as we can only experience properties in this way by having expectations regarding the objects, and given that these expectations are dependent on prior bodily interactions with them, the properties we happen to experience are far from arbitrary. In the case of synaesthesia proper, as we have seen, the properties subjects happen to experience—the concurrents—are arbitrarily related to their inducers. The experience does not reveal properties that

[20] Although testimony might be a source of expectations regarding the properties of an object, it does not seem plausible to say that one might have a quasi-sensory experience of a property, without a corresponding stimulus, just on the basis of an expectation originated in testimony.

objects in the world do have but which happen to be hidden from subjects in a given moment, nor does it depend on expectations given prior exposure.

Thus, given these two hallmarks of synaesthesia proper—perceptual reality, from the subject's point of view, and arbitrariness—it just seems to fall outside the net of Merleau-Ponty's account.

7.4 Crossmodal correspondences, crossmodal mental imagery, and sensorimotor crossmodality

If Merleau-Ponty's account is unsuitable to deal with synaesthesia proper, can it deal with crossmodal correspondences instead? Well, as we have briefly remarked, typical cases of such correspondences also seem to fall outside of Merleau-Ponty's net. Take, for instance, a tendency of subjects to match lower-pitched sounds with larger objects. It can be explained in terms of exposure to a co-occurrence in nature: larger objects tend to resonate at lower frequencies (Marks et al., 1987: 52). This tendency manifests itself in that subjects, when asked, more often than not relate larger objects to lower, and not higher, pitched sounds. It need not be—and typically is not—a matter of one having a quasi-sensory experience of a low-pitched sound given a visual presentation of a large object.

So, Merleau-Ponty's account is not suitable to deal with such cases. Nor is it suitable to deal with cases such as the bouba/kiki effect. Again, this reveals a tendency of subjects to match the speech sound 'bouba' with round shapes, and the speech sound 'kiki' with jagged ones. When shown the words and the shapes, the subjects tend to match them in such a way. It need not be—and typically is not—a matter of one having a quasi-sensory experience of the shape when hearing the word.

Merleau-Ponty's account is thus not suitable to deal with typical cases of crossmodal correspondences. In fact, given that crossmodal correspondences are a matter of subjects having a tendency to match sensory features in different modalities, and not of subjects having quasi-sensory experiences in the absence of a corresponding stimulus as a result of bodily preparation for action, Merleau-Ponty's account is not suitable to deal with crossmodal correspondences in general.[21]

Closer to Merleau-Ponty's account is a phenomenon recently discussed by Spence and Deroy (2013) under the label 'crossmodal mental imagery'. These are cases "of mental imagery occurring in one sensory modality as the result of the presentation of a physical stimulus in another (or possibly even of an imagined experience in that modality)" (Spence and Deroy, 2013: 160). One example of crossmodal mental

[21] As quoted earlier, Merleau-Ponty writes that "we speak appropriately of a 'soft', 'dull' or 'sharp' sound" (2002: 267). Insofar as we understand such cases in terms of us having a tendency to match, for instance, certain sounds with things which happen to instantiate the property of softness, and not in terms of us having quasi-sensory experiences of softness when hearing certain sounds, they also fall outside the net of Merleau-Ponty's account.

imagery is that of silent lipreading, in which by attentively watching a speaker's lips move in the absence of actual speech sounds—such as in watching a movie with the sound off—a subject might have a quasi-auditory experience of what is being said; that is, a subject might *almost* hear what is being said.[22] Such an experience fits the definition of crossmodal mental imagery if we understand mental imagery along the lines suggested by Richardson (1969: 2): "Mental imagery refers to all those quasi-sensory or quasi-perceptual experiences of which we are self-consciously aware, and which exist for us in the absence of those stimulus conditions that are known to produce their genuine sensory or perceptual counterparts". If we thus understand mental imagery, then, in silent lipreading, we have a visual experience—watching the speaker's lips—leading to auditory mental imagery—to a quasi-auditory experience of what is being said. We thus have a case of crossmodal mental imagery.

Now, insofar as Merleau-Ponty's account is one in which quasi-sensory experiences are involved—mental imagery, in Richardson's sense—we might be tempted to take it as being suitable to deal with cases of crossmodal mental imagery.[23] This would be a mistake, however. After all, in Merleau-Ponty's account, quasi-sensory experiences result from us having our bodies in preparation to take up perceived opportunities for action. It is an account focused on the consequences of us being in preparation for bodily interactions with the world. In this respect, it is quite unsuitable to deal with cases of crossmodal mental imagery, in which quasi-sensory experiences related to a given modality result from the physical presentation of a stimulus in a different one. Having the body in preparation for taking up perceived opportunities for action does not seem to play any role here.

So, if Merleau-Ponty's account is unsuitable to deal with cases of synaesthesia proper, crossmodal correspondences and crossmodal mental imagery, what *does* he have to offer us after all? It might seem at this point that Merleau-Ponty's account is less than interesting, and deserving of the neglect it has received. But here we should pause. The fact that the account fails in dealing with different forms of sensory union does not mean that it is hopeless. It is not, because in his discussion Merleau-Ponty happens to identify cases which have not been the focus of research on forms of sensory union up to this point, ones in which by perceiving objects in a given modality as offering opportunities for action, subjects might be led to have quasi-sensory experiences related to another modality without a corresponding stimulus. More interestingly still, Merleau-Ponty is telling us that we might undergo such experiences even in the absence of acts of imagination. It suffices that, in perceiving

[22] There is in fact evidence suggesting that silent lipreading is sufficient for auditory cortex activation. See, for instance, Calvert et al. (1997).

[23] Imagination might involve imagery, in Richardson's sense, but not all cases of imagery are cases of imagination. Thus, Merleau-Ponty's account might involve imagery without involving imagination. I think that is the case.

objects as offering opportunities for action, our bodies are set in a state of potential movement towards them, or in preparation for movement.

In a few words, I wish to defend that Merleau-Ponty has to offer the identification and an account of a hitherto neglected form of sensory union, one we may call *sensorimotor crossmodality*. This is, of course, not what Merleau-Ponty takes himself to be offering. He wishes to offer more than that: a phenomenological account of synaesthesia in its including sense. This more ambitious project is, I think, a failure. But behind this failure there is an interesting and, I think, correct account of a neglected form of sensory union.

We should also notice that Merleau-Ponty is silent regarding the mechanisms that might underlie what I am calling sensorimotor crossmodality. He is, after all, looking to present a phenomenological, personal-level account of synaesthesia in its including sense. This does not mean, however, that no account of such mechanisms is in the offer. Experimental work by Tucker and Ellis (1998) and Grèzes and Decety (2002), for instance, suggests that the perception of objects may automatically involve the detection of opportunities for action and the activation of motor representations of these actions, prior to and independently of the formation of explicit intentions to act. These representations would underlie bodily preparation for action. We are here talking of, for example, representations of the movements to be realized in taking up a perceived opportunity for action—if one perceives a cup as offering the opportunity for grasping, one would subpersonally represent the movements needed to reach it and the adequate hand position to grasp it. To have a story along these lines regarding the mechanisms that underlie sensorimotor crossmodality, one would have to show how the activation of subpersonal motor representations might lead to quasi-sensory experiences related to a given modality in the absence of a corresponding stimulus. There seems to be no reason in principle why this could not be done.

Would such an account be in harmony with Merleau-Ponty's? The answer to this question depends on whether one takes him as being averse to any talk of representations in a discussion of perceiving objects as offering opportunities for action and having one's body in preparation to take up these opportunities—a reading favoured by Dreyfus (2002)—or only being focused on personal-level, phenomenological descriptions of these experiences, and thus wishing to remain silent regarding the mechanisms that underlie them—a reading that seems to be favoured by people such as Romdehn-Romluc (2013). If one favours the latter reading, Merleau-Ponty would be eager to stress that no personal-level, explicit representations need be involved in perceiving objects as offering opportunities for action and having one's body in preparation to take up these opportunities, but he would wish to remain silent on the issue of whether subpersonal representations are involved in the mechanisms that underlie these experiences. Although I myself tend to favour the latter reading, we need not engage this debate here. I only wish to point out that there are stories available regarding the mechanisms that underlie perceiving objects as offering opportunities for action and having the body in preparation for taking up these opportunities, and these stories can in principle be developed to deal with the mechanisms that underlie sensorimotor crossmodality, opening up a new avenue of empirical research.

7.5 Conclusion

In this chapter, I presented Merleau-Ponty's so-called solution to the problem of synaesthesia. In the reading I favoured, the problem of synaesthesia is solved (or begins to be solved) once we recognize that, in perceiving objects as offering opportunities for action, subjects might be in a state of bodily preparation to take up these opportunities. This might lead to quasi-sensory experiences related to a given modality without a corresponding stimulus. I argued that Merleau-Ponty fails to provide a solution to the problem of synaesthesia proper, but that he manages to identify and provide an account for a hitherto neglected form of sensory union, which I named sensorimotor crossmodality.

Let me end by returning to a controversial quote from Merleau-Ponty: "Synaesthetic perception is the rule" (2002: 266). By this he means that we are all synaesthetes, at least potentially so. Synaesthesia proper is certainly not the rule in this sense. But once we take Merleau-Ponty as offering an account of sensorimotor crossmodality, we can ask: Is sensorimotor crossmodality the rule? Here it seems correct to answer 'yes'.

References

Calvert, G. A., Bullmore, E. T., Brammer, M. J., Campbell, R., Williams, S. C., McGuire, P. K., Woodruff, P. W., Iversen, S. D., & David, A. S. (1997). Activation of auditory cortex during silent lipreading. *Science*, 276, 593–6.

Crisinel, A. S. & Spence, C. (2011). Crossmodal associations between flavoured milk solutions and musical notes. *Acta Psychologica*, 138, 155–61.

Cytowic, R. E. (1997). Synaesthesia: phenomenology and neuropsychology: A review of current knowledge. In S. Baron-Cohen & J. E. Harrison (Eds.), *Synaesthesia: Classic and Contemporary Readings* (pp. 17–39). London: Basil Blackwell.

Deroy, O. & Spence, C. (2013). Why we are not all synesthetes (not even weakly so). *Psychonomic Bulletin & Review*, 20, 1–22.

Dillon, M. C. (1988). *Merleau-Ponty's Ontology*. Bloomington and Indianapolis: Indiana University Press.

Dreyfus, H. (2002). Intelligence without representation—Merleau-Ponty's critique of mental representation and the relevance of phenomenology to scientific explanation. *Phenomenology and the Cognitive Sciences*, 1/4, 367–83.

Dreyfus, H. (2005). Overcoming the myth of the mental: how philosophers can profit from the phenomenology of everyday expertise. *Proceedings and Addresses of the American Philosophical Association*, 79/2, 47–65.

Evans, K. K. & Treisman, A. (2010). Natural cross-modal mappings between visual and auditory features. *Journal of Vision*, 10, 1–12.

Fish, W. (2008). Disjunctivism, indistinguishability, and the nature of hallucination. In A. Haddock & F. Macpherson (eds.) *Disjunctivism: Perception, Action, Knowledge* (pp. 144–67). Oxford: Oxford University Press.

Gibson, J. J. (1977). The theory of affordances. In R. Shaw & J. Bransford (eds.) *Perceiving, Acting, and Knowing: Toward an Ecological Psychology* (pp. 67–82). Hillsdale, NJ: Erlbaum.

Gilbert, A. N., Martin, R., & Kemp, S. E. (1996). Cross-modal correspondence between vision and olfaction: the color of smells. *The American Journal of Psychology*, 109, 335–51.

Grèzes, J. & Decety, J. (2002). Does visual perception afford action? Evidence from a neuroimaging study. *Neuropsychologia*, 40, 1597–607.

Johnson, G. A. (1993). Structures and painting: "Indirect language and the voices of silence". In G.A. Johnson (ed.) *The Merleau-Ponty Aesthetics Reader: Philosophy and Painting* (pp. 14–34). Evanston, IL: Northwestern University Press.

Marks, L. E. (1975). On colored-hearing synesthesia: cross-modal translations of sensory dimensions. *Psychological Bulletin*, 82, 303–31.

Marks, L. E., Hammeal, R. J., & Bornstein, M. H. (1987). Perceiving similarity and comprehending metaphor. *Monographs of the Society for Research in Child Development*, 52, 1–102.

Martino, G. & Marks, L. E. (2001). Synesthesia: strong and weak. *Current Directions in Psychological Science*, 10, 61–5.

Merleau-Ponty, M. (1964). Indirect language and the voices of silence. In G.A. Johnson (ed.) *The Merleau-Ponty Aesthetics Reader: Philosophy and Painting* (pp. 76–120). Evanston, IL: Northwestern University Press.

Merleau-Ponty, M. (1968). *The Visible and the Invisible.* Translated by A. Lingis. Evanston, IL: Northwestern University Press.

Merleau-Ponty, M. (2002). *Phenomenology of Perception—Second Edition.* Translated by C. Smith. London: Routledge.

Ramachandran, V. S. & Hubbard, E. M. (2001). Psychophysical investigations into the neural basis of synaesthesia. *Proceedings of the Royal Society London* B, 268, 979–83.

Richardson, A. (1969). *Mental Imagery.* London: Routledge & Kegan Paul.

Romdehn-Romluc, K. (2012). Thought in action. In D. Zahavi (ed.) *Oxford Handbook of Phenomenology* (pp. 198–215). Oxford: Oxford University Press.

Romdehn-Romluc, K. (2013). Habit and attention. In D. Moran & R. T. Jensen (eds.) *The Phenomenology of Embodied Subjectivity.* Philadelphia: Springer.

Spence, C. (2011). Crossmodal correspondences: a tutorial review. *Attention, Perception, & Psychophysics*, 73, 971–95.

Spence, C. & Deroy, O. (2013). Crossmodal mental imagery. In S. Lacey & R. Lawson (eds.) *Multisensory Imagery: Theory and Applications* (pp. 157–83). Philadelphia: Springer.

Tucker, M. & Ellis, R. (1998). On the relations between seen objects and components of potential actions. *Journal of Experimental Psychology: Human Perception and Performance*, 24, 830–46.

Yablo, S. (1993). Is conceivability a guide to possibility? *Philosophy and Phenomenological Research*, 53/1, 1–42.

8

When is Synaesthesia Perception?

Mohan Matthen

My thesis in this chapter is that under certain conditions, synaesthesia would properly be understood as perception, i.e. as experience that affords the subject a true and accurate imagistic representation of the world. I shall attempt to outline the conditions that must be met for this to be so. It is an empirical question whether these conditions are standardly, or even *ever*, met. I shall not attempt to say anything about this empirical question.

In the literature, there is considerable disagreement about the status of synaesthesia. Some claim that it is perceptual in nature (for example, Rich and Mattingley, 2002), though these researchers do not concern themselves with the *accuracy* or *truth* of synaesthetic experience. Others claim that it cannot, on pain of inconsistency, be taken to be true perception (Macpherson, 2007). To adjudicate such disagreements, it is essential to be explicit about the criteria used to decide the question. In what follows, therefore, I shall lay out some important characteristics of perception, and define a variety of synaesthesia, which I call *direct synaesthesia*, in which these essential characteristics of perception are present. I do not claim that direct synaesthesia actually exists, though some descriptions of some types of synaesthesia suggest that it might. My interest is to provide a basis for distinguishing among synaesthetic phenomena. This would actually help, as synaesthesia is probably construed in too unified a manner in the literature, without allowances for the many different kinds and varieties thereof. (See Marks, Chapter 1 of this volume, for other suggestions that synaesthesia is not all of one kind.)

8.1 What is perception?

Let us begin with a characterization of perception. (I'll explain each clause in what follows.)

A perception is an experience that is (a) imagistic, (b) of the situation that obtains *here* (i.e., in the region of space around the perceiver, presented relative to the perceiver) and *now*, and (c) true.

Additionally, (d) it provides the perceiver with an unmediated reason to believe that the here-and-now situation conforms to the image that it presents.

Whether synaesthesia is perception turns on whether it conforms to these conditions. (I have said that perception is *experience*-based. We do not need to worry about unconscious perception in what follows. We can consider synaesthesia in its conscious form here, and extend the analysis to unconscious forms in ways that parallel the extension of conscious perception to the unconscious.)

Let me now explain the clauses in the above definition.

(a) An imagistic experience is a presentation of objects and/or features arrayed in a continuous region of space. When you use your eyes, you *experience* objects and backgrounds, each located in the visual field. Each of these objects and backgrounds is experienced as possessing visual features. Everything you experience visually appears located relative to everything else. Similarly, when you hear, you hear sounds and their features; they too are *experienced* as possessing location, and though auditory locations are coarser in grain than visual ones, sounds are located relative both to one another and to visual objects. Touch gives you awareness of external objects and of such features as hardness, heat, and sharpness, as well as of parts of your own body and what is happening to them. Taste tells you of things in your mouth; smell of the character of odours *here*. Every object or feature sensed in one modality is located relative to objects and features sensed by every other modality. Taken together, perception gives the subject a *multimodal* image.

(b) Memory can give you imagistic experience; so can mental imagery and anticipation. Perception is different because it purports to represent the world as it is *here* (in the broad sense of 'here' indicated above: all locations presented relative to where the subject is), and *now*, i.e. around the time of the perception itself. (I use the vague term 'around' so as to accommodate the 'specious present', i.e. the brief but finite spread in time over which events appear to be simultaneous.)

(b') A close relative of the 'here-and-now' condition is suggested by extrapolation from Susanna Siegel (2006). Perceptual experience presents itself as perspective-dependent; that is, it contains the idea that if conditions of observation or perceiver point of view were to change, so also, in predicable ways, would the perceptual experience. I see my keyboard under my fingers immediately in front of me, but were I to move to the right, it would be to my left. My experience of the keyboard 'contains', as it were, the potentiality of such movement and its effect on experience. Similarly, I taste the lemonade that I am sipping. This perception is freighted with the idea that I do so because it is in my mouth; if I had left it in the tumbler, I would have had a different experience—the experience is a consequence of my perspective on the lemonade. In short, the perceiver's own body is implicitly a part of any scene she perceptually experiences, and the *other* things she experiences are presented as located relative to her own body and its orientation. Filled out in this way, Siegel's perspective-dependency condition is closely related to the here-and-now condition.

(c) Perception must be true, but for a relatively uninteresting reason. It is because the verb 'perceive' is 'factive'. That is, to say that I *perceive* the redness of a rose is to imply that there is a rose for me to perceive, and, further, that it is red. If the rose were a hallucination or if it was green, it would be a linguistic solecism to say that I perceived it to be green. Factiveness is a rather shallow point about language, and tells us very little about the nature of perceptual processes. However, it is accommodated with minimal inconvenience. One can distinguish between perceptions *proper*, which must be true, by virtue of the meaning of the term, and *perceptual experiences*, which seem to the subject to be true, but may not be.

Perceptual experiences are imagistic experiences that present themselves as of the here and now.

Perceptual experiences present themselves as true. This is closely connected with the here-and-now condition. When I have a perceptual experience as of a red rose, it seems to me that there really is *now* a red rose in a location that I can identify relative to myself. This object, if it were there, would make my visual state *true*.

(d) Finally, perceptual experience has a role in rational belief-fixation. By itself, and with no additional supplementation—i.e., unmediatedly—it is a reason for the perceiver to *believe* that her here-and-now situation conforms to the image that her perceptual experience presents. Suppose I have a perceptual experience of something as blue or high-pitched or hard. This, all by itself, gives me a reason for believing that this thing is blue or high-pitched or hard. I do not have to figure this out; I do not treat my perceptual experience as a sign or indication of external conditions that has to be further assessed. I do not investigate correlations between experience and the world. All of these further investigations would, in any case, rely to some extent on perception, and so they would not increase the credibility of perception. (On the other hand, perception or previously gained knowledge could undermine or defeat the epistemic force of my current perceptual state, since it could be inconsistent with it. I might, for instance, learn that I am astigmatic, and that the things I see are therefore distorted in shape. The reasons for belief that perception provides are in this way *defeasible*.) In virtue of perceiving, the subject is simply and directly in a position to arrive at perceptual knowledge. (See Pollock, 1974 and Pryor, 2000 for canonical discussions of the reason-giving role of perceptual experience.)

8.2 What is synaesthesia?

With this characterization of perceptual experience and perception in place, let us turn now to synaesthesia.

Synaesthesia is a condition in which 'normal' perception is (almost) invariably accompanied by an additional sensory appearance—consistently the same additional experience for the same 'normal' experience—in the absence of the stimulus that would be appropriate for a *normal* occurrence of the additional experience. For example, some synaesthetes experience a certain colour whenever they appear to hear a particular tone—always the same colour for the same tone; others experience a colour when they see a certain letter—same letter, same colour; others see numbers, or dates, as possessing a consistent location in space, and so on. The important point here is that they have the same 'normal' experience that most others would have in the same situation, and that this normal experience is consistently accompanied by a different experience that most other subjects do not experience in that situation.

Synaesthesia consists, then, of two distinct but associated experiences. The first is the *inducer* which is what normal as well as synaesthetic subjects experience in the circumstance—for example, a visual experience as of 'A' in the presence of an 'A'. The second is the *concurrent* experience that only synaesthetes are subject to—for example, an experience of *red* when looking at the 'A'.

The above description is standard, but it is somewhat misleading, as Malika Auvray and Ophelia Deroy (2015) have recently argued. They point out that, in the first place, there are incongruent concurrents: "Take the report that the letter E is loud", they write (where a written 'E' is the inducer). "How can one have a sensation of loudness in the absence of other perceived properties such as pitch and timbre, which are not attributed to E?" As well, the loudness of the 'E' does not drown out the softness that is concurrent with another letter. In these and other cases of synaesthesia, the concurrent experience does not possess the characteristics of an *independent* perceptual experience. A synaesthete may experience the letter 'E' as loud *in some sense*, but not in the same way as she experiences a chord played on a piano as loud. The latter is a stand-alone experience; the synaesthete's concurrent experience is not.

Second, and notwithstanding the lack of independence, there are noticeable interactions between the inducing and the concurrent experiences. For example, consider synaesthetes who experience colour concurrently with graphemes. Let's say that a grapheme, '4', induces an experience of blue. It is reported that such synaesthetes identify '4' more slowly against a blue background. In the same way, synaesthetic musicians (such as Hélène Grimaud) find it easier to learn pieces because they have more than one experiential cue to hook into memory.

A third important point for my purpose here is that the concurrent quality does not completely obscure the inducing stimulus. A synaesthete may, for example, see a black 'A' as black and still concurrently experience redness when she looks at an 'A'. The concurrent quality is more or less tightly associated with the object that bears the inducing property. For instance, when a black 'A' induces the colour red, so-called 'projector' synaesthetes will experience the colour as co-located with the letter in some fashion; for instance, as a mask or filter. (This is relevant to the previous point about interaction: projector synaesthetes somehow associate redness with the 'A' but still see the colour in which that 'A' is written.) But not all synaesthetes are projectors; most are 'associators', who "experience the atypical colour in an internal space, or in the 'mind's eye'", to quote Auvray and Deroy again.

Now, regardless of whether they are projectors or associators, synaesthetes draw from their experience the awareness that the *inducer* is present, but none is inclined to think that the concurrent feature is. Thus, in intra-modal cases, there is (as emphasized above) no confusion between the actual colour in which a letter is printed, and the concurrent colour—a black 'A' is seen as black despite the concurrent maroon. And the same is true for cross-modal cases: when a musical note, say middle C, induces colour experience, say maroon, it is unmediatedly clear to the synaesthete that the concurrent maroon colour she experiences is associated with the middle C. Nonetheless, she experiences no confusion between *this* maroon appearance and the appearances of actually maroon things that might also happen to be present.

Or suppose that a numeral-location synaesthete sees the inscription '6+4' written on a board. Her grasp of the meaning of this expression might lead her to experience the *numeral* six as having a certain position in space, and the *operation* plus-four as linking the position of six to that of ten (as shown below). But she typically has no tendency whatsoever to experience the numeral ten as written on the board.

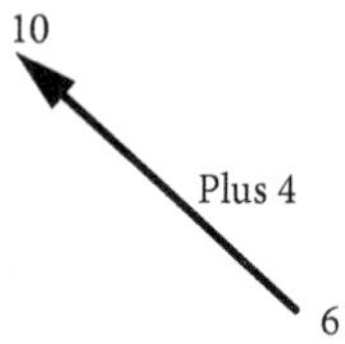

8.3 Direct synaesthesia

Now suppose that the synaesthetic experience of the inducer is, *at least sometimes*, unmediated. That is, suppose that there are synaesthetes who know *without prior investigation or learning* that their concurrent experience *betokens the inducer*. Just as the normal perceiver knows immediately and without investigation that her experience of blue gives her reason to believe that something blue is present, so also this type of synaesthete—call her the *direct synaesthete*—knows immediately and without investigation that her concurrent experience (for instance, the experience of red) gives her reason to believe that a certain mark is the numeral '5'.

I am not making a claim here about what proportion of synaesthetes are direct synaesthetes, or even that *any* are. It may be that in most or all actual cases, the concurrent experience is discounted because prior experience has shown it to be unreliable. These are matters of empirical investigation and discovery. What *is* empirically clear, for the reasons given in the previous section, is that the synaesthete's concurrent experience does not have the same character as that of the inducing perceptual experience. It can be loud without being of the same pitch; it can be over to the left without seeming to be co-located with other objects over to the left; it can be red and the same place as an 'A' without obscuring the black colour of the 'A'. Because the concurrent experience is distinct in these ways, it is at the very least *possible* that there might be direct synaesthetes. At the very least, it seems to me that this is a possibility worth investigating (perhaps by a meta-analysis that reviews published descriptions of synaesthesia).

Regardless of whether there actually are any direct synaesthetes, my claim is simply that *direct synaesthesia is perception*. In the empirical literature, the directness criterion is not discussed and this is why it is unknown whether there actually are any direct synaesthetes. My claim is that the possibility of direct synaesthesia is important for the discussion of synaesthesia as perception. Once again: it is a question worth investigating.

8.4 Synaesthesia and information

As a preliminary to investigating whether and to what degree synaesthesia meets the necessary conditions on perception mentioned earlier, let us note that the concurrent experience is information-carrying in the same sense as perception. A normal perceiver experiences a chord as a fifth, let us say. Her experience carries the information that the chord *is* a fifth. That is, given that she has this experience, the probability is (or is close to) unity that it is so. The information carried by a perceptual experience may not be directly available to the perceiver; it is based on an *objective* probability. Thus, information theory does not give us a direct insight into the epistemic significance of perceptual experience. Nonetheless, the information carried by a perceptual experience is an important background condition to understanding what it tells us.

Now suppose that a synaesthete has a concurrent impression of maroon whenever he experiences a fifth. His concurrent experience of maroon carries the information that the chord heard was a fifth. His synaesthetic experience of maroon carries information by exactly the same test as before. That is, given that he is concurrently experiencing red, the probability is (or is close to) unity that the chord is a fifth. In fact, the concurrent experience could, in certain synaesthetic perceivers, carry *more* information than the inducing perception. Suppose that the person does not have very good tone discrimination in auditory terms. I know nothing that *prohibits* his having finer discrimination in the concurrent field. If a chord is very slightly off a fifth, the perceiver's inducing auditory experience might not be sufficient to reveal that this is so; however, the concurrent maroon might shift to a bluer shade of red.

One of the functions of perception is to carry information about the subject's surroundings. Synaesthesia fulfils this function. Clearly, however, this is not enough to make it perception. My experience of something as green 'carries the information' (R) that an object of a certain reflectance profile is in my vicinity, and (V) that a certain cell in my brain's visual area V4 is activated. That is, given that I visually experience the thing as green, the propositions (R) and (V) have probability close to unity. But seeing that the thing is green does not make the information (R) or (V) *available to me*. Perception gives me *extracted* information that is unmediatedly available for my use; my visual state represents extracted information that the thing in my vicinity is green, but though it *carries* other information, it does not present all of this other information to me for my use.

I stipulate (by definition) that in direct synaesthesia, the concurrent experience carries the same *extracted information* as the inducer experience.

8.5 Locating the concurrent feature

Our earlier discussion shows how synaesthesia at least sometimes presents the subject with extracted information from the incoming signal for the use of the subject. In the hypothetical case of the direct synaesthete, it provides the subject with a concurrent experience, which she, the subject, is immediately and without further supplementation able to use as a reason for believing that the *inducing* property is present.

This point has sometimes been overlooked or wrongly treated. William Lycan, for example, writes about the 'interesting example of synaesthesia' (which derives from a thought experiment in Wager, 1999):

> Cynthia is a synaesthete who hears colors: When middle C is played, she has the normal auditory experience, but she also experiences, in her visual field, 'a six inch high by one inch wide bar of some determinate shade of red.' Cynthia and her normal counterpart Norma have (obviously) experiences with different qualitative contents. Yet, [some authors] want to say, all that is represented by the visual component of Cynthia's synaesthetic experience is middle C, which is already represented by the normal auditory components; difference in qualia without difference in intentional content.
>
> The obvious rejoinder is that Cynthia's visual component is representing redness; vision is telling her that there is redness dead ahead.

As may be obvious by now, I am one of those who want to say that all that is represented by Cynthia's concurrent visual experience is middle C. Lycan's rejoinder is simply not right. The synaesthete's experience tells her (either directly or mediatedly) that the *inducing* feature is present—middle C, in Cynthia's case. If Cynthia seemed to see that there was redness dead ahead—i.e., the concurrent feature—then she would take this as a prima facie reason to *believe* that there is redness dead ahead, and that it was in front of or behind or coincident with other things that are seen dead ahead. (Note that Cynthia is a projector synaesthete; her experience is of red, the location of which gives information about the location of the middle C.) But synaesthetes have no tendency to believe that the concurrent feature is present. The redness they see dead ahead is a kind of phantom; it is not seen as *really* located relative to other things in their field of view; if they were to count the maroon things in their vicinity, they would not count the maroon bar as one of them. If Cynthia was a *direct* synaesthete, her vision would *not* be 'telling her that there is redness dead ahead'. It would rather give her unmediated reason to believe that one of the tones she was hearing was a middle C coming from somewhere in the purported location of the red bar.

Here, the point made by Auvray and Deroy about the conjointness of synaesthetic experience is important. Synaesthetes experience the concurrent quality differently from this 'same' quality when it is presented normally. Concurrent maroon supplements and heightens Cynthia's experience of middle C. (This, by the way, is how Hélène Grimaud's synaesthetic experience is described in various journalistic accounts.) Cynthia's concurrent experience does not present, for her epistemic employment, *false* news of colours in her environment. At least, not if she is a direct synaesthete.

This point is important in coming to a fuller understanding of a point raised by Fiona Macpherson (2007).

> In grapheme-colour synaesthesia, we are supposing that a numeral '5', say, provokes a perception-like synaesthetic experience as of red. It is often claimed that the experience is such that the numeral looks to have the synaesthetic colour. At the same time, however, synaesthetes can tell what the colour of the ink is that such numerals are printed in, say, black. It is tempting to suppose that they can do this because the '5' looks black to them. Thus, it is tempting to think that the experience is such that the numeral looks to be both black and red at the same time! Indeed, introspective reports of projector synaesthetes back up this conclusion: 'When probed about the locations of the two colors, A.D. reported that she didn't know how to explain it, but that both appeared on the shape in the same location at the same time'.

A. D. is, as Macpherson describes her, a projector synaesthete: her visual system projects the concurrent feature out to the location of the object to which the inducing feature belongs. But, contrary to what Macpherson suggests, we are *not* told that the concurrent feature is perceived as belonging to the inscription '5'; nor does A. D. say that it is.

I think that the correct description of A. D.'s experience is this: red appears *in the same location* as the '5' but the '5' itself looks black, not red—black is bound to the '5', but red is bound only to the location in which the '5' happens to be. (Sagiv and Robertson, 2005, from whom Macpherson takes the example of A. D., explicitly use a location-binding model, not an object-binding model, of feature-placing.)

Co-location of colours is actually a very common phenomenon: when you see something reflected in a pane of transparent glass, a reflection can appear to be in the same location as something you see *through* the glass. For example, you might see your own face reflected in the pane in the same location as a white wall beyond. The colour of your face is bound to the reflection of your face; the colour of the wall is bound to the wall; they are both in the same visual location, but in different objects. In such cases, the reflection can make it difficult to discern the exact visual features of the thing beyond the glass, but it is normally not seen as belonging to the thing beyond. As well, it doesn't appear real; the reflection is seen as in a place, but in a way that intimates that something else (or sometimes nothing) is in that place.

(Another example, mentioned to me by Berit Brogaard in correspondence, is that of coloured after-images: these may appear in the same location as objects that have different colours, but they are not bound to these objects, and they don't look real.)

Here I am speculating somewhat, but I would imagine that A. D. shows no tendency to think that the redness of the concurrent experience is the colour of anything actually present. She is fully aware that her impression of red is induced by the fact that the inscription she is viewing is a '5', and she is fully able to distinguish between the kind of redness that '5' induces from the kind of redness that she sees when she encounters a '5' written in red ink. Unfortunately, I have not found an explicit statement of this in the literature, but I venture that when synaesthetes make errors such as taking the black '5' to be red, the psychologists who work with them would have mentioned it explicitly. I can only hope that my speculative assertion will lead to further investigation, and confirmation or refutation.

8.6 Sensory encoding

Let me now present, in a context different from synaesthesia, a view about the significance of sensory experience. I believe it gives us an appropriate framework for understanding synaesthesia. (For more details, see Matthen, 2005, 2010.)

Consider the perception of the 'unique hues': blue with no reddish or greenish admixture is 'unique blue'; green with no blue or yellow is 'unique green', and so on. All trichromats experience unique hues, which represent cross-comparable singularities in the continuum of hue experience. In other words, your unique green is, in an interesting way, the same experience type as my unique green. Yet it appears that there is substantial variation in the physical colours (for example, wavelength) that different people experience as unique green. That is, the wavelength of light that I see as unique green can be quite a bit different from that which you so experience.

Now, there are many ways of understanding this variability. Some are inclined to think that unique green is a physical property independent of any observer. Thus, they think that there is a wavelength that is *really and truly* unique green, and that the aforementioned disagreement exists because many colour perceivers *misperceive*. Thus, there is one wavelength that is truly unique green, and in the above example, at least one of you and I get it wrong. The problem of this way of understanding the issue is that not only is it impossible to say what wavelength is truly unique green, but, further, it is unclear what it would be for a particular wavelength to be *really and truly* unique green. *Green* is not a physical category; rather, it arises out of opponent processing in the vertebrate visual system. As such, it is hard to know what it could mean to say that a physical wavelength is truly unique green, independently of a particular visual system.

Here is one way to think of *red*, *green*, and the other colours. The light incident upon our eyes has a wavelength-intensity profile—an intensity value for each wavelength. The light affects the colour-sensitive cone cells according to this profile—for example, light that is more intense in long wavelengths will activate the long-wavelength cone cells more than light that is less intense in long wavelengths. Opponent processing *encodes* the activation of cone cells in a certain way (which we need not go into here). This encoding is presented to our consciousness as a combination of values in three dimensions: red-green, blue-yellow, and bright-dark. These values are not properties of light as such; rather, they are the system's encodings of properties of light. (The same encoding is used for light-related properties such as reflectances of surfaces, etc.)

The situation with respect to the colours is comparable to that of expressing mass in kilograms. I am not *intrinsically* 75 kg; rather, a particular physical property (i.e., mass) of my body is 75 kg relative to a particular system of measurement. *75 kg* is a second-order relational property of a physical property. The kilogram system encodes mass in terms of numbers. This encoding is a second-order relational property. Similarly, nothing is *intrinsically* green; rather, it is green relative to a particular visual system's method of extracting colour information and encoding it in terms of visual experience. *Green* is a second-order encoding-relational property of a certain physical property of light.

In this way of understanding the colours, it is no mystery that different wavelengths are unique green for different people. Different people have visual systems that vary from one another in small ways. These differences express themselves in slightly different measurements of the properties of light. Thus, my unique green is a slightly different second-order relational property of light than your unique green is. It is a different encoding.

8.7 Synaesthesia as non-normal sensory encoding

It is relatively obvious how the sensory-encoding thesis would apply to synaesthesia, so I'll be brief about it. Middle C is usually encoded by an auditory experience. But in some people it is encoded simultaneously by a colour experience.

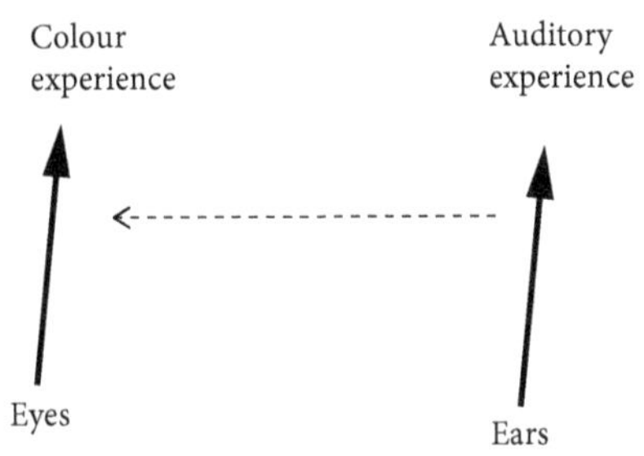

In synaesthesia, there is some sort of non-standard data-pathway that flows from the auditory data-stream to the visual data-stream. When auditory data enter the visual stream, they are treated there as if they are visual, and they end up producing visual experience. Note that the synaesthetic data-pathway is different from the visual one, though it overlaps with the latter.

We can imagine a random leakage from one stream to another. This would produce random visual effects related to ambient sound. Or it could lead to visual effects that are systematically related to auditory input, though the perceiver is unaware of it. However, in the case of *direct* synaesthesia, auditory information not only transfers over into the visual stream, but presents itself to the perceiver as content that betokens auditory input.

This analysis allows us to define *direct* synaesthesia.

> *Direct synaesthesia* consists of a concurrent experience that encodes information about the inducing stimulus in a manner that affords the perceiver unmediated reasons for *the same* belief as does the inducing experience.

So understood, the concurrent experience can be interpreted as a non-standard encoding of the inducing stimulus. Just as in the case of the unique hues, encoding can vary from person to person. The direct synaesthete is subject to two distinct experiential encodings of the same sensory stimulus.

8.8 Synaesthesia and perception

Let me now return to the conditions on perception that I laid out above. Does synaesthesia understood as above sit well with those conditions?

First, is synaesthesia imagistic? One can imagine (at least) three cases.

a. The first is where the concurrent feature is experienced as *real* and possessing definite location relative to other things experienced at the same time. For example, Cynthia (mentioned above) might experience her red bar as a real thing directly in front of her.
b. The second is that the red bar might be experienced as a phantom that non-inferentially betokens the occurrence of a middle C. Cynthia sees it as in front of her, but, somewhat in the manner of an after-image, she does not see it as a real red object, but rather as a reason for believing that middle C has been sounded.
c. Some concurrent features may not seem to have location at all; they may be experienced instead as occurring in an internal space. The loudness of 'E' might be an example—it might not seem that the 'E' itself is loud, but rather that there is an internal experience of loudness in the 'mind's ear'. Such internally located loudness is not experienced as possessing location relative to the 'E' (which is seen).

The direct synaesthesia case that I am imagining corresponds to b; a is Lycan's gloss on the Cynthia case. She perceives a middle C through her visual experience of red, as well as through her auditory experience of middle C. Her experience gives her unmediated reason to believe that the middle C occurs where it occurs, and it gives her no reason to believe that the red that she seems to see directly in front of her exists anywhere.

In case c, the loudness is not located. Hence it is not perceptual. This suggests that the experiences of associator synaesthetes is not perceptual. I take it that in the case of direct projector synaesthesia, the inducing feature is unproblematically perceived as occurring here and now, and the perception presents itself as true. As well, the non-inferential reasons condition is met.

8.9 Conclusions

I have posited a form of synaesthesia that seems, under the sensory-encoding formulation of section 8.4, to be perceptual. In this form of synaesthesia, which I call *direct projector synaesthesia*, the subject has an additional experience, which she takes to be a non-inferential reason for believing that the inducing feature is present. I take this to be a non-standard perceptual encoding of the inducing feature. As I have said, I do not know for sure that direct synaesthesia exists. However, some philosophers write as if the mere existence of a non-standard concurrent experience is so weird as to show that synaesthesia is non-perceptual. The possibility of direct synaesthesia shows that this is not so. Finally, my analysis highlights the sensory-encoding thesis for further discussion.

References

Auvray, Malika and Deroy, Ophelia (2015) "Synaesthesia," in M. Matthen (ed.) *Oxford Handbook of the Philosophy of Perception*. Oxford: Oxford University Press, 640–58.

Lycan, William (2008) "Representational Theories of Consciousness", E. Zalta (ed.) *Stanford Encyclopedia of Philosophy*, <http://plato.stanford.edu/archives/fall2008/entries/consciousness-representational/>.

Macpherson, Fiona (2007) "Synaesthesia, Functionalism and Phenomenology," in M. De Caro, F. Ferretti, and M. Marraffa (eds.) *Cartographies of the Mind: Philosophy and Psychology in Intersection*. Dordrecht: Springer, 65–80.

Matthen, Mohan (2005) *Seeing, Doing, and Knowing: A Philosophical Theory of Sense-Perception*. Oxford: Clarendon Press.

Matthen, Mohan (2010) "Color Experience: A Semantic Theory," in J. Cohen and M. Matthen (eds.) *Color Science and Color Ontology*. Cambridge MA: MIT Press, 67–90.

Pollock, John (1974) *Knowledge and Justification*. Princeton: Princeton University Press.

Pryor, James (2000) "The Skeptic and the Dogmatist," *Noûs* 34: 517–49.

Rich, Anina N. and Mattingley, Jason B. (2002) "Anomalous Perception in Synaesthesia: A Cognitive Neuroscience Perspective," *Nature Reviews Neuroscience* 3.1: 43–52.

Sagiv, Noam and Robertson, Lynn C. (2005) "Synesthesia and the Binding Problem," in L. C. Robertson and N. Sagiv (eds.) *Synesthesia: Perspectives from Neuroscience* Oxford: Oxford University Press, 90–107.

Siegel, Susanna (2006) "Subject and Object in the Contents of Visual Experience," *Philosophical Review* 115: 355–88.

Smilek, D., Dixon, M. J., Cudahy, C., and Merikle, P. M. (2001) "Synaesthetic Photisms Influence Visual Perception," *Journal of Cognitive Neuroscience* 13: 930–6.

Wager, A. (1999) "The Extra Qualia Problem: Synaesthesia and Representationism," *Philosophical Psychology* 12: 263–81.

9

Can Synaesthesia Present the World as it Really Is?

Michael Sollberger

Can some synaesthetic experiences be treated as veridical perceptual experiences, i.e. as conscious mental states in which worldly objects and their features perceptually appear *as they really are*? Most empirical scientists and philosophers working on synaesthesia answer this question in the negative. Received wisdom has it that synaesthetic experiences, such as 'seeing' sounds as colours or 'hearing' letters as sounds, always involve some form of *error* or misrepresentation. Synaesthetic phenomena are treated either as merely sensational mental states which are not in the business of informing the synaesthete about the actual layout of her environment at all (Segal, 1997: 218), or as illusory or hallucinatory perceptual states which misinform their bearer about her surroundings (Fish, 2010: 132–4; Gray, 2001: 79; Lycan, 2006).

Contrary to this prevailing opinion, Mohan Matthen's 'When is Synaesthesia Perception?' (Chapter 8 of this volume) argues that such a dismissive approach to the epistemic properties of synaesthetic experiences is not mandatory. Matthen claims that there is conceptual room for a more tolerant approach according to which at least one variety of synaesthesia, which he calls *direct synaesthesia*, is epistemically on a par with everyday non-synaesthetic perception. The idea is that direct synaesthesia is free of error at the perceptual level; in addition, direct synaesthetes are said to be in a position to arrive at perceptual knowledge in virtue of their unusual synaesthetic experiences alone. Given our current scientific knowledge on synaesthesia, it is an open empirical question whether some of the synaesthetes around us qualify as direct synaesthetes. But if some of them do, then they would be in an epistemically privileged position vis-à-vis non-synaesthetes, since they would have an additional synaesthetic way of coming to know about the outside world.

Clearly, these are intriguing claims which deserve further attention. I fully agree with Matthen that the *epistemic properties* of synaesthesia have not got the attention they deserve so far. His chapter is a step towards filling in this lacuna. The aim of this short chapter is to evaluate the idea of direct synaesthesia and to assess whether the accepted dogma that synaesthesia is always prone to error has to go.

The central claim of Matthen's chapter is that under certain specific conditions, *synaesthetic experiences can qualify as veridical perceptions.*[1] To get a grip on this claim, we need to know three things: i) the conditions under which a conscious mental state counts as a veridical perceptual experience; ii) the distinctive features of synaesthetic experiences; iii) whether synaesthetic experiences might satisfy the conditions for veridical perception. Let's start with i).

Matthen lays down the following four necessary conditions for veridical perception: a mental state counts as a veridical perceptual experience if it a) is imagistic, b) is of the here and now, c) is true, and d) provides the subject with non-inferential reasons for empirical belief. Summarizing points a) and b), the suggestion is that veridical perceptions are experiences which make the subject directly aware of presently existing worldly objects and their features, such as round tables, rainbows, pieces of music, specific flavours and odours, or what have you. These worldly objects and features experientially appear to be located in outer physical space, and their existence does not seem to be causally or ontologically dependent on the perceiving subject. Much more would have to be said to pinpoint the phenomenological features of veridical perception, to be sure, but for present purposes it is sufficient to work with this rough-and-ready characterization.

The gist of condition c) can be spelled out as follows: for a perceptual experience to count as veridical, worldly things and their properties *really are as they experientially appear to the subject to be.*[2] Leaving subtleties about causation aside, my perceptual experience of, say, a round table in front of me is veridical if the table in front of me is round. It is well known that objects do not always appear as they are. In illusions, objects appear to possess properties they objectively lack, and hallucinations are mental states where the subject seems to be perceptually aware of objects that do not exist here and now. Condition c) ensures that no perceptual state can count as a veridical perception unless worldly objects and their features experientially appear as they are.

Condition d) is linked to condition c) in the following way: a perceptual experience of such-and-such provides the subject with a reason to believe that things are such-and-such. This means that I am usually in a position to form the true belief 'There is a round table in front of me' solely in virtue of perceiving a round table in front of me.[3] This kind of *perceptual reason* for empirical belief is taken to be direct or unmediated

[1] The terms 'veridical perception' and 'veridical perceptual experience' will be used interchangeably throughout this chapter. Also, when talking about perception and perceptual states, I will always be referring to conscious or experiential mental states, i.e. perceptual states there is something it is like for the subject to be in (Nagel, 1974).

[2] Instead of 'true' I use the term 'veridical' for a perceptual experience which presents worldly objects and their features as they really are. This is to mark the contrast with propositions, which are either true or false.

[3] I couch the reason-providing role of perceptual experience in dispositional terms to allow cases where perceptual experiences present the empirical world as it is yet the subject fails to form true beliefs because she is drunk, inattentive, confused, mentally ill, or otherwise cognitively impaired.

in the sense of not being inferential, i.e. not being based upon any kind of psychological or epistemic inference.[4] The idea is intuitively compelling: it is in virtue of seeing the table as round that I directly or non-inferentially form the belief that the table is round. More generally, a subject forms the belief 'O is F' precisely because O looks F to her. As pointed out before, condition c) makes sure that the world is as it perceptually appears. Therefore, if the subject veridically perceives an object O to be F and forms the belief 'O is F' on the basis of the veridical perceptual experience, then her belief usually amounts to perceptual knowledge.

To better understand in what sense such perceptual reasons for belief are distinctively direct or non-inferential, it is instructive to contrast them with an example where reasons might be based upon perception but be inferential. Consider the case of smoke and fire: upon seeing smoke, you might form the true belief that there is a fire. That is, you might come to know that there is a fire in virtue of having a veridical perception of the smoke. Clearly, although one might be willing to call your reason for your fire-belief perceptual or perceptually based, it cannot be non-inferential in the way outlined above. The reason is that you need to activate a connecting state of the kind 'Fire reliably causes smoke' to get from the veridical perception to your belief, 'There is a fire'. It is not necessary that the activation of such an inferential connection holding between two of your mental states is conscious or psychologically salient to you. But it is *epistemically* needed for your fire-belief to count as justified, and that you have the connecting belief also *explains* why you come to think that there is a fire. Summing up, the reason for your fire-belief is epistemically indirect or inferential because it is based upon the perceptual experience plus a further connecting belief. Condition d) is thus not satisfied.

A second contrasting example is this: a diabetic person may come to form the true belief that her body is in a hypoglycaemic state upon feeling dizzy. That is, she might form the justified true belief that the content of glucose in her blood is abnormally diminished in virtue of feeling dizzy. However, just as in the example above, the feeling of dizziness is to be treated as a *sign* for hypoglycaemia, since it is not in virtue of experiencing her blood as having an abnormally diminished glucose content that the diabetic forms the belief that her body is hypoglycaemic. Rather, she already knew that her bodily experiences of dizziness are reliably caused by states of hypoglycaemia. Knowledge of this cause-effect correlation is what enables her to use her feeling of dizziness as a reason to *infer* that her glucose content is diminished, even though this inference needn't be psychologically salient to her. As before, the connecting state has to be *epistemically activated* for the diabetic's belief to be warranted, so the reason for her hypoglycaemia-belief turns out to be inferential.

These examples are meant to show that there is more than one way that perceptual experiences can be said to provide the subject with reasons for empirical belief.

[4] See McNeill (2012) for a discussion of the distinction between psychological and epistemic inference.

According to condition d), what is truly distinctive about veridical perception, however, is that the subject is in a position to form the belief that O is F *solely* in virtue of the fact that she has an experience in which O perceptually looks F to her. The smoke-fire and hypoglycaemia cases are supposed to highlight ways of affording the subject inferential reasons for empirical belief. This is why they are not in line with d).

Certainly, there are alternative ways of characterizing the reason-providing role of perceptual experiences (see Heck, 2000 for a discussion). Furthermore, one may have doubts about whether all of the aforementioned conditions a) to d) are truly necessary, or about whether conditions a) to d) are jointly sufficient for an experience to be conceptualized as a veridical perception.[5] To digress into these discussions here, however, would take us too far afield. My goal is to stay faithful to how I understand Matthen's account, so I will work with conditions a) to d) as specified above. Given this, let's now tackle ii) and see how he conceives of synaesthetic experiences.

There is now ample evidence that synaesthesia is a tremendously *heterogeneous* and idiosyncratic condition. There appear to be considerable biological, behavioural, and experiential differences among people diagnosed with synaesthesia. This means that synaesthetes are not only manifestly different from the general population, but they are also different to each other (Cohen, Chapter 3 of this volume; Deroy and Spence, Chapter 10 of this volume; Simner, 2013; Ward et al., 2007). One should therefore not expect a theory of synaesthesia to apply to all cases of synaesthesia across the board, even if one's analysis is confined to the experiential aspect of synaesthesia alone. Matthen's main argument is in line with this insight, for he concentrates on a particular type of synaesthesia which he calls *direct synaesthesia*. Before spelling out his argument, however, some more words about synaesthesia are in order.

To a first approximation, synaesthetes are people in which 'stimulation of one sensory modality automatically triggers a perception in a second modality, in the absence of any direct stimulation to this second modality' (Harrison and Baron-Cohen, 1997). Although sketchy and incomplete as it stands, this definition captures one key element of synaesthesia: *some sensory qualities are reliably elicited in response to certain stimuli which are not elicited in 'normal' non-synaesthetic subjects.* Visual qualities may be triggered by digits, letters, or words, in either their written (grapheme-colour synaesthesia) or spoken (phoneme-colour synaesthesia) form, and sounds may trigger olfactory qualities in addition to the customary auditory qualities. I will follow common practice and use the terms 'inducer' to refer to the stimulus that triggers the

[5] Some may contend that a veridical perception typically provides guidance for action with respect to worldly objects and their features (Anderson and Rosenberg, 2008). Others may maintain that the causal link between the perceptual experience and its object must be 'appropriate' (Lewis, 1980). Accordingly, the action-guiding role and/or appropriate causation might be taken to present further conditions which are necessary for veridical perception. Be that as it may, I will argue below that 'direct synaesthesia' does not satisfy condition d). If this is correct, then it follows that direct synaesthesia is not an instance of veridical perception regardless of whether the necessary conditions a) to d) are jointly sufficient or not.

synaesthetic experience and 'concurrent' to refer to the synaesthetically induced sensory qualities (Grossenbacher and Lovelace, 2001; see Deroy, in press, for a discussion).

To illustrate direct synaesthesia, Matthen refers to the synaesthete Cynthia.[6] Here is how Cynthia's coloured-hearing synaesthesia is supposed to work: upon hearing middle C, she visually experiences a kind of red patch in addition to the customary auditory experience she has when middle C is played. The redness (the concurrent) is experienced as somehow bound to middle C (the inducer). To be more precise, the concurrent appears to be bound to the *location* in which middle C auditorily appears to be. Moreover, Cynthia does not confuse the concurrent with a normal red entity in her vicinity. That is, she is not inclined to think that there is some red patch in front of her. Finally, the concurrent is taken to betoken the inducer in such a way as to enable Cynthia to directly form the belief that middle C is played upon being synaesthetically aware of redness. According to Matthen, this is possible because awareness of the concurrent provides Cynthia with an unmediated reason to believe that middle C has been sounded.

It is crucial to note that Cynthia is not a *real-world* person whose synaesthesia has been investigated in the lab. However, this does not mean that Cynthia is no more than the leading actress of an eccentric philosophical thought-experiment with no significance for empirical research whatsoever. Rather, Matthen takes Cynthia's direct synaesthesia to highlight a way of characterizing some synaesthetic experiences which sits well with anecdotal reports given by some actual synaesthetes. Hence his suggestion is that we have reason to believe that some real-world synaesthetes are, or at least can be, like Cynthia in relevant experiential and epistemic respects.

Cynthia illustrates what is distinctive of direct synaesthesia: the concurrent appears to be bound to the physical location in which the inducer perceptually appears; the direct synaesthete does not mistake the concurrent for a real property of the inducer; and being aware of the concurrent provides the synaesthete with a non-inferential reason to believe that the inducer is present. Furthermore, Matthen argues that Cynthia is aware of the concurrent as something unreal, similar to a kind of ghostly *after-image* which does not even purport to make the subject perceptually aware of a worldly object. This explains why direct synaesthetes like Cynthia are not inclined to misattribute their concurrents to any worldly object.

These, then, are the main features which Matthen takes to be definitional of direct synaesthesia. What about iii)? Is direct synaesthesia an instance of veridical perception? He claims it is. According to him, direct synaesthesia satisfies a) to d). As far as I understand it, conditions a), b), and c) are meant to be satisfied because direct synaesthetes have a normal perceptual experience which is only *qualitatively enriched*

[6] The discussion of 'Cynthia-examples' in the philosophical literature started with Wager (1999, 2001).

by the concurrent, and the concurrent is bound to the location in which the inducer perceptually appears but does not present direct synaesthetes with new *illusory properties* of empirical objects.[7] Condition d) is satisfied as well because the concurrent provides the synaesthete with a non-inferential reason to believe that the inducer is present. If this is right, then it follows that there is no error involved in direct synaesthesia. So, according to Matthen, the final upshot is that synaesthetic experiences afford direct synaesthetes non-inferential reasons for belief *in just the same way* as do normal experiences.

In the remainder of this chapter, I will focus on what I think are the two most serious difficulties associated with the foregoing argument. My first concern goes as follows: although it is very interesting, Matthen's proposal of comparing concurrents to after-images brings its own problems with it. For instance, it is far from clear whether after-images are ever *experientially* given to the subject *as something unreal* or purely subjective. Phillips (2013) has argued at great length that we are not experientially aware of after-images as sensational entities. Based upon empirical data, he claims instead that after-images can be fully characterized in terms of the ways in which apparent worldly objects and their features are presented to us. After-image experiences are thus entirely *intentional*, i.e. they are in the business of presenting the subject with empirical objects. Thus conceived, after-image experiences are experiences which fail to present the empirical world as it is—i.e., such experiences are always illusory or hallucinatory. Therefore, if concurrents are assimilated to after-images, it follows that there is *error* at the level of perceptual consciousness, and direct synaesthesia cannot, pace Matthen, be of the same species as veridical perception.

For the sake of argument, let's suppose that Phillips is wrong and allow that the subject can be aware of after-images as something purely sensational or unreal (Block, 2003). Does this proposal fare any better than the previous one? On this assumption, one tension that comes to mind is between two ways the concurrent is thought to be experientially given to Cynthia. On the one hand, she is aware of redness as something *unreal* and, let's accept, something purely subjective or sensational. On the other hand, she is also aware of it as *being bound to the physical location* in which the inducer, i.e. the sound middle C, auditorily appears. Given this, the problem is that 'being located in outer physical space' and 'being unreal' are two properties which seem to be incompatible with each other. After all, having a location

[7] It is unclear whether the concurrents are to be treated as qualitative enrichments of normal experiences or whether they count as additional experiences which are autonomous with respect to the normal experience (see Auvray and Deroy, 2014 for a discussion). Matthen opts for the first: the enrichment thesis. Note, however, that there is the case of the blind coloured-hearing synaesthete JF who nevertheless has synaesthetically evoked colour experiences (Steven et al., 2006). At first sight, JF's case seems to strongly support the idea that the concurrents are autonomous with respect to the normal experience. Space precludes a more thoroughgoing discussion of this important topic here.

in physical space is a paradigmatic property of empirical objects. But unreal objects arguably lack this property. So the worry is that concurrents cannot be experienced both as unreal and bound to the inducer-location at the same time.

Against this, Matthen may counter that although objects cannot really instantiate both properties at the same time, it can nonetheless *seem* to us in experience as if they did. I am not sure whether this idea can be made to work. Appearing in some sort of subjective, private mental space seems to me a very good candidate for explaining why after-images are experientially given to the subject as unreal. In any case, much more would have to be said about these issues. For now, I think it is fair to insist that we are owed a story about how it is possible that Cynthia experiences the redness both as unreal and as bound to the physical location in which middle C appears.

My second worry, which is largely independent of the first one, is that Cynthia's synaesthesia-based belief about the inducer fails to satisfy d). To begin with, it is important to realize that Cynthia does not form the belief 'middle C is played' upon having an experience in which middle C *appears as being played*. She is supposed to form that true belief upon being synaesthetically aware of redness, and it is plain that after-image-like redness is not experientially given to her as middle C being played. This is a problem, since it shows that Cynthia's synaesthetic way of arriving at perceptual beliefs must be *fundamentally distinct* from the normal way of arriving at perceptual beliefs, as it was formulated in d).

This is not yet a knockdown objection. For even if Cynthia's reason for belief fails to satisfy d) in some respects, it might still count as truly non-inferential. I take it that this is what Matthen has in mind when he stresses that Cynthia directly forms the belief that middle C is played upon *experiencing redness as a reason to believe that middle C is played*. That is to say, direct synaesthetes are supposed to have reasons to believe that the inducer is present solely in virtue of the fact that the concurrent is experientially given to them *as a reason to believe that the inducer is present*. For the sake of argument, I will admit that this way of forming inducer-related beliefs would count as non-inferential, even though it would obviously differ from the usual reason-providing schema 'One forms the belief that O is F solely in virtue of the fact that O is experientially given to one as F'.

However, I contend that the idea is a non-starter. How could reasons to believe that a particular inducer is present be properties which figure in synaesthetic experiences? It seems plain that properties which are that *cognitively complex* cannot be proper parts of the *experiential* aspect of veridical perceptions. It has been pointed out that a corridor which reliably gives one a strong headache every time one enters it could eventually be experienced as 'headachy' (Farkas, 2013). If so, couldn't reasons to believe that a particular inducer is present be explained along similar lines? The answer is 'No', since headachy-corridor-scenarios are about externalizing experiential properties like headaches which, at first glance, seem to be purely sensational. If anything, examples like the headachy corridor and their cognates might be used to bolster the idea that synaesthetes experience the concurrent as a real feature of the inducer itself.[8] Yet this idea does not fit with Matthen's construal of direct synaesthesia.

Or suppose you are a hard-core liberal about the kinds of properties which can figure in perceptual experiences. As a liberal, you are happy to accept that in addition to low-level properties like shapes, colours, motion, and so on, perceptual experiences can also involve natural kind properties, causal properties, and other high-level categories (Bayne, 2009). But I guess that even for you, accepting that concurrents, which are said to share important experiential features with ghostly after-images, can be experienced as reasons for beliefs about their own inducers would be too extreme. In the end, I just see no way of making sense of the idea that synaesthetes *could be* perceptually aware of the concurrents as reasons to believe that their inducers are present. If we want to hold on to the idea that synaesthetes can somehow form true beliefs about the inducers in virtue of being aware of their concurrents, there must be another story to tell.

Well, I believe there is such a story: Cynthia thinks that the inducer is present because she has learned to associate her concurrents with the inducers through previous encounters. Cynthia knows that the inducer-concurrent pairing is causally reliable. That Cynthia has that connecting belief explains why she comes to think that middle C is played. The scenario is analogous to the fire-smoke and hypoglycaemia examples discussed at the outset: Cynthia cannot non-inferentially form the belief that middle C has been sounded solely on the basis of how the concurrent experientially appears to her. Rather, she can use the concurrent as a *sign* for the presence of the inducer. It is true that Cynthia might have become so familiar with her synaesthesia that she infers the presence of the inducer from the awareness of the concurrent without engaging in any conscious activity. Nevertheless, activating her background knowledge is essential from an epistemic point of view. To sum up: Cynthia's synaesthetically acquired belief must be based upon an epistemic inference because she can neither be perceptually aware of the inducer as such, nor can she be aware of the concurrent as a reason to believe that it is present.

In the long run, this is why I think there is no way for Cynthia to satisfy condition d). Direct synaesthesia is therefore *not* an instance of veridical perception.

Despite this negative conclusion, it is worth noting that Cynthia is still in an epistemically *privileged* position, for she can come to know about the inducers by making appropriate use of her concurrents. This is an idiosyncratic way of coming to know which non-synaesthetes lack. In this respect, then, direct synaesthesia is epistemically *beneficial*, even though the means of arriving at beliefs synaesthetically and non-synaesthetically are fundamentally distinct.

[8] There are synaesthetes, i.e. so-called 'surface-projectors', who report experiencing the concurrents as features of the inducers (Ward et al., 2007). I will not here examine whether corridors that appear headachy and middle Cs that appear red might be explicable in terms of shared underlying mechanisms.

Finally, I would like to stress that although I have argued in this chapter that direct synaesthesia and veridical perception do not belong to the same species, I have argued elsewhere that some instances of synaesthetic experiences might be veridical under certain conditions (Sollberger, 2013). So I share with Matthen the key idea that synaesthetic experiences are not necessarily prone to error.[9] This idea is controversial and may not square with our commonsensical intuitions. But we should not forget that synaesthesia has a long history of being treated with incredulity, prejudice, scorn, or social disbelief (Day, 2005). It is only recently that most researchers have started to acknowledge synaesthesia as a real condition which is worth being investigated in the lab. The currently widespread assumption that synaesthetic experiences must always be illusory or hallucinatory may be just one further prejudice that we have to abandon eventually.

References

Anderson, Michael L., and Gregg Rosenberg. 2008. Content and action: the guidance theory of representation. *The Journal of Mind and Behavior* 29 (1/2): 55–86.

Auvray, Malika, and Ophelia Deroy. 2014. How do synesthetes experience the world? In *Oxford Handbook of Philosophy of Perception*, ed. M. Matthen. Oxford: Oxford University Press.

Bayne, Tim. 2009. Perception and the reach of phenomenal content. *The Philosophical Quarterly* 59 (236): 385–404.

Block, Ned. 2003. Mental paint. In *Reflections and Replies: Essays on the Philosophy of Tyler Burge*, eds. M. Hahn and B. Ramberg. Cambridge, MA: MIT Press.

Day, Sean. 2005. Some demographic and socio-cultural aspects of synesthesia. In *Synesthesia: Perspectives From Cognitive Neuroscience*, eds. L. C. Robertson and N. Sagiv, 11–33. New York: Oxford University Press.

Deroy, Ophelia. in press. Can sounds be red? A new account of synaesthesia as enriched experience. In *Phenomenal Qualities*, eds. P. Coates and S. Coleman. Oxford: Oxford University Press.

Farkas, Katalin. 2013. Constructing a world for the senses. In *Phenomenal Intentionality*, ed. U. Kriegel, 99–115. New York: Oxford University Press.

Fish, William. 2010. *Philosophy of Perception: A Contemporary Introduction*. New York: Routledge.

Gray, Richard. 2001. Cognitive modules, synaesthesia and the constitution of psychological natural kinds. *Philosophical Psychology* 14 (1): 65–82.

Grossenbacher, Peter G., and Christopher T. Lovelace. 2001. Mechanisms of synesthesia: cognitive and physiological constraints. *Trends in Cognitive Sciences* 5 (1): 36–41.

[9] See also Cohen (Chapter 3 of this volume) for the idea that synaesthesia is continuous with normal perception. Note that Cohen's account is not primarily concerned with the experiential dimension of synaesthetic and non-synaesthetic perception. However, his account can be seen as a further contribution to the overall idea that synaesthesia is not as error-prone as it is usually assumed to be.

Harrison, John E., and Simon Baron-Cohen. 1997. Synaesthesia: a review of psychological theories. In *Synaesthesia: Classic and Contemporary Readings*, eds. S. Baron-Cohen and J. E. Harrison, 109–22. Oxford: Blackwell.

Heck, Richard G. Jr. 2000. Nonconceptual content and the 'space of reason'. *The Philosophical Review* 109 (4): 483–523.

Lewis, David. 1980. Veridical hallucination and prosthetic vision. *Australasian Journal of Philosophy* 58 (3): 239–49.

Lycan, William. 2006. Representational theories of consciousness. In *The Stanford Encyclopedia of Philosophy*, ed E. N. Zalta, <http://plato.stanford.edu/archives/win2006/entries/consciousness-representational/>.

McNeill, W. E. S. 2012. On seeing that someone is angry. *European Journal of Philosophy* 20 (4): 575–97.

Nagel, Thomas. 1974. What is it like to be a bat? *The Philosophical Review* 83 (4): 435–50.

Phillips, Ian. 2013. Afterimages and sensation. *Philosophy and Phenomenological Research* 87 (2): 417–53.

Segal, Gabriel M. A. 1997. Synaesthesia: implications for modularity of mind. In *Synaesthesia: Classic and Contemporary Readings*, eds. S. Baron-Cohen and J. E. Harrison, 211–23. Oxford: Blackwell.

Simner, Julia. 2013. Why are there different types of synesthete? *Frontiers in Psychology* 4 (558): doi: 10.3389/fpsyg.2013.00558.

Sollberger, Michael. 2013. Rethinking synesthesia. *Philosophical Psychology* 26 (2): 171–87.

Steven, Megan S., Peter C. Hansen, and Colin Blakemore. 2006. Activation of color selective areas of visual cortex in a blind synesthete. *Cortex* 42 (2): 304–8.

Wager, Adam. 1999. The extra qualia problem: synaesthesia and representation. *Philosophical Psychology* 12 (3): 263–81.

Wager, Adam. 2001. Synaesthesia misrepresented. *Philosophical Psychology* 14 (3): 347–51.

Ward, Jamie, Ryan Li, Shireen Salih, and Noam Sagiv. 2007. Varieties of grapheme-colour synaesthesia: a new theory of phenomenological and behavioural differences. *Consciousness and Cognition* 16: 913–31.

PART III

Boundaries of Synaesthesia: Unconscious, Acquired, and Social Varieties of Sensory Unions

10

Questioning the Continuity Claim

What Difference Does Consciousness Make?

Ophelia Deroy and Charles Spence

In the present state of our knowledge we are not in a position to offer any satisfactory explanation of this singular anomaly of vision. That its seat is not in the eye but in the sensorium is however most probable.

(White Cooper, 1852: 1462, on synaesthesia)

10.1 Introduction

Are high-pitched sounds bright or dark? Our spontaneous response will certainly be to find them bright, although we know that such sounds do not literally have brightness, nor do we necessarily believe that they are regularly accompanied by bright visual stimuli. We also consider high-pitched sounds as going together better with higher spatial elevations than sounds having a lower pitch, once again without any subjectively good reason. What's more, certain vowels, like 'i' or 'e', will make us think of smaller, brighter, and more angular objects, especially if accompanied by the right consonants (Köhler, 1929, 1947; Sapir, 1929; Ramachandran and Hubbard, 2001; see also Aveyard, 2012; Nielsen and Rendall, 2011, 2013; Figure 10.1).

These connections between apparently disconnected sensory dimensions, such as pitch and brightness or speech sounds and shapes, are by no means isolated: We also agree on some consistent pairings of musical notes and odours, colours and pieces of music, or flavours and speeds.[1] This range of sensory combinations does not seem to have much in common except for the fact that they seem, at least initially, arbitrary: They do not seem to be explained by the regular associations of properties in objects or events, or in the environment (but see Parise et al., 2014, on the pitch and elevation correspondence). In this respect, they differ from the other well-documented cross-modal matchings between felt and seen shapes, or certain sounds and visual textures,

[1] See Deroy, Crisinel, and Spence (2013) and Spence (2011) for reviews.

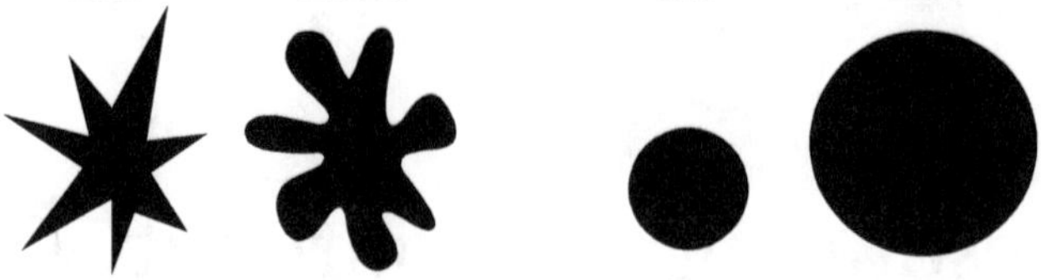

Figure 10.1. People consistently match meaningless speech words, such as 'kiki' or 'mil', with angular and small visual shapes (see Köhler, 1929, 1947; Sapir, 1929; Ramachandran and Hubbard, 2001). These crossmodal correspondences also appear in the literature on 'sound symbolism'.

which can be explained by an obvious common physical property or regularity that is present 'out there' in the environment. The distinctively surprising character of certain crossmodal matches explains why they have been singled out as 'crossmodal correspondences', referencing the poetic and mystical notion of correspondences inherited from Baudelaire and Swedenborg (see Wilkinson, 1996). At that time, and even more nowadays, it has become usual to link our sensitivity to these surprising crossmodal matchings to an unusual union of the senses, or synaesthesia. That crossmodal correspondences have sometimes been referred to as 'synaesthetic associations' (Parise and Spence, 2008; Wagner and Dobkins, 2011; see also Gallace and Spence, 2006) and 'synaesthetic correspondences' (Braaten, 1993; Martino and Marks, 2000; Melara and O'Brien, 1987; Parise and Spence, 2009; Walker et al., 2010) could be innocuous, if the terminology did not mean that correspondences were therefore related to other cases also known as synaesthesia, where the presentation of a stimulus is not simply matched to another sensory element but induces an additional atypical experience as well. Cases of crossmodal correspondences have also been documented alongside such cases, without a clear distinction, and labelled 'synaesthesia' *tout court* (Calkins, 1893), or 'synaesthetic thinking' (Karwoski et al., 1942; Odbert et al., 1942). Certainly, whether crossmodal correspondences and conscious cases of synaesthesia deserve to be related should not be left to terminological choices, or to the broad meaning of a 'union of the senses'. The arbitrariness of an audiovisual correspondence between pitch and brightness can perhaps easily make one think of stranger cases of coloured-hearing synaesthesia, whereby certain auditory stimuli elicit unusual visual experiences of colours. In both cases, an auditory element is matched or associated in a surprising way with a visual element.

Is the relation between crossmodal correspondences and synaesthesia so straightforward and unproblematic, though? The seemingly similar surprising character of synaesthetic experiences and crossmodal correspondences and the difficulty of finding a satisfactory explanation for the presence of synaesthetic experiences in some individuals mean that many researchers have turned to correspondences as a possibly common root for both of these phenomena, and see them as part of a broader family of synaesthetic tendencies. However, one should not forget that the legitimacy of synaesthesia as a genuine condition has been won by establishing its difference from other arbitrary associations: Reports of surprising associations and experiences between sensory features, such as the ones coming from the seventy-six college students who reported forms or colours associated with numbers, letters, and sounds in Mary Calkins' (1893) article, were for long not seen as sufficient to recognize a special condition of 'synaesthesia', as they could manifest a mere tendency to associate sensory features in a seemingly arbitrary manner (which is the case in crossmodal correspondences). The so-called 'consistency test', which was originally introduced more than a century ago (Holden, 1885; see also Jordan, 1917) and which is still used today in different variants to screen for synaesthesia (Baron-Cohen, Wyke, and Binnie, 1987; see also Asher et al., 2006), is meant to build on the hypothesized difference between mere associations and synaesthesia: Only those individuals who have systematic synaesthetic conscious experiences (or concurrents) when presented with letters can provide fast, precise, and consistent responses about their letter-colour associations, whereas those who have simply memorized such associations are likely to be less consistent, slower, and less specific. In other words, if it is the conscious manifestation that makes synaesthetes special,[2] it seems inappropriate to confuse them with individuals who don't have this kind of conscious manifestation.

The scientific respectability of synaesthesia as a distinct psychological kind therefore pulls in opposite directions: towards differentiation, as synaesthesia needs to be contrasted with crossmodal correspondences for its distinct conscious manifestation; and towards assimilation, as synaesthesia seems related to crossmodal correspondences because of its origins and contents. An increasingly popular tendency, and a seemingly reasonable way in which to reconcile differentiation and assimilation, is to consider synaesthesia as a continuum, with distinctively conscious cases representing one extreme end of a tendency that is present in everyone (see Figure 10.2a). In this way, these rare conscious cases remain different, but they can share the same underlying mechanism, and explanation, as the more widespread crossmodal correspondences. The hypothesis of a synaesthetic continuum has either been explicitly embraced or else implicitly endorsed by a number of researchers following Martino and Marks' (2001) suggestion that crossmodal correspondences constitute a form of 'weak synaesthesia' while the canonical cases of conscious synaesthesia constitute a form of 'strong synaesthesia'. However, the consequences of acknowledging a genuine continuum, with individual cases varying from weaker to stronger, rather than a

[2] In Baron-Cohen, Harrison, Goldstein, and Wyke's (1993) study, individuals who were pre-selected on the basis of their questionnaire results as coloured-hearing synaesthetes gave a mean of 90 per cent identical reports of their colour experiences elicited by words when retested a year later. This robust pattern of results was observed even in the absence of any previous warning that they were going to be retested. By contrast, the reports of a control group retested, with warning, after just a month only matched their original choice for 30–40 per cent of the stimuli.

strictly bipolar distribution, with individuals being either weak or strong synaesthetes but no one falling in the middle, are rarely considered.

There is more than one reason to want to examine this question in greater detail. A central motivation is certainly to decide on whether we should all be counted as synaesthetes (Cohen, Chapter 3 of this volume; but see Deroy and Spence, 2013a). This question also goes to the heart of how much difference consciousness makes, or at least how much difference we are ready to grant to consciousness. What happens when the most relevant difference between two sets of cases amounts to differences in consciousness? Are differences in conscious manifestation sufficient to recognize a discontinuity between the two sets of cases, or should a difference in conscious manifestation be considered too subjective and variable a difference? Can we conclude that a single condition is at stake, with a conscious and unconscious side, and can we make sense of intermediate cases? Raised in the abstract, these questions might end up being too general, and the case of synaesthesia might here help in getting a better grip on them, and deliver some more specific conclusions on the status of consciousness (e.g., Ward et al., 2007; see also Myrtopolos and Ro, Chapter 5 of this volume).

The current state of knowledge is insufficient to conclude that synaesthesia and crossmodal correspondences are identical in terms of their function, content, or neurological implementation: As detailed in section 10.2, even when good evidence has been obtained, it reveals similarities that can lead to conflicting interpretations

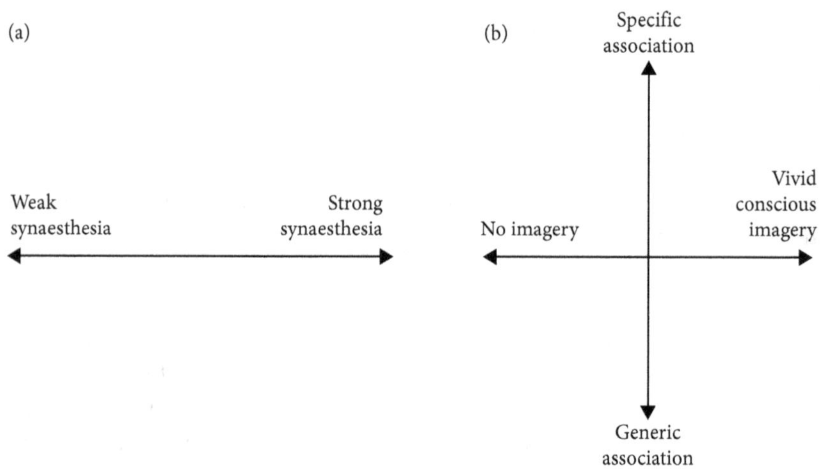

Figure 10.2. Two ways of recognizing a continuity between cases of non-conscious crossmodal matchings known as crossmodal correspondences and cases of systematic unusual conscious experiences known as synaesthesia: (a) Inherited from Martino and Marks (2001), this view merely acknowledges that a shared mechanism can lead continuously from non-conscious matchings all the way through to conscious joint experiences; (b) Adapted from Rader and Tellegen (1987), the latter view postulates two dimensions of variation (specificity and the vividness of concurrent).

and verdicts. One interpretation, examined in section 10.3, is that the differences between canonical cases of synaesthesia and crossmodal correspondences are due to the strength or degree that one occupies on a synaesthetic continuum: The main challenge for this hypothesis is, then, to identify the dimension, or dimensions, along which individuals should gradually differ from one end of this synaesthetic continuum to the other (see Figure 10.2).

The hypothesis of a synaesthetic continuum also needs to demonstrate that cases are distributed in an even manner, without gaps or clusters that might suggest some kind of discontinuity of processing. Section 10.4 reviews a range of conscious cases that would appear to constitute the best candidates for being intermediate between the mere intuitions and behavioural effects highlighted in the cases of crossmodal correspondences and the striking cases of systematically induced conscious synaesthesia. The evidence, as we argue below, still falls some way short of demonstrating the existence of a synaesthetic continuum. Rather, what is shown are some clusters of criteria which the continuum hypothesis seemingly cannot account for. In section 10.5, and to conclude, the continuity hypothesis seems to miss some important discontinuities between the cases at stake: The conscious manifestations which characterize synaesthesia cannot be reconciled with other occasional manifestations observed with crossmodal correspondences.

10.2 The synaesthetic continuum hypothesis

According to many researchers, there is room to believe that the very same cross- or intra-modal matching process is at stake in those individuals usually known as synaesthetes who report vivid and specific conscious experiences when presented with specific stimuli and in those who only report more general feelings of congruence between pairs of stimuli, either physically present, or merely imagined (e.g., Bien et al., 2012; Ludwig et al., 2011; Mulvenna and Walsh, 2006; Sagiv and Ward, 2006). Tracing things back, this idea would appear to derive from an influential review paper published by Martino and Marks back in 2001 in which the authors attempted to distinguish between weak and strong forms of synaesthesia. According to the latter researchers: 'Strong synaesthesia is characterized by a vivid image in one sensory modality in response to stimulation in another one. Weak synaesthesia is characterized by cross-sensory correspondences expressed through language, perceptual similarity and perceptual interactions during information processing' (Martino and Marks, 2001: 61). This claim implies that the strong (or what we suggest to call 'canonical') form of synaesthesia and what is more often called crossmodal correspondences constitute a single psychological kind, and suggests that they lie on the opposite ends of one and the same continuum: These authors go on to conclude that, 'in both types of synesthesia, cross-modal correspondences are evident, suggesting that the neural processes underlying strong and weak synesthesia, although not wholly identical, nonetheless may have a common core' (Martino and Marks, 2001: 62).[3]

According to Deroy and Spence (2013a), the claim that sensory associations and canonical synaesthesia constitute a single psychological kind comes from rather superficial resemblances: Both look arbitrary and resistant to straightforward explanations in terms of learning from the statistics of the environment. Three less superficial criteria are typically used in philosophy—sometimes in conjunction, sometimes independently—to decide whether two sets of mental states or processes deserve to be grouped into a single kind: To belong to the same mental kind, the states under examination should present the same function, contents, and/or underlying process. To check whether crossmodal correspondences and canonical synaesthesia satisfy these three criteria, it is probably simpler to restrict the discussion to two well-documented examples involving the same sensory modalities; that is, a typical case of audiovisual correspondence, such as pitch-brightness, and a typical case of conscious synaesthesia, such as coloured hearing.

10.2.1 The functional criterion

The idea that a similarity in mental kind should derive from a similarity in function dominates the fields of philosophy and cognitive science: States that belong to the same psychological kind are those serving the same role, and taking similar inputs to compute them in a similar manner. They also lead to similar outputs (see Levinson, 2013, for a review). What the functional criterion requires, and what we need to examine, is whether the crossmodal correspondences between pitch and brightness and coloured hearing are functionally equivalent; that is, they take similar inputs and lead to similar outputs. Is such a claim empirically verified?

The similarities in behavioural outputs are often stressed by the supporters of the continuity claim, noticeably because of similar Stroop-like interference effects having been documented when the two dimensions or features that are associated happen to be presented together. For instance, people are comparatively slower to identify a dark visual target when it happens to be accompanied by a high-pitched sound rather than by a low-pitched sound (Ludwig et al., 2011; see also Walker and Smith, 1984); coloured-hearing synaesthetes are comparatively slower to identify the inducer when accompanied by a colour that happens to be different from their synaesthetic concurrent than when the synaesthetically congruent colour is presented (e.g., Mills, 1999).

Concluding that there is a similarity of behavioural outputs, however, is the result of a biased perspective: It is by no means clear that the Stroop-like interference effects that have been documented in those individuals with the conscious form of

[3] The word 'type' is a bit confusing here, if it is taken as a synonym of 'kind': The continuum hypothesis presented here recognizes that crossmodal correspondences and canonical cases of conscious synaesthesia are two forms or extremes of a single psychological kind or type.

synaesthesia are of the same kind as those demonstrated by others given the underdetermined nature of the interference effects, which can be grounded in a conflict in experience or in decisional processes (see MacLeod, 1991, for a review). In coloured hearing, the interference is likely to be perceptual in nature: The presentation of a musical note, middle C say, elicits a conscious experience of a specific colour, let's say red, and the experience of red interferes with the synaesthete's capacity to identify the colour that has been presented. The difference in reaction time, then, corresponds to the need to attend to a different content of experience—not the synaesthetically induced red, but the physically present colour. With the pitch-brightness correspondence, however, the interference is less likely to be perceptual in nature: If the presentation of a high-pitched sound is insufficient to elicit a conscious experience of a bright surface, there is no reason to believe that one's slower response to a dark surface results from the need to attend to this physically presented dark surface, and ignore the other bright visual content. The interference here is likely to be semantic and decisional in nature.[4]

Even if one considers that these differences are not evidenced by the behavioural results that have been documented to date, and accepts that the two outputs are really of the same kind, this similarity is still insufficient to conclude that there is a similarity in function, because of the potential confound regarding inputs. Experiments using Stroop-interference focus on a narrow set of cases where two inputs are present: The protocol relies on the joint presentation of the visual and auditory stimuli, for instance a dark visual surface and a high-pitched sound, or a coloured surface and a musical note. What is crucial, though, in the case of coloured hearing and canonical cases of synaesthesia is that interference effects will also occur when *only one* of the stimuli is present. To the best of our knowledge, this has only been tested with coloured numbers, as Dixon and colleagues have shown that the presentation of a colour patch, one that happens to be incongruent with a synaesthete's colour-number pairing, would slow down the speed with which the synaesthete could name the numerical result of a simple arithmetic operation (Dixon et al., 2000). That is, the presence of one element (the colour) is sufficient to prime the second and interfere with the processing or naming of the second element (the number) even if the latter is not physically present. Similarly, the presentation of a colour patch should interfere with one's ability to name the forthcoming note of a well-known melody, even if the sound is not physically present. More importantly, the presentation of a single element might be sufficient to lead to a variety of facilitatory outcomes in memory and visual search (Pritchard et al., 2013; Rich and Karstoft, 2013; Rothen et al., 2012; but see Rothen and Meier, 2009).

In the area of crossmodal correspondences, evidence regarding the presentation of a single dimension, and the effects on the processing of the second associated

[4] One cannot exclude the possibility that mental images interfere with the task and compete for the participant's attention.

dimension, are more nuanced. There is, for instance, no evidence that presenting a bright surface impacts the further processing of sounds of varying pitch. The closest cases have been documented in exogenous spatial cuing tasks (Chiou and Rich, 2012), where the crossmodal correspondence between high (low) pitch and high (low) elevation modulates the orienting of spatial attention. Another example here comes from versions of the Implicit Association Task, where the successive presentation of stimuli has been shown to lead to faster responses when 'corresponding' stimuli happen to have been paired with the same response key (Parise and Spence, 2012).

Looking, then, at the input-output function, all of the available evidence would appear to converge in defining coloured hearing as a case in which the presence of one input (the auditory inducer) leads to an additional conscious output (the visual concurrent) along with the conscious auditory one. By contrast, the crossmodal correspondence between pitch and brightness constitutes a case in which the joint presence of two inputs (a sound and a visual stimulus) modulates the processing of distinct visual and auditory outputs, leaving the conscious character and content of both experiences unaffected.

10.2.2 The content criterion

The discovery of so-called 'common trends' among synaesthetes on the one hand, and between synaesthetes and non-synaesthetes on the other, has led to a profound change in theorizing about synaesthesia (see Deroy and Spence, 2013a, b, for recent reviews). This brings us to the second criterion, i.e. the similarity of content. To be relevant, the notion of content here needs to be adjusted to fit the pair of contents which characterize crossmodal correspondences, the key argument being that the correlation of elements that figure in crossmodal correspondences such as between brightness and pitch, for instance, is also present in canonical cases of synaesthesia.

For many years, researchers had thought that synaesthetic repertoires were highly idiosyncratic. Recently, however, it has been shown that the associations reported by synaesthetes converge on the same specific associations between inducers and conscious concurrents (for instance, A, red, B, blue, C, yellow, to name but a few for coloured-grapheme cases). Synaesthetic pairings have also been shown to be broadly consistent with the rules of pairings that apply across sensory dimensions in non-synaesthetes, for instance between higher-pitched sounds and brighter visual targets (e.g., Evans and Treisman, 2010). Large-scale studies of the visual concurrents that are elicited by higher-pitched sounds in synaesthetes are of generally brighter colours and more angular shapes (e.g., Cohen Kadosh et al., 2007; Zigler, 1930). Indeed, when Ward et al. (2006) compared a group of individuals identified as synaesthetes with controls, they were led to the conclusion that there were indeed certain similarities between their hue-to-timbre mappings.

The criterion of content, though, is not entirely satisfied given the difference between generic and specific contents: Most of the commonalities tested do hold not between specific objects or properties (such as a bright crimson patch or a middle C) but between dimensions common to all the sensory experiences occurring in a certain modality (such as brightness for visual experiences and pitch for sounds). The specific contents of the association, like the experience of a bright crimson red and middle C, remain idiosyncratic (see also Elias et al., 2003). As such, the large-scale studies are compatible with the fact that synaesthetes and non-synaesthetes share the same crossmodal mappings, but that conscious synaesthesia implies a further conscious specification of content which is present only in very few individuals and remains idiosyncratic.[5]

10.2.3 *The neurological criterion*

As documented above, neither the functionalist nor the content criterion straightforwardly leads to the conclusion that crossmodal correspondences, such as between brightness and pitch, and synaesthetic cases, such as coloured hearing, belong to one and the same psychological kind. Although these criteria dominate the philosophical literature, the key criterion used in the debates on the continuity between synaesthesia and crossmodal correspondences is one that philosophers have often criticized, or even abandoned. According to this physicalist criterion, similarities in the physical (that is, neurological) implementation count as evidence that processes belong to the same mental kind. Is there evidence, then, of a similar neural basis underlying canonical synaesthesia and crossmodal correspondences?

The range of regions involved in synaesthesia (see Rouw et al., 2011, Yokoyama et al., 2014) and the individual differences between synaesthetes (Hubbard et al., 2005; Rouw and Scholte, 2010) and kinds of synaesthesia (Novich et al., 2011) make the comparison with crossmodal correspondences difficult. Focusing on localization, the evidence concerns only overlapping areas, and does not entirely satisfy the physicalist demand: Both synaesthesia and crossmodal correspondences can be disturbed by the application of transcranial magnetic stimulation over overlapping brain areas. Specifically, a disturbance of colour-grapheme synaesthesia has been reported following the disruption of neural activity in the right parieto-occipital junction (Muggleton et al., 2007). By contrast, disturbance of the crossmodal correspondence between pitch and size in a study by Bien et al. (2012) targeted the intraparietal sulcus instead (see Spence and Parise, 2012).

The idea of a single neurological profile has also been defended in connection with the claim that synaesthesia results from some form of hyper-connectivity, and from a lack of pruning of abundant connections that are present at birth (Maurer et al., 2013; see Deroy and Spence, 2013b, for a critical discussion of this idea). This hypothesis

[5] Several recent studies have examined these similarities in contents: Simner et al. (2005), for example, reported commonalities between the colour-grapheme associations reported by synaesthetes and non-synaesthetes. What is more, and contrary to the visual or audiovisual cases presented here, it is difficult to find correspondences whose contents echo some particularly rare forms of synaesthesia: That is, people do not spontaneously associate words and colours, or proper names and tastes, whereas word-colour and word-taste synaesthesia have been documented (Day, 2005).

makes room for differences in the degree of pruning, and therefore of synaesthesia. What still needs to be provided, though, is support for the idea that there is a continuously graded pruning between the individuals in a given population, leaving them with a continuum of synaesthetic connections.

10.2.4 Interim conclusions

The review of the existing evidence and our review of the criteria that are used to individuate mental kinds outlined here deliver a mixed verdict with regard to the hypothesis that crossmodal correspondences, such as those between pitch and brightness, and conscious cases documented as synaesthesia, such as coloured hearing, form a single mental kind. The hypothesis only holds if one is willing to recognize that some documented differences—in the outputs, the specificity of contents, and the neurological profile—are insufficient to draw a distinction between different kinds of processes. While these differences can simply be ignored, a better way is then to relate them to differences in degrees or strength in the manifestation of a single condition.

10.3 Refining the conscious continuum hypothesis

10.3.1 A continuum of specificity and vividness

One way to reconcile differences between crossmodal correspondences and canonical synaesthesia is to read these differences as a sign of a continuum of variations, where correspondences and synaesthesia are distributed along certain key dimensions. Rader and Tellegen (1987) were, to our knowledge, the first to argue that the difference between generic and specific associations for certain pairs of sensory contents, detailed in section 10.2.2, was to be considered not as a dichotomy but as a space of variation: Generic pairings of pitch and brightness would gradually evolve into more and more specific associations, and finally into the kind of sound-colour associations characteristic of canonical synaesthesia. This claim, which was not found so attractive at the time, finds some support in the recent surveys showing that, on average, synaesthetic associations respect the generic correspondence whereby higher-pitched sounds are paired with brighter visual objects. However, the claims go further than seeing a connection and claims that individual associations would be continuously distributed on a continuum of growing specificity: Does this growing specificity mean that individuals have a few and then more and more specific associations up until they reach a full synaesthetic repertoire for all the notes and timbres? Or does it mean instead that their whole repertoire would have more and more specific contents, for instance having more and more specific hues and saturation along with more and more specific levels of brightness for notes, corresponding to more and more distinctive sounds? The response was not clear in Rader and

Tellegen's (1987) original paper but the two interpretations can make sense of a continuous dimension of variation.

Rader and Tellegen (1987) also recognized the need for another dimension of variation, regarding this time the vividness of the conscious experience elicited in the presence of a single stimulus. This dimension combined with the previous one allows one to construct a two-dimensional space, as represented in Figure 10.2b. The second axis meant that while some individuals would have no visual concurrent experience or else a non-vivid one when presented with a sound, others would have a very vivid visual concurrent experience (see also Domino, 1989).

However, the notion of a continuum of vividness proves more difficult than the notion of a continuum of specificity. The word 'vividness' is often used in the literature on synaesthesia or mental imagery, but remains difficult to define, as authors often resort to contrast and metaphors to capture it: They talk about a 'distinctive and strong' aspect of perceptual experience (Campana and Tallon-Baudry, 2013: 1053), or like William James, about the fact that mental images are 'devoid of pungency and tang' (James, 1890). The very idea of a continuous variation of vividness suggests that consciousness is not an on-and-off phenomenon but comes as a matter of degree—a claim which is rather controversial (see Kouider et al., 2010; Overgaard et al., 2006; Sergent and Dehaene, 2004).

A more important question is to know how to reconcile the idea that vividness changes continuously by degrees with the idea of that synaesthetic concurrents are never taken for mental images: According to reports, synaesthetic concurrents are subjectively indiscriminable from other contents of perceptual experience. Is there then one tipping point where the vividness of the experience crucially determines whether it is imagistic or perceptual? Doesn't the continuum hypothesis require a grey area in the middle, and does it mean that the conscious manifestation of mental imagery and of perception might blur, at least for some? Isn't maintaining a subjectively manifest difference functional to tell dreams and imaginations apart from reality (e.g., Symons, 1993)?

One problem here comes from the fact that synaesthetes maintain such a difference between their perceptual and imagistic experiences, in other sensory domains: Although they report more vivid mental imagery (Barnett and Newell, 2008), they do not report mental images to be perceptually real outside the narrow set of experiences which constitute their synaesthesia.

General explanations, such as the fact that mental imagery and perception share neural representations (Cichy et al., 2012)[6] and that a high degree of overlap or activity could then explain the similarities between their manifestations (Jones et al., 2011), would predict that synaesthetes with colour concurrents would also confuse

[6] However, differences in contents between visual imagery and visual perception have also been found (Arterberry et al., 2002).

mental images of colours with perceptual experiences, outside their synaesthetic repertoire (see Craver-Lemley and Reeves, 2013, for discussion).

Taking number-space as an example, there is now growing evidence to suggest that this hypothesis could be valid and that at least some of the individuals classified as number-space synaesthetes might just have a particularly vivid and consistent form of spatial imagery, which can be tested for independently (see Price, 2009). Price has, for instance, demonstrated that many of those participants identified as 'number-space' synaesthetes because of their spontaneous subjective reports of experiencing numbers in space can be made to perform in a manner that is similar to other participants with particularly vivid visual mental imagery in congruent and incongruent imagery instructions. Price goes on to suggest that instead of synaesthesia, odd case reports of seeing numbers in space could perhaps be explained in terms of 'the interaction between (i) a predisposition for exaggerated and sometimes distorted spatial coding of numerical or temporal sequences, and (ii) the strong visual imagery needed to make these representations salient and explicit' (Price, 2009: 1239).

However, a couple of neuroimaging studies have suggested a difference, in a given visual-olfactory synaesthete, between synaesthetic experiences and vivid imagery episodes (Chan et al., 2014). Another difference, documented by Van Leeuwen et al. (2010), shows that synaesthetic experiences differ from mental images as they do not show a BOLD suppression effect after the repeated presentation of the stimulus. Whereas all neural responses tend to show adaptation effects and be lowered when the stimulus is repeated with very short intervals (e.g., Grill-Spector et al., 1999), mental imagery and perception have been shown to be associated with different patterns of adaptation (i.e., N170/VPP enhancement for imagery but suppression for perception) which makes them distinguishable using ERP (Ganis and Schendan, 2008). Adaptation is therefore likely to provide a robust criterion with which to distinguish between imagery and synaesthetic occurrences. What is more, the criterion could also help to draw a distinction between the synaesthetic experience and the perceptual experience of the same element as synaesthetic concurrents apparently do not show brightness contrast or chromatic adaptation effects, contrary to normal perception (Hong and Blake, 2008). Altogether, this evidence argues against the idea that one could bridge synaesthetic experiences and mental imagery only through an increase in subjective vividness, without missing important underlying discontinuities.

The conclusion also applies to those solutions which consider that the difference between less vivid mental images and more vivid perceptual experience actually maps onto differences in degrees regarding the strength of belief they generated. Hume, who famously considered that conscious experiences could be broadly ranked according to their degree of vividness, certainly meant by this that they would force themselves onto belief with different degrees of strength (Hume, 1739/2000): Perceptual experiences, which are supposed to be very vivid, demand to be taken to be true and actual, whereas imagined or remembered experiences are less vivid, not taken to be actual, and less spontaneously taken to be true. Synaesthetes and non-synaesthetes could be on a continuum regarding the degree of belief they grant to certain experiences, but there would be a distinction between cases where the degree of belief is justified and where it is not.

The idea of a continuous variation ranging from less to more vivid experiences remains hard to convert into robust measurable variations.

10.3.2 A three-dimensional space of variation

As the hypothesis of a continuum of vividness remains difficult to assess, we would recommend adding other dimensions to account for the variations in conscious manifestations. One obvious difference here consists of a difference in the *frequency* of conscious manifestations: Only a few individuals report experiencing a conscious concurrent every time a certain stimulus is presented, one they find impossible to turn off. The other manifestations, if any, seem then to be less frequent, which suggests that, if there is a continuum, it should vary from very rare to very frequent, all the way up to systematic conscious manifestations.

Several authors have underscored that the idea that synaesthesia needs to be consistent over long periods of time should perhaps be relaxed (e.g., Simner, 2012). This relaxation can, though, go in two ways: The conscious concurrent might not always be a consistent content (varying, for example, from red on one occasion to brown on another), or there could not always be a certain content. Individuals would not only differ regarding the specificity of the content but also regarding the frequency of conscious occurrences.

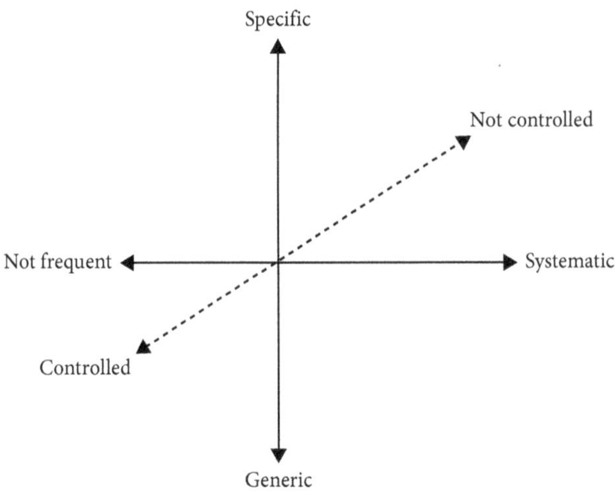

Figure 10.3. An alternative hypothesis positing that variations between crossmodal correspondences and synaesthesia vary along three dimensions (specificity, frequency, and control of the concurrent(s)).

Another dimension is needed here to account for the change in contents, as well as the occurrence of a conscious concurrent. It relates to the fact that the occurrence and content of the concurrent experience might be more or less under the individual's control: Whereas some individuals can suppress their conscious experience or change its contents, some just can't help having one. The involuntariness of synaesthesia is here very different from certain kinds of mental imagery (see Spence and Deroy, 2013, for a discussion).

With these two new dimensions in mind, we can schematically represent the hypothesis of a continuous 'space' of synaesthesia as shown in Figure 10.3:

10.4 Reviewing the evidence

Below, we review some of the evidence that has been taken to suggest that crossmodal correspondences, and sensory associations in general, can occasionally give rise to conscious concurrents, and we examine whether they present the sort of continuous variations that would be needed to support the continuum hypothesis. Thinking in terms of the three dimensions mentioned above, we will focus on two cases which potentially exist across a vast number of individuals: reports of olfactorily induced taste experiences, which have been claimed to be a universal phenomenon, and visual or proprioceptive sensations elicited in many people when they listen to music.

10.4.1 Frequency

The hypothesis of a continuum seems to posit that conscious concurrents vary in terms of their frequency, from those individuals who always have a conscious experience in one sensory modality when presented with a stimulus in another, to those individuals who have it on an occasional basis, all the way down to individuals who might almost never have a conscious experience of the sort. Music-induced visual concurrents provide just such an instance: Besides coloured-hearing synaesthetes who report systematic visual experiences when listening to specific notes, some people report occasional conscious experiences, whereby the sound of a flute produces the sensation of intense azure blue or of the French horn, purple (e.g., Krohn, 1892: 22), or where a certain melody traces a line going 'upward' or evokes a 'beautiful landscape' (Juslin and Västfjäll, 2008). Musical imagery is widely used as therapy, and conscious experiences are frequently reported in the study of these therapies (see Gold et al., 2009, for a review). Cases documented as synaesthesia appear similar to or at least only a step removed from these conscious concurrents experienced by many individuals in terms of their frequency.

One other area to look at first would perhaps be the induction of conscious taste concurrents by certain smells. Tastes, by which we mean gustatory sensations or oral-somatosensory sensations, are frequently reported in association with the presentation of orthonasal odours: Certain smells are reported as being sweet, sour, salty, and bitter (note that, strictly speaking, these are all taste-attributes; Stevenson and

Boakes, 2004), fat-like (an oral-somatosensory sensation, with a taste component; Sundqvist, Stevenson, and Bishop, 2006), or thick and viscous (a tactile attribute; see Stevenson and Mahmut, 2011). Stevenson and Tomiczek (2007) have argued that such cases correspond to the induction of taste or texture concurrents by smells, and could therefore provide an unrecognized example of a universal form of synaesthesia. This contrasts with what is found elsewhere in the literature: Day (2005), for example, only found one case of smell-to-taste synaesthesia from his set of self-reported cases; thus, to the extent that his list is representative, giving it an incidence of 0.1 per cent of all cases of synaesthesia. Stevenson and Tomiczek's synaesthetic hypothesis is meant to make sense of other documented phenomena, besides the use of taste (gustatory) and tactile adjectives to characterize olfactory stimuli: for instance, why certain odorants (e.g., vanilla) can enhance the perceived sweetness of specific solutions (e.g., see Djordjevic et al., 2004; Spence, 2012). The existence of consciously experienced tastes along with the presentation of olfactory stimuli is supposed to explain why orthonasal olfaction influences the perception of sweetness in foods and beverages. However, a non-phenomenally conscious representation could presumably have the same effect.

Cases such as musical imagery or smell-induced tastes might bring support to the idea that a certain crossmodal association could lead to more or less frequent conscious manifestations. One problem with these conscious phenomena, though, is that no precise quantification of their exact frequency has yet been reported, and it is plausible that the variations in frequencies are not evenly distributed on a continuum.

10.4.2 Specific and generic contents

Reflecting on the previous cases, it is important to see whether the conscious concurrents that are reported are always specific: Cases of musical imagery here resemble the kind of concurrents that have been documented in coloured hearing or seem even more specific (with full scenes occasionally being reported); olfactory-induced tastes would also seem to be specific.

Of course, subjective reports should always be handled with care. There are cases where people report hearing, or rather almost hearing, speech sounds when watching silent lip movements. The existence of auditory imagery has been backed up by various studies highlighting the activation of the auditory cortex when seeing silent speech-like lip movements (e.g., Hertrich et al., 2011, for a review), and confirmed by patterns of facilitation and interference in subsequent speech-recognition tasks (see Rosenblum, 2008, for a review). That being said, how specific the conscious experience is in these cases is difficult to assess: Do people hear distinct speech sounds, or only generic contents varying in pitch or loudness? In the case of musical imagery, for instance, there is, as yet, no evidence of bright images having been induced by high-pitched sounds: What is reported is rather specific images (of specific colours and shapes) whose brightness might well be modulated by variations in pitch.

10.4.3 Control over content

Focusing on musical imagery, taste-induced smells, and their synaesthetic analogues such as coloured-hearing, it seems difficult to assess whether these cases also present continuous variations regarding the control over the content of the induced image. The lack of voluntary control over the synaesthetic concurrent is often considered a key aspect of the condition while control over content is supposed to be characteristic of other cases of mental imagery. Some cases of crossmodal mental imagery—starting perhaps with tastes induced by smells—seem to escape the voluntary control of the subject, but the evidence needs to be further assessed (see Spence and Deroy, 2013). It is likely that these cases remain under a form of control, as this aspect of automaticity probably comes in a graded form. As such, strictly involuntary contents are the exception, and only exist in synaesthetes.

Is the argument sufficient? Another argument made by certain researchers here comes from the fact that even those individuals who are not synesthetic may, on occasion, have strange crossmodal experiences that they cannot control. Such experiences have, for example, sometimes been reported under the influence of psychotropes. These experiences are then argued to resemble those that have been reported by synaesthetes (e.g., MacDougal, 1898; Simpson and McKellar, 1955), leading to the idea that 'the potential to experience synaesthetically may lay latent within everyone' (Marks et al., 1987: 4; Grossenbacher and Lovelace, 2001; see Luke and Terhune, 2013, for a review). Not mentioning the problematic character of the evidence reported (i.e., people might not find it possible to identify the nature of their drug-induced experience; see Deroy and Spence, 2013c), it is difficult to see whether the lack of control over the conscious content exhibited in this case is really similar to the one exhibited in synaesthetes.

10.4.4 Interim summary

To summarize, it is indeed not impossible to find cases where crossmodal correspondences seem to be accompanied by conscious manifestations. In fact, the same is also true for other kinds of associations that have also been assimilated to synaesthesia (such as mirror touch; see De Vignemont, Chapter 13 of this volume). One problem with these conscious phenomena, as noted above, is that no precise quantification of the occurrence of the phenomenon has been reported to date. Elsewhere, we have argued that in the absence of robust evidence, it was difficult to use the presence of a conscious concurrent in other cases than synaesthesia to widen the category of synaesthesia (Deroy and Spence, 2013a). To go one step further, even while we wait for a more precise quantification, we want to suggest that there is a possible lesson to be learned from the gaps among the kind of conscious manifestations singled out above:

First, generic conscious concurrents do not seem to occur, even occasionally. For instance, no conscious experience of brightness is reported when hearing high-

Table 10.1. Summary of the different dimensions along which a continuity between crossmodal correspondences and canonical synaesthesia can be articulated. The evidence quoted for each hides the existence of clusters of cases.

Dimension of variation from correspondences to canonical synaesthesia	Quoted evidence	Problem
From less to more vivid	Subjective reports, neuro-imaging data	Misses the objective differences between synaesthetic experiences and mental imagery
From generic to specific	Common trends in associations between non-synaesthetes and synaesthetes	Lack of instances of conscious generic concurrents
From less to more frequent	Cases of occasional, more or less frequent, conscious experiences (e.g. musical imagery)	Lack of precise quantification
From more to less controlled	More or less automatic forms of crossmodal mental imagery	Bipartition between mental images, under various degrees voluntary control, and synaesthesia, completely beyond voluntary control

pitched sounds. If crossmodal correspondences concern such generic concurrents, then it seems to follow that there is no direct conscious manifestation of crossmodal correspondences. What seems rather to occur is that crossmodal correspondences can influence the kind of specific content which becomes conscious—for instance, pitch-brightness correspondence can influence the coloured hues and scenes occurring in musical imagery.

Second, when concurrents are systematically experienced, their contents also appear to be out of the subject's voluntary control. By contrast, more voluntarily controlled concurrents seem to occur less frequently, and perhaps also in a more strategic manner. There is seldom any report of coloured-hearing synaesthetes being able to control the kind of colour they experience when they hear a certain note or of people being able to change the conscious experience of vanilla as being sweet (see Table 10.1).

10.5 Conclusion: learning from the discontinuities

Much remains to be done regarding the occasional conscious manifestations of crossmodal correspondences, and how they can, for instance, influence crossmodal mental imagery (see Spence and Deroy, 2013). We think that attention should also be given to those cases which are not evidenced, and therefore where conscious manifestations seem impossible. The first of these apparent impossibilities concerns generic conscious concurrents. The lack of good empirical evidence can be reinforced here by a conceptual argument, as it seems impossible to be conscious of a pitch or a level of brightness in isolation: One can only be conscious of a sound, having a certain loudness, duration, and timbre (not to mention location) as well as pitch; and one can only be conscious of a certain colour patch, having a given spatial extension, saturation, and brightness, not to mention a possible hue. This said, the absence of a conscious generic content is compatible with the idea that such contents, even if phenomenally conscious, cannot be accessed (see Block, 2011).

The second series of cases which are not evidenced are cases of systematic concurrents with voluntary control over the content. Interestingly, being systematic and with no control is exactly the opposite of mental imagery, which is said to occur mostly for strategic goals (and not systematically) and to be under voluntary control (as illustrated by research on the mental rotation task; Shepard and Metzler, 1971). This opposition points towards a link between the systematic aspect of conscious manifestations and the involuntariness of the experienced content. A key question that remains to be addressed, then, is why the content of a mental image seems to escape control when its induction is systematic and more automatic.

The present chapter constitutes an attempt to spell out the hypothesis of a synaesthetic continuum. This hypothesis has grown out of an increasingly large body of behavioural evidence showing that we are all sensitive to crossmodal correspondences which are reminiscent of the kind of seemingly arbitrary associations that are seen in canonical cases of synaesthesia. By contrast with the idea that synaesthetes form a distinct group, the continuum hypothesis claims that they only reveal extreme manifestations of a process which can be evidenced in everyone. It is, in this sense, different from the claim that there are two distinct groups, one of weak synaesthetes and another of strong synaesthetes (Martino and Marks, 2001), and consists instead of claiming that everyone is more or less strongly synaesthetic. As reviewed here, it is difficult to make sense of the idea of a single psychological kind underlying all cases unless one accepts that there are variations in the conscious manifestations of this single synaesthetic process: Manifestations obviously differ regarding the specificity of the content (from generic dimensions to specific percepts), the frequency of conscious manifestations (from rare to systematic), and the voluntary control over the content (from an absence of control to a form of control). In those cases that are canonically listed as 'synaesthesia', the manifestation is specific, systematic, and involuntary. Cases of crossmodal correspondences, especially when they guide mental imagery, might lead to more or less frequent, more or less specific, and more or less voluntary manifestations, which need to be more specifically documented. This said, the range of conscious manifestations under review shows a breach in continuity when it comes to systematic conscious concurrents: Nowhere can we find evidence of generic concurrents or of concurrents being systematic and whose content remains under voluntary control. As such, the claim that the presence of a key difference between different kinds of phenomena, linked to the nature of their conscious manifestations, still stands. The main question is whether it is sufficient to be used as an argument for their discontinuity (Deroy and Spence, 2013a) and whether recent demonstrations of the potential to train adults to acquire synaesthetic experiences (as measured by subjective reports and, more importantly, conditioning) show that individuals can be moved along a continuum or led to acquire, for a short duration, a totally distinct kind of condition (Bor et al., 2014; see Deroy and Spence, 2013c, for a discussion).

Acknowledgements

OD and CS would like to thank the AHRC grant entitled 'Rethinking the senses' (AH/L007053/1) for supporting this research.

References

Arterberry, M. E., Craver-Lemley, C., & Reeves, A. (2002). Visual imagery is not always like visual perception. *Behavioral and Brain Sciences*, **25**, 183–4.

Asher, J., Aitken, M. R. F., Farooqi, N., Kurmani, S., & Baron-Cohen, S. (2006). Diagnosing and phenotyping visual synaesthesia: A preliminary evaluation of the revised test of genuineness (TOG-R). *Cortex*, **42**, 137–46.

Aveyard, M. E. (2012). Some consonants sound curvy: Effects of sound symbolism on object recognition. *Memory & Cognition*, **40**(1), 83–92. doi: 10.3758/s13421-011-0139-3.

Barnett, K. J., & Newell, F. N. (2008). Synaesthesia is associated with enhanced, self-rated visual imagery. *Consciousness and Cognition*, **17**, 1032–9.

Baron-Cohen, S., Harrison, J., Goldstein, L. H., & Wyke, M. (1993). Coloured speech perception: Is synaesthesia what happens when modularity breaks down? *Perception*, **22**, 419–26.

Baron-Cohen, S., Wyke, M., & Binne, C. (1987). Hearing words and seeing colours: An experimental investigation of a case of synaesthesia. *Perception*, **16**, 761–7.

Bien, N., ten Oever, S., Goebel, R., & Sack, A. T. (2012). The sound of size: Crossmodal binding in pitch-size synesthesia: A combined TMS, EEG and psychophysics study. *NeuroImage*, **59**, 663–72.

Block, N. (2011). Perceptual consciousness overflows cognitive access. *Trends in Cognitive Sciences*, **15**, 567–75.

Bor, D., Rothen, N., Schwartzman, D. J., Clayton, S., & Seth, A. K. (2014). Adults can be trained to acquire synesthetic experiences. *Scientific Reports*, **4**: 7089.

Braaten, R. (1993). *Synesthetic correspondence between visual location and auditory pitch in infants*. Paper presented at the Annual Meeting of the Psychonomic Society.

Calkins, M. W. (1893). A statistical study of pseudo-chromesthesia and of mental-forms. *The American Journal of Psychology*, **5**, 439–64.

Campana, F., & Tallon-Baudry, C. (2013). Anchoring visual subjective experience in a neural model: The coarse vividness hypothesis. *Neuropsychologia*, **51**, 1050–60.

Chan, J. S., van den Bosch, J. J., Theves, S., Hardt, S., Pflanz, P., Lötsch, J., Naumer, M. J. et al. (2014). Synaesthesia or vivid imagery? A single case fMRI study of visually induced olfactory perception. *Multisensory Research*, **27**, 225–46.

Chara, P. J. (1992). Some concluding thoughts on the debate about the Vividness of Visual Imagery Questionnaire. *Perceptual and Motor Skills*, **75**, 947–54.

Chiou, R., & Rich, A. N. (2012). Cross-modality correspondence between pitch and spatial location modulates attentional orienting. *Perception*, **41**, 339–53.

Cichy, R. M., Heinzle, J., & Haynes, J. D. (2012). Imagery and perception share cortical representations of content and location. *Cerebral Cortex*, **22**, 372–80.

Cohen Kadosh, R., Henik, A., & Walsh, V. (2007). Small is bright and big is dark in synaesthesia. *Current Biology*, **17**, 834–5.

Craver-Lemley, C., & Reeves, A. (2013). Is synaesthesia a form of mental imagery? In S. Lacey & R. Lawson (Eds.), *Multisensory imagery: Theory and applications* (pp. 185–206). New York, NY Springer.

Cytowic, R. E., & Eagleman, D. M. (2009). *Wednesday is indigo blue: Discovering the brain of synesthesia*. Cambridge, MA: MIT Press.

Day, S. (2005). Some demographic and socio-cultural aspects of synesthesia. In L. C. Robertson & N. Sagiv (Eds), *Synaesthesia: Perspectives from cognitive neuroscience* (pp. 11–33). New York, NY: Oxford University Press.

Deroy, O., Crisinel, A.-S., & Spence, C. (2013). Crossmodal correspondences between odors and contingent features: Odors, musical notes, and geometrical shapes. *Psychonomic Bulletin & Review*, **20**, 878–96.

Deroy, O., & Spence, C. (2013a). Why we are not all synesthetes (not even weakly so). *Psychonomic Bulletin & Review*, **20**, 643–64.

Deroy, O., & Spence, C. (2013b). Are we all born synaesthetic? Examining the neonatal synaesthesia hypothesis. *Neuroscience & Biobehavioral Reviews*, **37**, 1240–53.

Deroy, O., & Spence, C. (2013c). Training, hypnosis, and drugs: artificial synaesthesia, or artificial paradises? *Frontiers in Psychology*, **4**, 660.

Dixon, M. J., Smilek, D., Cudahy, C., & Merikle, P. M. (2000). Five plus two equals yellow. *Nature*, **406**, 365–5.

Djordjevic, J., Zatorre, R. J., & Jones-Gotman, M. (2004). Effects of perceived and imagined odors on taste detection. *Chemical Senses*, **29**, 199–208.

Domino, G. (1989). Synesthesia and creativity in fine arts students: An empirical look. *Creativity Research Journal*, **2**, 17–29.

Elias, L. J., Saucier, D. M., Hardie, C., & Sarty, G. E. (2003). Dissociating semantic and perceptual components of synaesthesia: Behavioural and functional neuroanatomical investigations. *Cognitive Brain Research*, **16**, 232–7.

Esterman, M., Verstynen, T., Ivry, R. B., & Robertson, L. C. (2006). Coming unbound: Disrupting automatic integration of synesthetic color and graphemes by transcranial magnetic stimulation of the right parietal lobe. *Journal of Cognitive Neuroscience*, **18**, 1570–6.

Evans, K. K., & Treisman, A. (2010). Natural cross-modal mappings between visual and auditory features. *Journal of Vision*, **10**, 1–12.

Gallace, A., & Spence, C. (2006). Multisensory synesthetic interactions in the speeded classification of visual size. *Perception & Psychophysics*, **68**, 1191–203.

Ganis, G., & Schendan, H. E. (2008). Visual mental imagery and perception produce opposite adaptation effects on early brain potentials. *NeuroImage*, **42**, 1714–27.

Gold, C., Solli, H. P., Krüger, V., & Lie, S. A. (2009). Dose-response relationship in music therapy for people with serious mental disorders: Systematic review and meta-analysis. *Clinical Psychology Review*, **29**, 193–207.

Grill-Spector, K., Kushnir, T., Edelman, S., Avidan, G., Itzchak, Y., & Malach, R. (1999). Differential processing of objects under various viewing conditions in the human lateral occipital complex. *Neuron*, **24**, 187–203.

Grill-Spector, K., Henson, R., & Martin, A. (2006). Repetition and the brain: Neural models of stimulus-specific effects. *Trends in Cognitive Sciences*, **10**, 14–23.

Grossenbacher, P. G., & Lovelace, C. T. (2001). Mechanisms of synesthesia: Cognitive and physiological constraints. *Trends in Cognitive Sciences*, **5**, 36–41.

Hertrich, I., Dietrich, S., & Ackermann, H. (2011). Cross-modal interactions during perception of audiovisual speech and nonspeech signals: An fMRI study. *Journal of Cognitive Neuroscience*, **23**, 221–37.

Holden, E. S. (1885). Color and other associations. *Science*, **6**, 242–3.

Hong, S. W., & Blake, R. (2008). Early visual mechanisms do not contribute to synesthetic color experience. *Vision Research*, **48**, 1018–26.

Hubbard, E. M., Arman, A. C., Ramachandran, V. S., & Boynton, G. M. (2005). Individual differences among grapheme-color synesthetes: Brain-behavior correlations. *Neuron*, **45**, 975–85.

Hume, D. (1739/2000). *A treatise of human nature*. Oxford, UK: Oxford University Press.

James, W. (1890). *Principles of psychology*. New York, NY: Henry Holt.

Jones, C. L., Gray, M. A., Minati, L., Simner, J., Critchley, H. D., & Ward, J. (2011). The neural basis of illusory gustatory sensations: Two rare cases of lexical-gustatory synaesthesia. *Journal of Neuropsychology*, **5**, 243–54.

Juslin, P. N., & Västfjäll, D. (2008). Emotional responses to music: The need to consider underlying mechanisms. *Behavioral and Brain Sciences*, **31**, 559–75.

Karwoski, T. F., Odbert, H. S., & Osgood, C. E. (1942). Studies in synesthetic thinking. II. The role of form in visual responses to music. *Journal of General Psychology*, **26**, 199–222.

Köhler, W. (1929). *Gestalt psychology*. New York, NY: Liveright.

Köhler, W. (1947). Gestalt psychology: An introduction to new concepts in modern psychology. New York, NY: Liveright.

Kouider, S., De Gardelle, V., Sackur, J., & Dupoux, E. (2010). How rich is consciousness? The partial awareness hypothesis. *Trends in Cognitive Sciences*, **14**, 301–7.

Krohn, W. O. (1892). Pseudo-chromesthesia, or the association of colors with words, letters and sounds. *The American Journal of Psychology*, **5**, 20–41.

Langfeld, H. (1914). Discussion: Note on a case of chromoaesthesia. *Psychological Bulletin*, **11**, 113–14.

Levinson, J. (2013). Functionalism. In E. N. Zalta (Ed.), *The Stanford encyclopaedia of philosophy* (Fall 2013 Edition, online only). <http://plato.stanford.edu/archives/fall2013/entries/functionalism/.

Ludwig, V. U., Adachi, I., & Matsuzawa, T. (2011). Visuoauditory mappings between high luminance and high pitch are shared by chimpanzees (Pan troglodytes) and humans. *Proceedings of the National Academy of Sciences of the USA*, **108**, 20661–5.

Luke, D. P., & Terhune, D. B. (2013). The induction of synaesthesia with chemical agents: A systematic review. *Frontiers in Psychology*, **4**, 753.

MacDougal, R. (1898). Music imagery: A confession of experience. *Psychological Review*, **5**, 463–76.

MacLeod, C. M. (1991). Half a century of research on the Stroop effect: An integrative review. *Psychological Bulletin*, **109**, 163–203.

Marks, L. E. (1978). *The unity of the senses: Interrelations among the modalities*. New York, NY: Academic Press.

Marks, L. E., Hammeal, R. J., & Bornstein, M. H. (1987). Perceiving similarity and comprehending metaphor. *Monographs of the Society for Research in Child Development*, **52** (215), 1–102.

Martino, G., & Marks, L. E. (2000). Cross-modal interaction between vision and touch: The role of synesthetic correspondence. *Perception*, **29**, 745–54.

Martino, G., & Marks, L. E. (2001). Synesthesia: Strong and weak. *Current Directions in Psychological Science*, **10**, 61–5.

Maurer, D., Gibson, L. C., & Spector, F. (2013). Synesthesia in infants and very young children. In J. Simner (Ed.), *Oxford handbook of synesthesia* (pp. 46–63). Oxford: Oxford University Press.

Melara, R. D., & O'Brien, T. P. (1987). Interactions between synesthetically corresponding dimensions. *Journal of Experimental Psychology: General*, **116**, 323–36.

Mills, C. B. (1999). Digit synaesthesia: A case study using a Stroop-type test. *Cognitive Neuropsychology*, **16**, 181–91.

Muggleton, N., Tsakanikos, E., Walsh, V., & Ward, J. (2007). Disruption of synaesthesia following TMS of the right posterior parietal cortex. *Neuropsychologia*, **45**, 1582–5.

Mulvenna, C. M., & Walsh, V. (2006). Synaesthesia: Supernormal integration? *Trends in Cognitive Sciences*, **10**, 350–2.

Nielsen, A., & Rendall, D. (2011). The sound of round: Evaluating the sound-symbolic role of consonants in the classic Takete-Maluma phenomenon. *Canadian Journal of Experimental Psychology/Revue canadienne de psychologie expérimentale*, **65**, 115–24.

Nielsen, A. K., & Rendall, D. (2013). Parsing the role of consonants versus vowels in the classic Takete-Maluma phenomenon. *Canadian Journal of Experimental Psychology*, **67**, 153–63.

Nikolić, D., Jürgens, U. M., Rothen, N., Meier, B., & Mroczko, A. (2011). Swimming-style synaesthesia. *Cortex*, **47**, 874–9.

Novich, S., Cheng, S., & Eagleman, D. M. (2011). Is synaesthesia one condition or many? A large-scale analysis reveals subgroups. *Journal of Neuropsychology*, **5**, 353–71.

Odbert, H. S., Karwoski, T. F., & Eckerson, A. B. (1942). Studies in synesthetic thinking. I. Musical and verbal associations of colour and mood. *Journal of General Psychology*, **26**, 153–73.

Overgaard, M., Rote, J., Mouridsen, K., & Ramsøy, T. Z. (2006). Is conscious perception gradual or dichotomous? A comparison of report methodologies during a visual task. *Consciousness and Cognition*, **15**, 700–8.

Parise, C. V., Knorre, K., & Ernst, M. O. (2014). Natural auditory scene statistics shapes human spatial hearing. *Proceedings of the National Academy of Sciences of the USA*, **111**, 6104–8.

Parise, C., & Spence, C. (2008). Synaesthetic congruency modulates the temporal ventriloquism effect. *Neuroscience Letters*, **442**, 257–61.

Parise, C., & Spence, C. (2009). 'When birds of a feather flock together': Synesthetic correspondences modulate audiovisual integration in non-synesthetes. *PLoS ONE* **4(5)**: e5664.

Parise, C. V., & Spence, C. (2012). Audiovisual crossmodal correspondences and sound symbolism: A study using the implicit association test. *Experimental Brain Research*, **220**, 319–33.

Price, M. C. (2009). Spatial forms and mental imagery. *Cortex*, **45**, 1229–45.

Pritchard, J., Rothen, N., Coolbear, D., & Ward, J. (2013). Enhanced associative memory for colour (but not shape or location) in synaesthesia. *Cognition*, **127**, 230–4.

Rader, C. M., & Tellegen, A. (1987). An investigation of synesthesia. *Journal of Personality and Social Psychology*, **52**, 981–7.

Ramachandran, V. S., & Hubbard, E. M. (2001). Synaesthesia – A window into perception, thought and language. *Journal of Consciousness Studies*, **8**, 3–34.

Rich, A. N., & Karstoft, K. I. (2013). Exploring the benefit of synaesthetic colours: Testing for "pop-out" in individuals with grapheme–colour synaesthesia. *Cognitive Neuropsychology*, **30**, 110–25.

Rosenblum, L. D. (2008). Speech perception as a multimodal phenomenon. *Current Directions in Psychological Science*, **17**, 405–9.

Rothen, N., & Meier, B. (2009). Do synesthetes have a general advantage in visual search and episodic memory? A case for group studies. *PLoS One*, **4**, e5037.

Rothen, N., Meier, B., & Ward, J. (2012). Enhanced memory ability: Insights from synaesthesia. *Neuroscience & Biobehavioral Reviews*, **36**, 1952–63.

Rouw, R., & Scholte, H. S. (2010). Neural basis of individual differences in synesthetic experiences. *Journal of Neuroscience*, **30**, 6205–13.

Rouw, R., Scholte, H. S., & Colizoli, O. (2011). Brain areas involved in synaesthesia: A review. *Journal of Neuropsychology*, **5**, 214–42.

Sagiv, N., & Ward, J. (2006). Crossmodal interactions: Lessons from synesthesia. *Progress in Brain Research*, **155**, 259–71.

Sapir, E. (1929). A study in phonetic symbolism. *Journal of Experimental Psychology*, **12**, 225–39.

Sergent, C., & Dehaene, S. (2004). Is consciousness a gradual phenomenon? Evidence for an all-or-none bifurcation during the attentional blink. *Psychological Science*, **15**, 720–8.

Shepard, R. N., & Metzler, J. (1971). Mental rotation of three-dimensional objects. *Science*, **19**, 701–3.

Simner, J. (2012). Defining synaesthesia. *British Journal of Psychology*, **103**, 1–15.

Simner, J., Ward, J., Lanz, M., Jansari, A., Noonan, K., Glover, L., & Oakley, D. A. (2005). Non-random associations of graphemes to colours in synaesthetic and non-synaesthetic populations. *Cognitive Neuropsychology*, **22**, 1069–85.

Simpson, L., & McKellar, P. (1955). Types of synaesthesia. *British Journal of Psychiatry*, **101**, 141–7.

Spence, C. (2011). Crossmodal correspondences: A tutorial review. *Attention, Perception, & Psychophysics*, **73**, 971–95.

Spence, C. (2012). Multi-sensory integration & the psychophysics of flavour perception. In J. Chen & L. Engelen (Eds.), *Food oral processing—Fundamentals of eating and sensory perception* (pp. 203–19). Oxford, UK: Blackwell.

Spence, C., & Deroy, O. (2012). Crossmodal correspondences: Innate or learned? *i-Perception*, **3**, 316–18.

Spence, C., & Deroy, O. (2013). Crossmodal mental imagery. In S. Lacey & R. Lawson (Eds.), *Multisensory imagery: Theory and applications* (pp. 157–83). New York, NY: Springer.

Spence, C., Deroy, O., & Bremner, A. (2013). Questioning the utility of the concept of amodality: Towards a revised framework for understanding crossmodal relations. *Multisensory Research*, **26 (Supple.)**, 57.

Spence, C., & Parise, C. V. (2012). The cognitive neuroscience of crossmodal correspondences. *i-Perception*, **3**, 410–12.

Stevenson, R. J., & Boakes, R. A. (2004). Sweet and sour smells: Learned synaesthesia between the senses of taste and smell. In G. A. Calvert, C. Spence, & B. E. Stein (Eds.), *The handbook of multisensory processing* (pp. 69–83). Cambridge, MA: MIT Press.

Stevenson, R. J., & Mahmut, M. K. (2011). Experience dependent changes in odour-viscosity perception. *Acta Psychologica*, **136**, 60–6.

Stevenson, R. J., & Tomiczek, C. (2007). Olfactory-induced synesthesias: A review and model. *Psychological Bulletin*, **133**, 294–309.

Sundqvist, N. C., Stevenson, R. J., & Bishop, I. R. (2006). Can odours acquire fat-like properties? *Appetite*, **47**, 91–9.

Symons, D. (1993). The stuff that dreams aren't made of: Why wake-state and dream-state sensory experiences differ. *Cognition*, **47**, 181–217.

Van Leeuwen, T. M., Petersson, K. M., & Hagoort, P. (2010). Synaesthetic colour in the brain: Beyond colour areas. A functional magnetic resonance imaging study of synaesthetes and matched controls. *PLoS ONE*, **5(8)**: e12074.

Wagner, K., & Dobkins, K. R. (2011). Synaesethetic associations decrease during infancy. *Psychological Science*, **22**, 1067–72.

Walker, P., Bremner, J. G., Mason, U., Spring, J., Mattock, K., Slater, A., & Johnson, S. P. (2010). Preverbal infants' sensitivity to synesthetic cross-modality correspondences. *Psychological Science*, **21**, 21–5.

Walker, P., & Smith, S. (1984). Stroop interference based on the synaesthetic qualities of auditory pitch. *Perception*, **13**, 75–81.

Ward, J., Huckstep, B., & Tsakanikos, E. (2006). Sound-colour synaesthesia: To what extent does it use cross-modal mechanisms common to us all? *Cortex*, **42**, 264–80.

Ward, J., Li, R., Salih, S., & Sagiv, N. (2007). Varieties of grapheme-colour synaesthesia: A new theory of phenomenological and behavioural differences. *Consciousness and Cognition*, **16**, 913–31.

White Cooper, W. (1852). Vision. In R. B. Todd (Ed.) *Encyclopaedia of anatomy and physiology* (pp. 1420–80). London, UK: Sherwood & Co.

Wilkinson, L. R. (1996). *The dream of an absolute language: Emanuel Swedenborg and French literary culture*. New York, NY: SUNY Press.

Yokoyama, T., Noguchi, Y., Koga, H., Tachibana, R., Saiki, J., Kakigi, R., & Kita, S. (2014). Multiple neural mechanisms for coloring words in synesthesia. *NeuroImage*, **94**, 360–71.

Zellner, D. A., McGarry, A., Mattern-McClory, R., & Abreu, D. (2008). Masculinity/femininity of fine fragrances affects color-odor correspondences: A case for cognitions influencing cross-modal correspondences. *Chemical Senses*, **33**, 211–22.

Zigler, M. J. (1930). Tone shapes: A novel type of synaesthesia. *The Journal of General Psychology*, **3**, 277–87.

11

The Induction of Synaesthesia in Non-Synaesthetes

Devin B. Terhune, David P. Luke, and Roi Cohen Kadosh

11.1 Introduction

Synaesthesia is an unusual but healthy neurological condition in which a stimulus, such as the number *7* or the note *E*, reliably and involuntarily elicits an atypical concurrent experience, such as the colour red (Ward, 2013). Synaesthesia occurs in a small minority of the population (~4 per cent; Simner et al., 2006) and has been shown to impact a wide range of cognitive and perceptual abilities from selective attention to episodic memory (Ward, 2013). In turn, uncovering the characteristics and mechanisms of this condition has the potential to inform our understanding of a diverse array of processes and functions including automaticity (Mattingley, 2009), conscious awareness (Cohen Kadosh and Henik, 2007), and memory (Rothen, Meier, and Ward, 2012).

Experimentally manipulating a phenomenon, such as by inducing, disrupting, or modulating it, can often yield information regarding both fundamental and ancillary characteristics as well as necessary and sufficient conditions for the expression of the phenomenon. Insofar as synaesthesia is relatively rare, there is interest in identifying methods by which it can be experimentally induced in the laboratory. The experimental induction of synaesthesia has the potential to shed light on the cognitive, neurophysiological, and neurochemical mechanisms that give rise to this condition (Cohen Kadosh, Henik, Catena, Walsh, and Fuentes, 2009; Luke, Terhune, and Friday, 2012). Induction methods also raise important questions regarding what can and should be considered synaesthesia and which demarcation criteria should be taken as paramount for discriminating synaesthesia from other conditions.

The present chapter reviews our current knowledge regarding the induction of synaesthesia in non-synaesthetes. First, we consider the criteria by which synaesthesia is currently defined with a view to using such criteria when we adjudicate whether different induced synaesthesias constitute genuine forms of this condition. We will describe three induction methods: *training*, *posthypnotic suggestion*, and *pharmacological agents*. In each case, we adopt a critical stance whether the phenomenon induced by a particular method meets consensus criteria for synaesthesia and draw attention to its prospects and limitations. We conclude by contrasting the different methods and considering the implications of the experimental induction of synaesthesia for our understanding of the cognitive and neural mechanisms of this condition.

11.2 Criteria and characteristics of synaesthesia

When considering induced synaesthesias, it is crucial to evaluate their veracity; that is, whether they represent the same or similar phenomenon as congenital synaesthesia. To do so, we need a set of criteria by which synaesthesia can be identified. In this section we describe first the consensus criteria by which synaesthesia can be demarcated from other phenomena. We next consider what synaesthesia *characteristics* should be expected to be present in induced synaesthesias. For the sake of convenience, we will throughout refer to different *induced synaesthesias* as synaesthesias, rather than qualifying this term (e.g., alleged synaesthesias) each time we use it. Nevertheless, we reserve judgement as to whether these phenomena meet accepted criteria for this condition.

11.2.1 Criteria

There is still debate about the criteria by which synaesthesia can be discriminated from other experiences or associations, such as crossmodal correspondences. For example, human non-synaesthetes, as well as chimpanzees (Ludwig, Adachi, and Matsuzawa, 2011), display pitch-luminance correspondences, with higher-pitch tones being associated with higher luminance; this phenomenon is highly prevalent in human non-synaesthetes and is not an accepted form of synaesthesia (Deroy and Spence, 2013). Nevertheless, there is an emerging set of criteria that are widely endorsed by the majority of synaesthesia researchers. Synaesthesia is often argued to be characterized by at least four criteria: 1) an atypical, ancillary conscious experience (e.g., colour) in response to a stimulus (e.g., a numeral); 2) a high degree of consistency in the inducer-concurrent associations; 3) a high degree of involuntariness (or automaticity) in the coupling of the inducer and concurrent and by which the concurrent breaches conscious awareness and impacts cognition; and 4) a high degree of specificity of the inducer and the concurrent (Deroy and Spence, 2013; Ward, 2013; Ward and Mattingley, 2006; see also Colizoli, Murre, and Rouw, 2014, for the application of demarcation criteria to trained synaesthesia).

A neglected question is whether induced synaesthesias should reasonably be expected to meet all of the foregoing criteria. That is, would we accept phenomena that meet certain criteria, but not others, as synaesthesia? For instance, if a synaesthete is not reliable over time in her inducer-concurrent associations but these associations are still automatic and accessible to consciousness, and perhaps even specific (at a particular time point), would we accept this as synaesthesia? This question is beyond the scope of the present chapter, but warrants attention (Simner, 2012). At present, it suffices to say that if one criterion is not met, we should not be too quick to discount a particular form of synaesthesia. Furthermore, certain criteria (conscious accessibility and automaticity) may be more fundamental than others (consistency and specificity).

Related to this question is the issue as to which criteria and characteristics should be expected in induced synaesthesias. This question has two strands: first, to what extent can the consensus criteria reviewed above be meaningfully applied to induced synaesthesias?; second, independent of these criteria, should induced synaesthesias be expected to also elicit other characteristics found in synaesthetes? With regard to the first question, it is useful to distinguish between characteristics of synaesthesia that originate with the initial experience of synaesthesia (synaesthesia-specific) and those that are produced by the consolidation process wherein synaesthetic associations are repeatedly associated and strengthened over time (consolidation-specific). This distinction has not been empirically addressed to the best of our knowledge, thus at present it is unclear which characteristics and criteria can discriminate synaesthesia and crossmodal correspondences at early (pre-consolidation) and later (post-consolidation) stages of synaesthesia.

Consider, for instance, the criterion of consistency. At an early developmental stage, when a congenital synaesthete first begins to experience synaesthesia, we might expect that her inducer-concurrent associations would not be as consistent as the corresponding associations of adult synaesthetes. In other words, it is plausible that consistency emerges through a consolidation process over time. Data by Simner and colleagues (Simner, Harrold, Creed, Monro, and Foulkes, 2009), which shows that synaesthete children become more consistent in their grapheme-colour associations over time, is consistent with this speculation. Thus, *early-stage* synaesthesia may not be expected to be as consistent as *late-stage* synaesthesia. This argument similarly applies also to the criterion of *specificity*, as inducer-concurrent pairings may become more specific or specialized as part of a consolidation process. On the other hand, *conscious access* and *automaticity* are not necessarily specific to late-stage synaesthesia although this has not yet been systematically studied to our knowledge.

Induced synaesthesias can be easily likened to early-stage synaesthesia. Accordingly, it might be that we shouldn't necessarily expect to observe consistency and specificity in induced synaesthesias, particularly in those where the inducer-concurrent pairings manifest on their own. When we contrast induced and congenital synaesthesias below, we take account of the four aforementioned criteria, as well as other characteristics of synaesthesia, but it is important to bear in mind that induced synaesthesias may more closely approximate early-stage synaesthesias and thus may not meet all of the criteria of late-stage synaesthesias.

11.2.2 Characteristics

Aside from the demarcation criteria of synaesthesia, it is important to consider whether induced synaesthesias should exhibit other characteristics observed in synaesthetes. Before doing so, we would like to draw a distinction between characteristics that are specific to the online experience of synaesthesia (e.g., grapheme-colour consistency) and those that are not, such as enhanced visual processing (Banissy, Walsh, and Ward, 2009; Banissy, Tester, Muggleton, Janik, Davenport, Franklin, Walsh, and Ward, 2013; Barnett et al., 2008; Terhune, Song, Duta, and Cohen Kadosh, 2014; Yaro and Ward, 2007) and memory (Rothen et al., 2012). Consistency and other demarcation criteria are specific to the online experience of synaesthesia, whereas the latter are largely independent of these experiences and seem to represent markers of broader differences in visual cortex associated with the synaesthesia phenotype (Rothen et al., 2012; see also Terhune, Rothen, and Cohen Kadosh, 2013). Accordingly, we should not expect to observe non-specific characteristics in induced synaesthesias.

There are certain characteristics of synaesthesia that are not used as demarcation criteria for this condition, but which may still be expected in induced synaesthesias if they are genuine. For instance, it has been shown that synaesthetes typically display implicit bidirectionality, wherein concurrent stimuli trigger implicit inducer representations (e.g., colours triggering numbers) (Cohen Kadosh and Henik, 2007). This effect may occur as a result of the consolidation process by which graphemes and colours get repeatedly bound and thus may not be present in early or induced synaesthesias. Nevertheless, it is worth investigating and, if observed, will surely strengthen the case for the veracity of induced synaesthesias. An additional characteristic of synaesthesia is that of colour opponency in synaesthetic photisms (Nikolić, Lichti, and Singer, 2007). Hue-selective neurons in different regions of visual cortex have colour-opponent receptive fields such that cells that are excited by a particular colour (e.g., red) are inhibited by its opponent colour (e.g., green) (e.g., Zeki, 1980). Nikolić and colleagues found that synaesthetes were slower to name the colour of incongruently coloured graphemes when the incongruent colour was in an opponent colour as opposed to when it was in a non-opponent colour. They argued that the results suggest the involvement of early visual processing, perhaps involving V1, and point to the perceptual basis of synaesthesia. If induced synaesthesia is genuine, we might expect it to relate to colour-opponency effects. Finally, synaesthetes have also been shown to vary in the perceived visuospatial location of colour photisms, with some synaesthetes experiencing colours as endogenous images or representations (*associators*) and others as vivid percepts that are spatially colocalized with the inducer (*projectors*) (Dixon, Smilek, and Merikle, 2004; Ward, Li, Salih, and Sagiv, 2007), with evidence for neurophysiological differences (Cohen, Weidacker, Tankink, Scholte, and Rouw, 2015; Rouw and Scholte, 2010; Terhune, Murray, Near, Stagg, Cowey, and Cohen Kadosh, 2015; van Leeuwen, den Ouden, and Hagoort, 2011). Although we might not expect such effects, observing individual differences among induced synaesthetes increases the likelihood that genuine synaesthesia has been produced. These represent a few examples of characteristics of synaesthesia that may or may not be expected to be present in induced synaesthesias.

11.3 Induced synaesthesias

Induced synaesthesias refer to instances in which synaesthesia or a synaesthesia-like phenomenon is *temporarily* elicited through exposure to an agent or manipulation. It is instructive to contrast these with *acquired* synaesthesias, which include those that develop in adulthood in the wake of some type of event (e.g., head injury) and which are experienced for an extended period of time. For instance, it has been shown that synaesthesias can be acquired through stroke (Fornazzari, Fischer, Ringer, and Schweizer, 2012; Ro et al., 2007) or perhaps sensory substitution (Ward and Wright, 2012) and have been reported to spontaneously occur during migraine (Alstadhaug and Benjaminsen, 2010). Below we describe three forms of induced synaesthesias: those that occur as a result of training, posthypnotic suggestion, and those that occur following the ingestion of pharmacological agents.

11.3.1 Training

A number of studies have explored the possibility of producing synaesthetic associations in non-synaesthetes through training and whether these associations qualify as genuine synaesthesia (for a review, see Rothen and Meier, 2014). These studies involve repeatedly pairing two sets of stimuli that are typically associated in a form of synaesthesia (e.g., graphemes and colours) and examining whether training leads to behavioural or physiological responses to the stimuli in a manner typical of synaesthesia. In addition to exploring the possible induction of synaesthesia, researchers have been motivated to use this approach to include *trained* participants as a control group for synaesthetes (Cohen Kadosh et al., 2005; Elias, Saucier, Hardie, and Sarty, 2003; Nunn et al., 2002) to examine whether synaesthetic effects are just a product of semantic associations or memory. Moreover, in a number of documented cases, synaesthetes' specific grapheme-colour pairs appear to have been determined by exposure to coloured graphemes in early childhood (Hancock, 2006; Witthoft and Winawer, 2006, 2013). Accordingly, investigating whether synaesthesia can be induced through training also has a direct bearing on the learning mechanisms at play in developmental synaesthesia.

Multiple studies have shown that grapheme-colour association training can reproduce the behavioural markers of grapheme-colour synaesthesia. In a nice early example of this, Elias and colleagues (2003) compared a single grapheme-colour synaesthete with a single *semantic*-control and untrained controls. This study is unique insofar as the semantic-control had spontaneously developed grapheme-colour associations through exposure over an eight-year period to a cross-stitching system in which a particular number signifies a particular thread colour. Strictly speaking, the development of the grapheme-colour associations in this case is spontaneous and not the product of an experimental manipulation as is the case with the training studies described below.

In this study, Elias and colleagues administered a series of behavioural tasks previously shown to discriminate controls and synaesthetes as well as multiple behavioural tasks during functional magnetic resonance imaging. The three tasks included a coloured grapheme Stroop task, a mathematical Stroop task, in which mathematical equations are followed by colour patches that are either congruent or incongruent with the correct answer (Dixon, Smilek, Cudahy, and Merikle, 2000), and a conscious priming task in which congruent or incongruent graphemes preceded colour patches in a colour-naming task (Mattingley, Rich, Yelland, and Bradshaw, 2001). Crucially, in all three tasks, the synaesthete and the semantic-control exhibited congruency effects characterized by slower responses on incongruent than congruent trials, whereas none of the untrained controls displayed such effects. Indeed, the semantic-control displayed comparably sized, or numerically larger, congruency effects relative to the synaesthete in all conditions. In contrast, in the fMRI paradigms, the synaesthete displayed activation in left parietal and extrastriate visual cortex during auditory and visual numerical processing, respectively, whereas no such effects were observed in the semantic-control. Although caution is required when interpreting single-case results, these findings suggest that trained semantic associations between graphemes and colours are not producing the same cortical activation patterns observed in synaesthesia, or the conscious, involuntary experience of colour photisms that is a hallmark phenomenological property of synaesthesia.

A subsequent study that included trained non-synaesthetes similarly shows that they do not exhibit behavioural effects observed in congenital synaesthesia (Cohen Kadosh et al., 2005). In this study, non-synaesthetes were trained over five sessions to associate specific digits and colours and evidenced clear learning effects. The authors sought to investigate whether colours implicitly activate numerical magnitude representations in synaesthetes and the trained group. Participants completed a magnitude comparison task in which they had to judge which of two numbers was numerically larger. The numbers were presented in their associated synaesthetic colours (*matched-colour* condition) or in colours that were associated with a larger numerical distance (*large-colour* condition). Crucially, grapheme-colour synaesthetes were faster in the large colour than in the matched-colour condition, indicating that colour implicitly triggers a numerical representation, even though synaesthetes are not consciously aware of this implicit association. Of special interest in the present context is that the trained control group did not display this effect, although they did display a normal congruency effect (faster responses for the matched-colour condition). This indicates that whilst non-synaesthetes can be trained to associate graphemes and colours, they not do not exhibit implicit bidirectionality, as is observed in congenital synaesthetes.

Meier and Rothen (2009) adopted a similar approach and investigated whether seven days of training would elicit the physiological concomitants of synaesthesia. After training, the trained controls completed a synaesthesia Stroop task and a synaesthesia conditioning task (Meier and Rothen, 2007). In the latter, a particular colour was paired with a startling sound, thereby producing a conditioned startle response to the colour, as measured by skin conductance response. The training produced a small, but significant, Stroop effect (23 ms); in contrast, unlike congenital synaesthetes (Meier and Rothen, 2007), the participants displayed a conditioning effect for colours, but *not* graphemes. One explanation for why this divergence arises is that the trained controls do not develop implicit bidirectional associations between colours and graphemes; that is, in synaesthetes, it may be that colour implicitly activates grapheme representations, which are then associated with the conditioned stimulus, whereas colour does not activate grapheme representations in trained controls (Cohen Kadosh et al., 2005).

A subsequent study by Rothen and colleagues (Rothen, Wantz, and Meier, 2011) sought to expand upon their previous study by contrasting two different types of training. In addition, the authors administered digit-colour and colour-digit priming tasks (Gebuis, Nijboer, and Van der Smagt, 2009) so as to examine bidirectionality effects in the wake of training as a follow-up to the studies described above. In a *non-adaptive* training schedule, participants judged whether digits were correctly or incorrectly coloured on the basis of predefined digit-colour associations. In contrast, the *adaptive* training schedule involved participants identifying the colour that was associated with an achromatic digit, according to the predefined associations. The digit was re-presented in the correct associated colour hue with altered luminance and participants had to judge whether the stimulus colour was brighter or darker than the colour associated with the digit. Feedback was given after both the initial digit as well as the coloured digit in the adaptive training schedule but not in the non-adaptive training schedule.

The authors found that participants displayed larger priming effects across both tasks after ten days of training. In addition, participants exhibited larger digit-colour than colour-digit priming effects, as might be expected given the results of Cohen Kadosh et al. (2005). Exploratory analyses further revealed that both groups displayed significant digit-colour priming effects post-training, whereas only the adaptive training group displayed a colour-digit priming effect. Importantly, as in other studies, none of the trained participants reported colour photisms in response to digits. Insofar as the authors found no differences across tasks as a function of the type of training, caution should be exerted in interpreting these results. Nevertheless, these findings suggest that the adaptive training schedule may give rise to bidirectionality effects observed in synaesthetes (Gebuis et al., 2009). At the same time, it should be noted that the largest digit-colour priming effect (observed in the adaptive training group; ~37 ms), and the largest colour-digit priming effect (observed in the non-adaptive training group; ~18 ms) stand in stark contrast to the far larger priming effects observed in synaesthetes (digit-colour priming: ~135 ms; colour-digit priming: ~134 ms; Gebuis et al., 2009). Given the results, it is unclear whether the adaptive training produces stronger effects and, because multiple components of the training were different across the two methods, it is difficult to determine which component(s) of training are crucial for any benefit with this method. Nevertheless, this study does suggest that adaptive training may be used to replicate behavioural markers of synaesthesia.

The remaining studies that we will describe adopt a more naturalistic approach by having participants complete tasks that should produce synaesthesia-like associations rather than explicitly attempting to train such associations. Colizoli and colleagues had participants read one or more books in which four letters were uniquely coloured (Colizoli, Murre, and Rouw, 2012). Participants subsequently completed multiple behavioural tasks that are potentially diagnostic of synaesthesia including a synaesthesia Stroop task, a perceptual crowding task, and a surprise letter-colour pair recollection test. The crowding task involved viewing a group of letters with one unique target letter embedded within the display and identifying the target letter; a control task involved untrained letters. The surprise test involved querying participants about the grapheme-colour associations four to six months after the conclusion of the study.

In line with some of the foregoing studies, Colizoli et al. (2012) observed that trained participants displayed a larger Stroop effect after training. A subset of participants who read multiple books displayed larger Stroop effects as more books were read, but the magnitude of this change was unrelated to the number of words read, nor was the number of words read related to the overall Stroop effect. Accordingly, this study provides mixed results regarding whether the amount of training is a determining factor of the magnitude of the post-training Stroop effect. One related notable finding is that there were marked individual differences in the magnitude of the Stroop effect after training with Stroop effects ranging from −26 to 185 ms: this points to considerable variability in the extent to which training elicits Stroop effects and suggests that certain individuals are more prone to these effects. Finally, the extent to which participants reported *experiencing* colours when seeing letters was unrelated to Stroop effects.

The results of the crowding and recall tests were less conclusive. Participants were unable to recall all of the letter-colour pairs in the recall test, but recalled with high accuracy the colours paired with each number. No controls were included in this task and thus it is unclear how remarkable this result is. Similarly, trained participants did not outperform controls on the crowding task, unlike synaesthetes (Ward, Jonas, Dienes, and Seth, 2010). Moreover, there is disagreement regarding the interpretation of superior performance among synaesthetes in this task (Ward et al., 2010), and so it is unclear whether training here is failing to reproduce a perceptual or attentional benefit conferred by synaesthesia. This study, as above, confirms that training can produce Stroop effects, but not other features of synaesthesia, and is equivocal regarding the extent to which training strengthens grapheme-colour associations.

Another study (Kusnir and Thut, 2012) shows that training can produce further behavioural effects that parallel those observed in synaesthetes. In this study, participants completed a letter-search task, in which they searched for target letters among an array and judged whether the target was to the left or the right of a central fixation cross. Certain target letters were more often associated with specific colours to facilitate statistical semantic learning over time; half of the participants were informed of the bias in the stimulus presentation. Participants' search times were faster for biased (congruent and incongruent) than unbiased stimuli, suggesting strong grapheme-colour binding. However, although the search time was faster over time, it did not vary over time for the different types of stimuli. In other words, the grapheme-colour binding effect appears to occur relatively early, although it is difficult to say when it became robust.

Stroop interference was associated with grapheme-colour binding strength in the aware group, but participants did not display an overall Stroop effect as a result of training, nor did the best learners exhibit the largest Stroop effect. An interesting result is that participants displayed larger interference in the search task when target colours were in opponent colours relative to the grapheme-colour association as opposed to non-opponent colours. For example, if *6* was paired with the colour *red*, participants were slower in responding when *6* was printed in *green* ink. This result is notable, because it is also displayed by synaesthetes (Nikolić et al., 2007) and because it implicates early visual processing, thereby suggesting a perceptual component to the processing of grapheme-colour associations (and potentially indirectly corroborating some of Colizoli et al.'s (2016)).

To summarize, as is the case with the other studies, this study produced somewhat equivocal results. Training did not elicit Stroop effects, but did elicit robust grapheme-colour binding and colour-opponency effects. The authors argue that explicit instructions such as those in Meier and Rothen (2009) may be more likely to produce associations at a more conceptual level, and thus larger Stroop effects, whereas implicit training may be more likely to elicit perceptual associations. However, this is at odds with the interpretation of synaesthetic Stroop effects by Nikolić and colleagues (2007), who argue that synaesthetic Stroop effects reflect a perceptual component, as exemplified by colour-opponency effects, as well as a smaller, semantic component. Further research is clearly needed to test these varying interpretations and to assess the extent to which the grapheme-colour associations induced in Kusnir and Thut's (2012) study resemble genuine synaesthesia.

It is plausible that behavioural tasks are insufficiently powerful in detecting induced synaesthesia and that neuroimaging methods may be more sensitive in capturing training-induced synaesthesia. Towards this end, Colizoli and colleagues recently investigated the neurophysiological effects of their coloured-letter training paradigm using fMRI (Colizoli, Murre, Scholte, van Es, Knapen, and Rouw, 2016). The authors found that training with coloured books over approximately 20 days did not produce grapheme-colour consistency at the level typically observed in developmental synaesthetes. Similarly, none of the participants subjectively reported experiencing colour photisms. As in some previous studies, training was associated with a significantly greater Stroop effect post-training relative to baseline; moreover, as commonly observed in this literature, the magnitude of post-training Stroop interference (~26 ms) was substantially lower than that observed in congenital synaesthetes and was unrelated to imagery and subjective colour experiences.

Functional correlates of these effects are difficult to interpret (Colizoli et al., 2016). The authors found that activation of V4, a region widely implicated in colour processing and synaesthesia (Ward, 2013), was greater for coloured (untrained) letters than trained and untrained (achromatic) letters, as would be expected. However, surprisingly, trained letters were characterized by less V4 activation than untrained letters and trained letters were also associated with a negative BOLD response relative to untrained letters in primary visual cortex. Moreover, visual cortex activation patterns were unrelated to Stroop effects, although there was some indication that the tendency to have associator experiences in response to graphemes was associated with greater V4 differences between trained and untrained letters. By implicating primary visual cortex in training of synaesthesia, these results are encouraging but preliminary. In particular, the results suggest that training grapheme-colour synaesthesia might elicit changes in the brain's response to graphemes but the meaning of these effects is somewhat equivocal, and it remains unclear how they may relate to, or inform our understanding of, developmental synaesthesia.

A final recent study suggests that the limited results of previous studies may be driven by insufficient training (Bor, Rothen, Schwartzman, Clayton, and Seth, 2014). This study aimed to couple greater ecological validity with a rigorous and diverse training schedule that changed over time. Fourteen participants underwent 9 weeks of training involving a range of cognitive tasks in which specific grapheme-colour pairs were repeatedly presented; they were also given "homework" consisting of books with coloured letters (Colizoli et al., 2012) and performance gains were reinforced with monetary compensation. After training, over 50 per cent of participants reported phenomenological associations resembling synaesthesia but only one participant reported projector-like perceptual experiences (these effects did not seem to be related to individual differences in imagery at baseline). Interestingly, nearly all participants spontaneously developed ordinal linguistic personification, in which certain characteristics (aggression) are tied to specific graphemes; these phenomena seem to closely resemble similar effects in congenital synaesthetes (Simner and Holenstein, 2007). Participants also displayed greater Stroop colour-naming effects post-training relative to baseline although this effect seemed to be specific to semantic associations. Critically, for the first time, to our knowledge, the authors also reported that participants displayed superior grapheme-colour consistency post-training than at baseline and at levels typically observed in developmental synaesthetes (Rothen et al., 2013), as well as other synaesthesia-specific effects (Bor et al., 2014).

The training studies undertaken to date clearly demonstrate that grapheme-colour *associations* can be induced in non-synaesthetes through training (Rothen and Meier, 2014). However, trained participants do not reliably display behavioural markers of synaesthesia, such as greater Stroop effects post-training (Kusnir and Thut, 2012; Rothen et al., 2011), implicit bidirectionality (Cohen Kadosh et al., 2005), or perceptual crowding (Colizoli et al., 2012). Moreover, when effects are observed, they do not display the same behavioural response patterns (Rothen et al., 2011), and/or they are smaller in magnitude than those observed in genuine synaesthetes (Dixon et al., 2004; Gebuis et al., 2009). For example, the largest Stroop effect in trained participants to the best of our knowledge was ~57 ms (Colizoli et al., 2012), which is comparable to that observed in congenital associator synaesthetes (Dixon et al., 2004; Ward et al., 2007). In contrast, when both associator and projector synaesthetes are included, the magnitude of the Stroop effect has been found to vary from ~90 ms (Dixon et al., 2004) to ~130 ms (Ward et al., 2007). Inconsistent or limited findings may stem from differences in training regimens across studies, with comprehensive training regimens seeming to produce the most compelling results (Bor et al., 2014). Moreover, only one study (Bor et al., 2014) has observed reports of conscious experiences of colour associations and even this was rare and transient. Three studies have shown that trained participants do not display the same patterns of neural (Elias et al., 2003; Nunn et al., 2002) or physiological (Meier and Rothen, 2009) effects as genuine synaesthetes, although preliminary research has implicated changes in primary visual cortex in trained synaesthesia (Colizoli et al., 2016). Whilst we do not want to dismiss the possibility that future training studies will successfully induce synaesthesia, we think it is prudent to interpret the present results as providing only tentative evidence for inducing certain features of synaesthesia (see also Rothen and Meier, 2014).

It is instructive to consider the trained associations relative to the demarcation criteria and characteristics of synaesthesia that we outlined above. First, there is evidence that training can produce consistency of grapheme-colour associations that rivals that observed in developmental synaesthetes (Bor et al., 2014) (other results are suggestive (Colizoli et al., 2012)). However, it could be argued that consistency is only a valuable measure when a sizeable number of grapheme-colour associations are trained because a small number of associations, as used in the training studies reviewed here, will be relatively easy to remember. Some studies to date have used canonical colours (Bor et al., 2014), which may further facilitate recall. Nevertheless, the criterion of consistency appears to have been met at least in a preliminary fashion. Similarly, we believe the criterion of automaticity has been met by training studies, but only to an extent. A number of studies have highlighted the fact that Stroop effects in trained groups are comparable to those in congenital synaesthetes (e.g., Elias et al., 2003) and/or that Stroop-type effects should not be used as diagnostic indicators of synaesthesia because they are unable to distinguish between semantic associations and those produced by involuntary colour photisms (Colizoli et al., 2012). We agree with this in part but it is important to recall that Stroop effects in trained groups of a comparable magnitude to those observed in synaesthetes do not always occur and no training study has observed Stroop effects comparable to those seen in projector synaesthetes (Dixon et al., 2004; Ward et al., 2007). One study has provided evidence that the criterion of conscious accessibility has been met as the majority of participants reported conscious experiences of colour photisms; however, insofar as only one participant reported projector-like experiences, there is not yet clear evidence for the individual differences typically observed in congenital synaesthetes. We revisit whether these results warrant revision of demarcation criteria later in this chapter.

When comparing congenital and induced synaesthetes, it is important to consider the confound of differential consolidation in this line of research. It is entirely possible that trained synaesthetes would display each of the behavioural, phenomenological, and neural markers of congenital synaesthesia if their associations were continuously reinforced (and consolidated) with long-term experience. Given the length of time that most synaesthetes have experienced this condition, this appears to be an insurmountable confound. The trained participant in Elias and colleagues' (2003) study exhibited grapheme-colour associations and underwent a form of training over eight years and still did not display the neural markers of synaesthesia, suggesting that long-term consolidation may not actually be sufficient to induce genuine synaesthesia. This was a case study and thus this result is far from conclusive. However, this confound should be considered when evaluating the authenticity of trained and other induced synaesthesias.

One approach to advancing research in this domain may be to couple training regimens with non-invasive brain stimulation techniques, which have been shown to enhance the impact of cognitive training (Krause and Cohen Kadosh, 2013). For example, we and others have consistently shown that concurrent application of transcranial electrical stimulation can be used to enhance the effects of training on a range of cognitive and perceptual functions, with long-lasting effects in specific cases (Fertonani, Pirulli, and Miniussi, 2011; Snowball, Tachtsidis, Popescu, Thompson, Delazer, Zamarian, Zhu, and Cohen Kadosh, 2013; Cappelletti, Gessaroli, Hithersay, Mitolo, Didino, Kanai, Cohen Kadosh, and Walsh, 2013; Looi, Duta, Brem, Huber, Nuerk, and Cohen Kadosh, 2016; Reis, Schambra, Cohen, Buch, Fritsch, Zarahn, Celnik, and Krakauer, 2009). Elsewhere, we have shown that synaesthetes display elevated cortical excitability in primary visual cortex (Terhune, Tai, Cowey, Popescu, and Cohen Kadosh, 2011; Terhune, Murray, Near, Stagg, Cowey, and Cohen Kadosh, 2015). Thus, specifically coupling non-invasive brain stimulation methods for enhancing excitability in primary visual cortex with rigorous cognitive training may provide an approach that is both methodologically robust but also grounded in contemporary knowledge of the neurophysiology of congenital synaesthesia.

11.3.2 Posthypnotic suggestion

A second method for the induction of synaesthesia involves the use of posthypnotic suggestion with highly suggestible individuals. Here we introduce a few of the hallmark features of hypnosis and posthypnotic suggestion and then review the studies that have used this approach to induce synaesthesia.

Hypnosis consists of a set of procedures including an induction and one or more suggestions (Oakley and Halligan, 2009; Terhune and Cohen Kadosh, 2012a). Inductions vary but generally involve instructions and suggestions to promote minimized awareness of one's environment, reduced metacognition, and perceived effortless attention towards the instructions of the experimenter (Brown, Antonova, Langley, and Oakley, 2001). Suggestions are verbal statements administered by an experimenter for *specific* changes in affective, cognitive, motor, or perceptual functions. They are typically conveyed in such a manner that they invite passive responses that are experienced as *happening* to an individual, rather than actions or representations that an individual willingly *performs* or *produces*, so as to augment the extra-volitional phenomenology of hypnotic responding (Bowers, 1981; Spanos and Gorassini, 1984). An example of a hypnotic suggestion for a visual hallucination may be, "When you open your eyes in a few moments, you will look at the computer monitor in front of you and see a red circle." Posthypnotic suggestions are suggestions for alterations in a particular function *following* a hypnotic de-induction. Although not originally intended for this purpose, most hypnosis researchers favour using such suggestions instead of regular hypnotic suggestions to dissociate the effects of the suggestion from those of the hypnotic induction. Specifically, it has been repeatedly shown that a hypnotic induction impairs attention in highly suggestible individuals (Egner and Raz, 2007), or at least a subset of highly suggestible individuals (Marcusson-Clavertz, Terhune, and Cardeña, 2012; Terhune, Cardeña, and Lindgren, 2011b). Posthypnotic suggestions circumvent the possible confound of impaired attention that may impact responding to hypnotic suggestions.

The most well established fact about hypnosis is that people display marked variability in their responsiveness to hypnotic suggestions (Hilgard, 1965). Hypnotic suggestibility varies widely in the general population with approximately 10–15 per cent of individuals displaying low hypnotic suggestibility, 10–15 per cent displaying high hypnotic suggestibility, and the remaining 70–80 per cent of the population exhibiting a moderate level of suggestibility (Laurence, Beaulieu-Prévost, and du Chéné, 2008). Hypnotic suggestibility is typically measured with one or more behavioural scales that comprise a series of hypnotic suggestions (for a review, see Woody and Barnier, 2008). These instruments are necessary for reliably screening participants and identifying individuals of different levels of hypnotic suggestibility, who cannot be differentiated by questionnaires or self-report. Most hypnosis research involves the use of highly suggestible individuals, including low-suggestible and/or medium-suggestible participants as a control group.

The first study demonstrating the posthypnotic induction of synaesthesia was reported by Cohen Kadosh and colleagues (Cohen Kadosh et al., 2009). In this study, the authors administered a posthypnotic suggestion to highly suggestible participants to experience *projector* grapheme-colour synaesthesia for six grapheme-colour pairs. Control participants received instructions for the same digit-colour associations but with no posthypnotic suggestions. Under the cover of the posthypnotic suggestion and in a control condition, participants completed a digit detection task in which they had to judge whether a digit was presented on a monitor or not (Smilek, Dixon, Cudahy, and Merikle, 2001). Digits were presented in black ink against a coloured background, which was either congruent or incongruent with the colour associated with the digit. A previous study found that congenital synaesthetes were poorer at detecting whether a digit was present during the congruent condition (Smilek et al., 2001). The induced synaesthetes, but not the control groups, displayed this same response pattern. In addition, whilst under the posthypnotic suggestion, they also reported experiencing colour photisms in response to graphemes outside of the laboratory. This study nicely demonstrates that both the behavioural and experiential markers of synaesthesia can be induced in the laboratory using posthypnotic suggestion.

Recently, a second study failed to observe behavioural markers of synaesthesia in non-synaesthetes given a posthypnotic suggestion for synaesthesia (Anderson, Seth, Dienes, and Ward, 2014). Null results are challenging to interpret and thus we can only speculate as to the reasons for their failure to observe induced synaesthesia. First, their procedure for screening participants was not as rigorous as most hypnosis studies, including that by Cohen Kadosh et al. (2009), which typically include two rounds of hypnotic suggestibility measurement to ensure that participants are sufficiently highly suggestible (Woody and Barnier, 2008). In addition, the participants were not screened prior to the experiment for their ability to respond to hallucination or synaesthesia suggestions. Highly suggestible individuals display pronounced variability in hypnotic responding and some are incapable of responding to hallucination suggestions (Szechtman, Woody, Bowers, and Nahmias, 1998). Combined, these two features already strongly suggest that only a small subset of the participant pool in this study would be responsive to such a suggestion. Finally, the authors used an embedded figures task, in which synaesthetic concurrent colours are presumed to facilitate "pop-out" of embedded higher-order stimuli in an array of stimuli. This task is problematic as synaesthetes have not been reliably shown to outperform controls in this task (for a review, see Ward et al., 2010). It is imperative that research attempting to assess the veracity of induced synaesthesia uses well-established tasks that reliably distinguish synaesthetes from controls.

In another study, we expanded upon the approach of Cohen Kadosh et al. (2009) and used posthypnotic suggestion to induce different phenomenological subtypes of synaesthesia (Terhune and Cohen Kadosh, 2012b). We were motivated to conduct this experiment because it remains unclear whether the observed behavioural markers of associator and projector synaesthesia (Dixon et al., 2004) are reliable (Hupé, Bordier, and Dojat, 2011; Ward et al., 2007) and are actually the product of individual differences in the perceived visuospatial location of colour photisms. We first doubly screened participants (Woody and Barnier, 2008) and then identified highly suggestible individuals who were *subjectively* responsive to hypnotic suggestions for either associator or projector grapheme-colour synaesthesia. Next, we administered posthypnotic suggestions to associate four numbers with four colours and to experience colours as either spatially colocalized with graphemes (projectors) or as mental images (associators) to the respective two subgroups who were responsive to these types of suggestions. Participants completed two Stroop colour-naming tasks previously shown to discriminate associators and projectors (Dixon et al., 2004): in the stimulus colour-naming task, they named the colour of the digit, whereas in the photism colour-naming task, they named the colour *associated* with the digit.

The behavioural and phenomenological responses of the induced synaesthetes in this study closely resemble those of the congenital synaesthetes. In both groups, projector synaesthetes displayed larger congruency effects in the stimulus colour-naming task than associator synaesthetes (Dixon et al., 2004), whereas the two groups did not differ in the photism colour-naming task. Attempting to identify the stimulus colour is presumably more difficult for projectors because their colour photisms are perceived to be spatially colocalized with the stimulus and thereby elicit greater response conflict when naming the stimulus colour. Across conditions, induced synaesthetes displayed comparable performance, as measured by response latencies, to congenital synaesthetes. Indeed, induced projectors actually displayed numerically, but not significantly, larger Stroop effects in the stimulus colour-naming task than congenital projectors. Below we maintain that this unexpected result is actually consistent with the induction of genuine synaesthesia. The phenomenological reports nicely complement the behavioural results. Congenital and induced synaesthetes reported similar subjective levels of both the involuntariness and the vividness of colour photisms *during* the Stroop tasks, but congenital synaesthetes actually reported experiencing colour photisms more often (some induced synaesthetes did report colour photisms on 100 per cent of the experimental trials, though). Two other effects are worth mentioning in the present context. Two highly suggestible participants reported *spontaneous* colour photisms for numbers that were *not* paired with a colour by posthypnotic suggestion and a single highly suggestible participant reported *explicit* bidirectionality such that colours triggered conscious experiences of the paired number. Insofar as these variables were not formally assessed in this experiment, the extent to which these experiences spontaneously occur is unclear; nevertheless, these effects highlight the range of synaesthetic effects that could potentially be induced using posthypnotic suggestion.

This study corroborates and extends the results of Cohen Kadosh and colleagues (2009). First, it replicates the previous result that posthypnotic suggestion can be used to induce synaesthesia-like behavioural and phenomenological response patterns. These studies indicate that the behavioural and phenomenological markers of synaesthesia can be reproduced using posthypnotic suggestion. Second, it extends the results of Cohen Kadosh and colleagues by showing that different phenomenological subtypes of synaesthesia can be induced. Finally, it demonstrates that variability in response patterns on Stroop tasks among synaesthetes is a product of individual differences in the perceived visuospatial location of colour photisms, and thereby provides valuable information regarding individual differences in grapheme-colour synaesthesia. Accordingly, these studies nicely complement other instrumental hypnosis research (Oakley and Halligan, 2009) and present a method by which synaesthesia can be experimentally modulated in the laboratory. The use of such a method has considerable potential in tackling a wide range of questions regarding the characteristics and mechanisms of synaesthesia.

These studies raise the question whether posthypnotic suggestion is producing genuine synaesthesia. The available evidence *suggests* the affirmative. Posthypnotic suggestion is capable of reproducing the behavioural and phenomenological markers of congenital synaesthesia. Posthypnotic synaesthetes also display behavioural effects of comparable magnitude, suggesting a similar degree of involuntariness, which is corroborated by the phenomenological reports. However, whether congenital and induced synaesthesia are occurring through similar or overlapping neural mechanisms remains an open question that needs to be addressed empirically. Hypnotic suggestions for colour hallucinations have previously been shown to produce greater activation in V4 (a region repeatedly implicated in the representation of synaesthetic colour photisms (Brang, Hubbard, Coulson, Huang, and Ramachandran, 2010; Hubbard, Arman, Ramachandran, and Boynton, 2005)) than colour imagery (Kosslyn, Thompson, Costantini-Ferrando, Alpert, and Spiegel, 2000; McGeown et al., 2012). This indicates that colour experiences associated with V4 activation can be produced using posthypnotic suggestion. One notable finding that is especially compelling here is that induced projector synaesthetes displayed numerically larger Stroop effects in the stimulus colour-naming task than congenital projector synaesthetes, suggesting elevated involuntariness of colour photisms relative to congenital projector synaesthetes (this was also found by Cohen Kadosh et al. (2009)). This finding seems peculiar at first glance but we think it actually provides further evidence for the authenticity of posthypnotically induced synaesthesia. Congenital synaesthetes are repeatedly exposed to incongruent grapheme colours pairs in product labels, street signs, web content, and so on. In turn, it is necessary for them to develop strategies to manage this conflict in their daily lives, which aids them when completing a synaesthesia Stroop task. In contrast, grapheme-colour associations are novel experiences for induced synaesthetes and this group will not have access to a repertoire of conflict management strategies to attenuate synaesthesia-specific response conflict, and in turn, Stroop effects. Indeed, many of our synaesthetes reported that the experience was so novel and unusual that the Stroop task was especially difficult. Accordingly, it may be that numerically greater Stroop effects in induced synaesthetes are a consequence of having only experienced grapheme-colour associations for a short duration.

The posthypnotic induction of synaesthesia has broader implications for the neural mechanisms underlying this condition. If posthypnotic suggestion is temporarily and instantaneously producing synaesthesia, these results are at odds with the position that synaesthesia is a direct result *of* greater anatomical connectivity between cortical structures supporting the processing of the inducer and the concurrent (cross-activation theory; Hubbard, 2007; Hubbard, Brang, and Ramachandran, 2011). It is highly unlikely that a posthypnotic suggestion is capable of producing excess structural brain connectivity within minutes, thus posthypnotic induction of synaesthesia suggests that theories postulating that anatomical connectivity plays a *causal* role in the development and online occurrence of synaesthesia are incorrect or at least incomplete (Cohen Kadosh et al., 2009).

If we momentarily accept that a posthypnotic suggestion is producing *genuine* synaesthesia, there are two plausible ways by which these results can be reconciled with cross-activation theory. One possibility is that there are two (or more) sets of mechanisms by which synaesthesia can be produced. On this account, synaesthesia can occur through both a genetic predisposition for enhanced connectivity, but also through a second mechanism, such as *cortical disinhibition* (Cohen Kadosh et al., 2009). According to this view, synaesthesia results from a disruption of cortical inhibition, producing conscious awareness of visual information that is normally inhibited (Cohen Kadosh and Walsh, 2008; Eagleman and Goodale, 2009). A second possibility is that both congenital and induced synaesthesia occur through disinhibition and that excess connectivity is a byproduct of the repeated binding of inducer and concurrent representations; that is, it is a *consequence*, rather than *cause*, of synaesthesia (Cohen Kadosh and Walsh, 2008). Determining which possibility is more plausible is ultimately an empirical issue. Nevertheless, coupled with other results that are at odds with cross-activation theory (Nikolić, Jurgens, Rothen, Meier, and Mroczko, 2011), the two studies described above call into question the viability of the cross-activation theory as a comprehensive account of synaesthesia.

One critique of this line of research is that the mechanisms underlying hypnosis are poorly understood and thus it remains unclear how hypnotic suggestion is effecting the synaesthetic response (Hubbard, 2011). We think that this line of argument sidesteps the value of the use of posthypnotic suggestion for studying synaesthesia. Although a comprehensive account of the neurocognitive mechanisms underlying hypnosis has yet to be advanced, there is emerging evidence that a *reduction* in prefrontal cortical activity (Dienes and Hutton, 2013) or a *decoupling* of prefrontal cortex with anterior cingulate cortex (Egner, Jamieson, and Gruzelier, 2005) or parietal cortex (Terhune, Cardeña, and Lindgren, 2011a) in highly suggestible individuals facilitates hypnotic responding, in particular the experience that responses are occurring extra-volitionally. A number of studies have also suggested candidate regions for the top-down modulation of alterations in conscious awareness following particular suggestions including orbitofrontal cortex and precuneus (Cojan et al., 2009; Mendelsohn, Chalamish, Solomonovich, and Dudai, 2008). Such regions, or perhaps other regions in the frontal-parietal network, most likely play a top-down role in producing activation in V4 and other regions involved in the synaesthetic experience (Cohen Kadosh et al., 2009).

11.3.3 Pharmacological agents

The context in which non-synaesthetes seem most often to spontaneously experience synaesthesia is arguably under the influence of pharmacological agents, such as recreational drugs. In turn, the administration of such agents provides a potentially valuable method for inducing synaesthesia in a controlled environment (Luke and Terhune, 2013). This method has a number of clear methodological advantages over training and posthypnotic suggestion methods. First, unlike training, pharmacological agents may be expected to elicit synaesthesia in a relatively short period of time. Second, unlike posthypnotic induction, this method is expected to be effective with a relatively large proportion of the population, perhaps as high as 60 per cent (Luke et al., 2012; Tart, 1975). Finally, insofar as much is known about the neurotransmitter systems affected by pharmacological agents (Carhart-Harris et al., 2012), their use for inducing synaesthesia may lend insights into the neurotransmitters implicated in the induction, modulation, and disruption of synaesthesia, as well as the neuro-developmental origins of congenital synaesthesia.

In some cases, the neurotransmitter systems targeted by particular drugs are well known, as with the classical tryptamine psychedelics such as psilocybin, which are selective $5HT_{2A}$ partial agonists (Lee and Roth, 2012). The neural mechanisms involved continue to be debated, but a recent fMRI study (Carhart-Harris et al., 2012) shows that, contrary to expectations, psilocybin decreases cerebral blood flow to key regions, specifically the thalamus, anterior and posterior cingulate cortex (ACC & PCC), and medial prefrontal cortex (mPFC), the latter two of which are primary regions in the default mode network (Raichle et al., 2001). Significantly, the usual positive coupling between the mPFC and the PCC is also reduced during the intake of psilocybin. At the same time, some chemicals, known as promiscuous drugs, modulate a variety of neurotransmitters, or their mode of action remains uncertain (*N, N*-dimethyltryptamine (DMT) is a good example of both (Ray, 2010; Wallach, 2009), thus the specific systems that mediate the induction of synaesthesia may be difficult to identify. However, a neurochemical taxonomy of action may be possible once more is known about the action of these chemicals and the specific types and features of synaesthesia they induce (Luke et al., 2012).

A wide range of pharmacological agents, especially those termed psychedelic, have been reported to induce synaesthetic experience, extending back to the earliest subjective accounts by scientists and explorers using mescaline (Ellis, 1898), LSD (Hofmann, 1983), and psilocybin (Wasson, 1978). A recent survey (Luke et al., 2012) corroborates the wide range of substances reported to induce synaesthesia and suggests that the prevalence of this experience among those using these substances is higher with certain classes of psychoactive substances than others, particularly the serotonergic tryptamines (e.g., LSD, psilocybin), then the largely serotonergic substituted phenethylamines (mescaline, 2CB), then the glutamatergic dissociatives (dextromethorphan, ketamine), and then other drugs to a lesser extent. Here we review the few experimental studies that have investigated the induction of synaesthesia using pharmacological agents and then describe other studies that have used questionnaire and survey methodologies.

Despite there being a long history of subjective reports of spontaneous experiences, direct experimental research of chemically induced synaesthesia is sparse and, until very recently, has not been conducted since the 1960s when prohibition effectively curtailed psychedelic research with humans for the next 30–40 years. In one of the first systematic studies (Simpson and McKellar, 1955), two non-synaesthete controls (the authors) and two congenital synaesthetes were each given four doses (0.3–0.5 mg) of mescaline on different occasions and presented with an array of possible inducer stimuli throughout the course of their drug-induced altered state (up to 12 hours). The experimenters recorded any synaesthetic impressions but did not attempt to train or repeat experiences. Participants collectively reported eight distinct types of novel synaesthesia; inducers varied considerably, whereas the concurrent was typically visual, with the most common type being auditory-visual, which was experienced by each participant in at least one session. The single congenital synaesthete who had multiple types of synaesthesia also reported enhancement of their ordinary auditory-tactile and visual-tactile synaesthesias. The researchers correctly predicted that mescaline would produce novel variants; however, given their roles as experimenters, the controls were not blind, or impartial, to the aims of the study. This study has a number of clear limitations, in particular the lack of measures of consistency and/or automaticity of inducer-concurrent associations, but points to the potential viability of experimentally inducing synaesthesia. It also suggests that the same pharmacological agents that induce synaesthesia in non-synaesthetes enhance synaesthesia in congenital synaesthetes, which was also found in a recent survey (Luke et al., 2012).

A second experimental study used a more rigorous approach and compared a range of different substances in the induction of synaesthesia (Hartman and Hollister, 1963). Hartman and Hollister administered mescaline, psilocybin, and LSD a week apart to eighteen participants who were blind to the type of drug. Participants listened to sixteen pure sonic tones at four set frequencies (between 500 and 4000 Hz) at relatively equal amplitudes at baseline and following the administration of each drug. Compared to baseline, the participants experienced significantly more colours and other visual effects (brightening of the visual field, shattering of patterns, and patterning of form) during the presentation of pure tones whilst under the influence of both LSD and mescaline. Psilocybin was associated with a non-significant increase in these experiences. This study expands upon the study of Simpson and McKellar (1955) by showing the induction of auditory-visual synaesthesia with controlled stimuli. It further highlights the role of serotonin agonists in the induction of synaesthesia, although the inclusion of a placebo would have strengthened the design. Recent survey research (Luke et al., 2012) similarly found LSD to be the most prevalent inducer of synesthesia as a percentage of those using the drug (55 per cent).

A number of studies have similarly administered psychedelic substances to examine neurocognitive processes more generally and have used altered-states questionnaires that include items pertaining to synaesthesia. These approaches are clearly less rigorous than experimental designs, but can potentially lend insights into the induction of synaesthesia, particularly when they reveal convergent effects. That such scales include synaesthesia is indicative of its consideration as an ordinary, if not relatively infrequent, feature of many altered states of consciousness (Dittrich and Scharfetter, 1987), as supported by the correlation between the synaesthesia subscale and all of the subscales of the *Altered State of Consciousness Rating Scale* (Studerus, Gamma, and Vollenweider, 2010) for psilocybin participants, ranging from elementary imagery, complex imagery, and experience of unity at one end to anxiety at the other.

Findings from studies employing a questionnaire approach highlight a wide range of pharmacological agents in the induction of synaesthesia. These studies suggest that the incidence of auditory-visual synaesthesia escalates linearly with psilocybin dosage (Griffiths et al., 2011; Studerus, 2013), and that reports of auditory-visual synaesthesia occur with decreasing prevalence from relatively equal doses of psilocybin (37 per cent), ketamine (27 per cent), and MDMA (10 per cent), as supported by prevalence figures from a survey of recreational users (Luke et al., 2012). Reports of auditory-visual synaesthesia with psilocybin are also evident from different laboratories (Carhart-Harris et al., 2011), although prevalence rates are lower (11 per cent). Laboratory studies of other psychedelic substances in humans also report the subjective experience of synaesthesia, such as auditory-visual synaesthesia with ayahuasca, evident in 28 per cent of participants (Riba, Anderer, Jane, Saletu, and Barbanoj, 2004), and with *Salvia divinorum*, which reportedly induced visual-somatic synaesthesia in 57 per cent of participants (Addy, 2010). Interestingly, the largest such laboratory database (Studerus, 2013), comprising 261 participants and 409 psilocybin administrations, indicates that induced auditory-visual synaesthesia is strongly predicted by drug dosage and the *Tellegen Absorption Scale* (Tellegen and Atkinson, 1974), and weakly predicted by alcohol consumption, and under-the-influence self-reports of sociability, emotional excitability, and activity. This finding is notable for two reasons. First, it identifies a possible moderating factor of individual differences in susceptibility to experiencing synaesthesia under the influence of psilocybin. Second, the construct of absorption is indiscriminable from that of fantasy-proneness (Rhue and Lynn, 1989) and the fantasizing component of empathy has been recently shown to be elevated in congenital synaesthesia (Banissy et al., 2013). This suggests that individuals who have a cognitive-perceptual personality profile similar to that of congenital synaesthetes may be more susceptible to drug-induced synaesthesia.

Collectively, these and other studies suggest that LSD and other serotonin agonists reliably produce spontaneous synaesthesia-like experiences (Luke and Terhune, 2013). Despite these promising, albeit preliminary, results, the available studies on drug-induced synaesthesia are severely methodologically limited. For example, none of the research studies of this phenomenon have used double-blind methods, placebo controls, or established behavioural markers of synaesthesia. To address this lacuna in contemporary knowledge, we recently conducted a double-blind placebo-controlled study investigating the effect of LSD on markers of synaesthesia (conscious accessibility, and inducer-concurrent consistency and specificity) in non-synaesthetes (Terhune, Luke, Kaelen, Bolstridge, Feilding, Nutt, Carhart-Harris, and Ward, 2016). After administration of placebo and LSD on separate days, participants rated the extent to which graphemes and sounds elicited conscious experience of colours and selected their first colour associations for these stimuli. Crucially, participants did not differ across the two conditions in the accessibility of colour concurrents, and their grapheme-colour associations did not differ in consistency or specificity. However, participants did report more spontaneous synaesthesia-like experiences in the LSD condition relative to the placebo condition. Although preliminary, this study clearly challenges the proposal that LSD produces genuine synaesthesia, as least according to the criteria by which we verify the occurrence of congenital synaesthesia.

Experimental and survey data, while sparse, indicate that spontaneous pharmacologically mediated synaesthesia is relatively reliable and widespread, especially with psychedelic agents (Luke et al., 2012; Luke and Terhune, 2013). Despite some researchers emphasizing the similarity between drug-induced and congenital synaesthesia in terms of their vividness, memorability, and emotionality (e.g., Cytowic, 1993; Cytowic, 2002; Cytowic and Eagleman, 2009), others have argued that they diverge in a number of important respects. Hubbard and Ramachandran (2003, 2005), for instance, maintain that pharmacologically induced synaesthesia lacks the specificity of congenital synaesthesia and is also more complex than the simple inducer-concurrent associations experienced by congenital synaesthetes. Our preliminary data supports this argument (Terhune et al., 2016). However, it could be argued that the complexity of psychedelic synaesthesia, while certainly reported by some (e.g., Klüver, 1966), is not obligatory (e.g., Simpson and McKellar, 1955). Sinke et al. (2012) further suggest that drug-induced synaesthesia lacks the automaticity and consistency of congenital synaesthesia, citing an older study which explored the consistency of sound-colour synaesthesia with mescaline (Beringer, 1927). Indeed, our study similarly found no effect of LSD on grapheme- or sound-colour consistency (Terhune et al., 2016). However, in one case, melatonin-induced grapheme-colour synaesthesia was shown to display consistency via a texture segregation behavioural test (Brang and Ramachandran, 2008). Interestingly, there is suggestive evidence that mescaline-induced synaesthesia can reproduce individual differences in synaesthetes. Klüver (1966: 93), for instance, notes that on mescaline, an "auditory stimulus may give rise to a sensation of color in some subjects, but in others the color, e.g., purple, is not actually seen. Instead, the subject experiences a 'feeling like purple' or a feeling 'as if purple'". It remains unclear whether this reflects broader individual differences in psychedelic experiences or something that is specific to the induction of synaesthesia.

A final difference between congenital and drug-induced synaesthesias may be in the types of inducers and concurrents. Sinke et al. (2012) note that congenital synaesthesias typically have graphemes as inducers, whereas drug-induced synaesthesias do not. Although it's true that graphemes are frequent inducers, there is evidence that music and sound stimuli function as inducers in more than 25 per cent of cases of congenital synaesthesia (Hochel and Milán, 2008). This is notable because sound-colour (or sound-visual) synaesthesia appears to be the most frequently observed type of drug-induced synaesthesia (Klüver, 1966; Luke et al., 2012; Pahnke and Richards, 1966; Simpson and McKellar, 1955; Sinke et al., 2012; for a review, see Luke and Terhune, 2013). Furthermore, approximately 1 per cent of recreational tryptamine psychedelic (e.g., psilocybin, LSD) users report spontaneous grapheme-colour synaesthesia (Luke et al., 2012) and at least one case of verified drug-induced grapheme-colour synaesthesia has been reported (Brang and Ramachandran, 2008). Moreover, the patterns of different synaesthesia types across congenital and drug-induced synaesthesias are most likely artefactual of the context in which people consume drugs. Specifically, during the consumption of psychedelic drugs, people are more likely to listen to music than to read and thus the prevalence rates of sound-colour and grapheme-colour synaesthesias under the influence of such drugs are very likely to be inflated and deflated, respectively.

Discerning the relationship between drug-induced and congenital synaesthesias is crucial because it may help us to identify the neurochemical markers of congenital synaesthesia and to discriminate between competing theories of synaesthesia. Disinhibition theories propose that the experience of synaesthesia is normally suppressed (Cohen Kadosh and Henik, 2007; Eagleman and Goodale, 2009; Grossenbacher, 1997) and thus these accounts can easily accommodate drug-induced synaesthesias. Disinhibition theories predict a reduction in GABA in visual cortex as a possible neurochemical mechanism underlying congenital synaesthesia. To date, no study has explicitly examined the influence of GABAergic agonists or antagonists on the experience of synaesthesia, although one study found that synaesthetes and controls don't differ in visual cortex GABA levels (Terhune et al., 2015), and thus there is as yet no direct evidence bearing on the implications of drug-induced synaesthesia for disinhibition theories of synaesthesia. Conversely, cross-activation theory suggests that congenital and drug-induced synaesthesias occur through disparate mechanisms (Hubbard et al., 2011).

Whether there are multiple aetiologies for synaesthesia or not, current theorizing proposes that serotonin-2A subtype agonism is fundamental to drug-induced synaesthesia (Brang and Ramachandran, 2008). In support of the $5HT_{2A}$ hypothesis, Brang and Ramachandran (2008) note that LSD largely operates via $5HT_{2A}$ agonism, that the presumed $5HT_{2A}$ inhibitors Prozac and Wellbutrin have been shown to inhibit congenital synaesthesia in case studies, and that melatonin was able to induce genuine grapheme-colour synaesthesia like a chemical switch, possibly via $5HT_1$ inhibition and subsequent $5HT_{2A}$ disinhibition. However, whole-gene linkage scan and family-based linkage analysis studies have as yet not found evidence for a $5HT_{2A}$-linked gene for synaesthesia, perhaps due to the low power of the studies or a polygenic aetiology (Brang and Ramachandran, 2011). Nevertheless, recent survey research (Luke et al., 2012) lends some support to the $5HT_{2A}$ agonism hypothesis, as serotonergic tryptamines (e.g., LSD, psilocybin) and the largely serotonergic substituted phenethylamines (mescaline, 2CB) were shown to be the most prevalent inducers of synaesthesia, although other classes of drugs were also reported to induce synaesthesia too, albeit to a lesser extent. Nevertheless, the psychedelic *Salvia divinorum*, which has no known serotonergic action, but known kappa opioid receptor activation only (Ray, 2010), was reported to induce synaesthesia with moderate prevalence in this survey (33 per cent) and in a laboratory study (57 per cent) (Addy, 2010). These results appear to challenge the serotoninergic hypothesis, but it is possible that kappa receptors regulate the serotonin system (Bruchas et al., 2011), giving rise to secondary serotonergic effects. Furthermore, not only do serotonergic psychedelics have the highest prevalence rates for inducing synaesthesias among non-synaesthetes, they also have the greatest tendency of any class of substances to enhance the existing synaesthesia of congenital synaesthetes (Luke et al., 2012), although caution is urged over the interpretation of self-report data from a self-selecting sample. Cumulatively, these results implicate serotonin in both the induction of synaesthesia in non-synaesthetes and its amelioration in congenital synaesthetes, but further research is clearly needed to corroborate these results with more rigorous experimental designs.

In summary, using pharmacological agents to induce and inhibit synaesthesia has advantages in that it can elicit effects quickly and with a large sample of people, and it also has the potential to illuminate the neurotransmitter systems involved in at least some subtypes of synaesthesia. However, little research has actually been conducted along these lines as yet, so current understanding is extremely limited and there is much to be learned. Our recent research suggests that LSD-induced synaesthesia does not meet standard criteria for synaesthesia (conscious accessibility and inducer-concurrent consistency and specificity) and thereby potentially calls into question this line of research (Terhune et al., 2016). By contrast, we are unaware of any investigation into the automaticity of inducer-concurrent associations. Nevertheless, as we noted earlier in this chapter, it may not be particularly meaningful to apply the criterion of consistency to early-stage synaesthesias. Given the relative paucity of data, we believe it remains premature to draw firm conclusions regarding the authenticity of drug-induced synaesthesias. Working with psychoactive substances can be challenging, but a growing interest in the neurobiological action of psychedelics makes this research more feasible now than previously. Nevertheless, despite group trends being somewhat well mapped, psychedelic agents produce largely unpredictable altered states of consciousness within individuals and effects other than synaesthesia will be produced that will need to be addressed. Despite these challenges, we believe that the use of pharmacological agents will be useful in helping to understand the neurobiology of synaesthesia.

11.4 Comparing methods

Here we briefly contrast the different methods of inducing synaesthesia. The studies conducted to date overwhelmingly demonstrate that posthypnotic suggestion is a more robust method for the experimental induction of synaesthesia than training approaches. Training is time-intensive (Bor et al., 2014; but see Kusnir and Thut, 2012), it does not reliably reproduce behavioural or phenomenological markers of synaesthesia, and it does not replicate the physiological and neurophysiological concomitants of synaesthesia. Furthermore, training has yet to reproduce individual differences in synaesthetic experience (Dixon et al., 2004; Ward et al., 2007). In contrast, posthypnotic suggestion can reliably reproduce the behavioural and phenomenological markers of synaesthesia, as well as individual differences therein, and it is effective in a relatively short time period. A further benefit of posthypnotic suggestion is that it can be used to modulate synaesthesia phenomenology in highly suggestible synaesthetes (see also Terhune, Cardeña, and Lindgren, 2010). We find it highly unlikely that training could accomplish this.

Nevertheless, the use of posthypnotic suggestion for the induction and modulation of synaesthesia has its limitations whilst training has other strengths. The posthypnotic induction of synaesthesia is hampered by the fact that posthypnotic suggestion is only reliably effective in highly suggestible individuals, who comprise a small minority of the population (Laurence et al., 2008), and extensive screening is required to identify these individuals (Woody and Barnier, 2008). We maintain that this explains failures to induce synaesthesia with suggestion (Anderson et al., 2014). Training, on the other hand, can be done with anyone, although there clearly seem to be important individual differences (Bor et al., 2014; Colizoli et al., 2012; Kusnir and Thut, 2012). Moreover, one might argue that training is more comparable to the real-life process by which inducer-concurrent associations are initially formed and consolidate over time. Posthypnotic suggestion, in contrast, does *not* present itself as a valuable method for studying the learning mechanisms underlying synaesthesia. Thus, whilst the available evidence reliably demonstrates that posthypnotic suggestion is a superior method for the induction of synaesthesia, training is clearly a better model for learning in synaesthesia. We hope to see both methods strengthened with further research. For instance, it would be valuable to undertake more rigorous screening of participants to exploit individual differences and identify participants who are most likely to develop strong associations from training, such as relatives of synaesthetes (Colizoli et al., 2016) or individuals with strong imagery (Bor et al., 2014).

In certain respects, psychedelic synaesthesias may present the closest model of genuine congenital synaesthesia. Synaesthesias experienced after the consumption of pharmacological agents are relatively common and thus this approach is likely to be more reliable than posthypnotic suggestion and more amenable to broad research. As in congenital synaesthesia, drug-induced synaesthesias appear to emerge relatively spontaneously. This is in contrast with training methods, which *require* an experimental manipulation to elicit concurrent experiences (posthypnotic suggestion) or grapheme-colour associations (training). Like posthypnotic suggestion, but unlike training, the induction of synaesthesia using pharmacological agents can also reproduce conscious awareness of synaesthetic concurrents. Taken together, these strengths suggest that this approach is the most viable for large-scale studies of induced synaesthesia. Drug-induced synaesthesias may potentially resemble early-stage synaesthesias that have not yet undergone consolidation. In addition, drug-induced synaesthesias provide a clearer framework for studying the neurochemical mechanisms of synaesthesia than do posthypnotic suggestion and training. However, despite the value of this approach, it does not afford the ability to carefully manipulate the phenomenology of synaesthesia, as does posthypnotic suggestion. Indeed, it has been argued that drug-induced synaesthesias are pervasive, inconsistent (Sinke et al., 2012), and non-specific (Hubbard et al., 2011), and thus may not be very amenable to research studies concerned with the characteristics and mechanisms of a specific form of synaesthesia. Ways of leveraging the strengths of this approach whilst circumventing these limitations would be to stratify participants by type of previous self-reported drug-induced synaesthesia and to explore the possibility of training inducer-concurrent associations after the consumption of pharmacological agents. Further exploring the combination of hypnosis and psychoactive substances could prove illuminating in experimental conditions, especially in light of the supposedly increased suggestibility of the psychedelic state (Sjoberg and Hollister, 1965; Carhart-Harris, Kaelen, Whalley, Bolstridge, Feilding, and Nutt, 2015) and the possibility of re-inducing such drug states via hypnotic suggestion (Hastings, 2006).

11.5 Implications and conclusions

The induction of synaesthesia using the methods described in this chapter has a number of significant implications. First, these approaches present potentially viable methods for experimental analogues of synaesthesia that can be used to aid our understanding of the cognitive and neural mechanisms of this condition. We hope to see further research exploring the induction of synaesthesia using these methods, but also research that uses such methods to answer questions about synaesthesia (Luke et al., 2012; Terhune and Cohen Kadosh, 2012b). The methods described here also have clear implications for the criteria by which synaesthesia is defined. Although none of the methods has been shown to meet all of the criteria of synaesthesia that we outlined at the beginning of this chapter, we are very confident that posthypnotic suggestion will be able to reproduce all of the hallmark features of synaesthesia. In turn, such research will have important implications regarding the utility of such criteria.

A diverse array of studies have explored the possibility that synaesthesia can be induced. These have included training, posthypnotic suggestion, and the administration of pharmacological agents. The foregoing review suggests that training can produce grapheme-colour associations, although the magnitude of these associations varies, as does the extent to which they impact different behavioural markers of synaesthesia. Crucially, training studies have so far been unable to reliably produce colour photisms although preliminary research is encouraging. In contrast, post-hypnotic suggestion is able to elicit both the behavioural and phenomenological markers of synaesthesia, as well as individual differences therein. Pharmacological agents have been shown to elicit the phenomenological features of synaesthesia, but the extent to which they reproduce the behavioural markers of this condition is unclear and preliminary research indicates that drug-induced synaesthesia is unlikely to meet standard criteria for synaesthesia. Multiple studies have shown that training does not reproduce the physiological and neural signatures of synaesthesia, whereas the impact of posthypnotic suggestion and pharmacological agents on these signatures has yet to be investigated. These different methods have their individual limitations but each can make unique contributions to our understanding of synaesthesia.

Acknowledgements

D.B.T. is supported by a Marie Curie Intra-European Fellowship within the 7th European Community Framework Programme and Bial Foundation bursary 344/14. D.P.L. is supported by University of Greenwich RAE grant R09469. R.C.K. is supported by the Wellcome Trust (WT88378).

References

Addy, P. H. (2010). *That deep internal voice: Controlled administration of Salvia divinorum.* Unpublished PhD thesis, Institute of Transpersonal Psychology, Palo Alto, CA.

Alstadhaug, K. B., & Benjaminsen, E. (2010). Synesthesia and migraine: Case report. *BMC Neurology, 10.* doi: 10.1186/1471-2377-10-121.

Anderson, H. P., Seth, A. K., Dienes, Z., & Ward, J. (2014). Can grapheme-color synesthesia be induced by hypnosis? *Frontiers in Human Neuroscience, 8*, 220. doi: 10.3389/fnhum.2014.00220.

Banissy, M. J., Holle, H., Cassell, J., Annett, L., Tsakanikos, E., Walsh, V., Ward, J. et al. (2013). Personality traits in people with synaesthesia: Do synaesthetes have an atypical personality profile? *Personality and Individual Differences, 54*, 828–31. doi: 10.1016/j.paid.2012.12.018.

Banissy, M. J., Tester, V., Muggleton, N. G., Janik, A. B., Davenport, A., Franklin, A., Walsh, V., & Ward, J. (2013). Synesthesia for color is linked to improved color perception but reduced motion perception. *Psychological Science, 24*, 2390–7. doi: 10.1177/0956797613492424.

Banissy, M. J., Walsh, V., & Ward, J. (2009). Enhanced sensory perception in synaesthesia. *Experimental Brain Research, 196*, 565–71. doi: 10.1007/s00221-009-1888-0.

Barnett, K. J., Foxe, J. J., Molholm, S., Kelly, S. P., Shalgi, S., Mitchell, K. J., & Newell, F. N. (2008). Differences in early sensory-perceptual processing in synesthesia: A visual evoked potential study. *NeuroImage, 43*, 605–13. doi: 10.1016/j.neuroimage.2008.07.028.

Beringer, K. (1927). *Der Meskalinrausch*. Berlin: Springer.

Bor, D., Rothen, N., Schwartzman, D. J., Clayton, S., & Seth, A. K. (2014). Adults can be trained to acquire synesthetic experiences. *Scientific Reports, 4*, 7089. doi: 10.1038/srep07089.

Bowers, K. S. (1981). Do the Stanford Scales tap the "classic suggestion effect"? *International Journal of Clinical and Experimental Hypnosis, 29*, 42–53.

Brang, D., Hubbard, E. M., Coulson, S., Huang, M., & Ramachandran, V. S. (2010). Magnetoencephalography reveals early activation of V4 in grapheme-color synesthesia. *Neuroimage, 53*, 268–74.

Brang, D., & Ramachandran, V. S. (2008). Psychopharmacology of synesthesia: The role of serotonin S2a receptor activation. *Medical Hypotheses, 70*, 903–4.

Brang, D., & Ramachandran, V. S. (2011). Survival of the synesthesia gene: Why do people hear colors and taste words? *PLoS Biology, 9*, e1001205. doi: 10.1371/journal.pbio.1001205.

Brown, R. J., Antonova, E., Langley, A., & Oakley, D. A. (2001). The effects of absorption and reduced critical thought on suggestibility in an hypnotic context. *Contemporary Hypnosis, 18*, 62–72.

Bruchas, M. R., Schindler, A. G., Shankar, H., Messinger, D. I., Miyatake, M., Land, B. B., Chavkin, C. et al. (2011). Selective p38alpha MAPK deletion in serotonergic neurons produces stress resilience in models of depression and addiction. *Neuron, 71*, 498–511. doi: 10.1016/j.neuron.2011.06.011.

Cappelletti, M., Gessaroli, E., Hithersay, R., Mitolo, M., Didino, D., Kanai, R., Cohen Kadosh, R., & Walsh, V. (2013). Transfer of cognitive training across magnitude dimensions achieved with concurrent brain stimulation of the parietal lobe. *Journal of Neuroscience, 33*, 14899-14907. doi: 10.1523/JNEUROSCI.1692-13.2013.

Carhart-Harris, R. L., Erritzoe, D., Williams, T., Stone, J. M., Reed, L. J., Colasanti, A., Nutt, D. J. et al. (2012). Neural correlates of the psychedelic state as determined by fMRI studies with psilocybin. *Proceedings of the National Academy of Sciences of the United States of America, 109*, 2138–43. doi: 10.1073/pnas.1119598109.

Carhart-Harris, R. L., Kaelen, M., Whalley, M. G., Bolstridge, M., Feilding, A., & Nutt, D. J. (2015). LSD enhances suggestibility in healthy volunteers. *Psychopharmacology* (Berlin), *232*, 785–94. doi: 10.1007/s00213-014-3714-z.

Carhart-Harris, R. L., Williams, T. M., Sessa, B., Tyacke, R. J., Rich, A. S., Feilding, A., & Nutt, D. J. (2011). The administration of psilocybin to healthy, hallucinogen-experienced volunteers in a mock-functional magnetic resonance imaging environment: A preliminary investigation of tolerability. *Journal of Psychopharmacology, 25*, 1562–7. doi: 10.1177/0269881 110367445.

Cohen, M. X., Weidacker, K., Tankink, J., Scholte, H. S., & Rouw, R. (2015). Grapheme-color synesthesia subtypes: Stable individual differences reflected in posterior alpha-band oscillations. *Cognitive Neuroscience, 6*, 56–67. doi: 10.1080/17588928.2015.1017450.

Cohen Kadosh, R., & Henik, A. (2007). Can synaesthesia research inform cognitive science? *Trends in Cognitive Sciences, 11*, 177–84.

Cohen Kadosh, R., Henik, A., Catena, A., Walsh, V., & Fuentes, L. J. (2009). Induced cross-modal synaesthetic experience without abnormal neuronal connections. *Psychological Science, 20*, 258–65. doi: 10.1111/j.1467-9280.2009.02286.x.

Cohen Kadosh, R., Sagiv, N., Linden, D. E., Robertson, L. C., Elinger, G., & Henik, A. (2005). When blue is larger than red: Colors influence numerical cognition in synesthesia. *Journal of Cognitive Neuroscience, 17*, 1766–73. doi: 10.1162/089892905774589181.

Cohen Kadosh, R., & Walsh, V. (2008). Synaesthesia and cortical connections: Cause or correlation? *Trends in Neurosciences, 31*, 549–50.

Cojan, Y., Waber, L., Schwartz, S., Rossier, L., Forster, A., & Vuilleumier, P. (2009). The brain under self-control: Modulation of inhibitory and monitoring cortical networks during hypnotic paralysis. *Neuron, 62*, 862–75. doi: 10.1016/j.neuron.2009.05.021.

Colizoli, O., Murre, J. M., & Rouw, R. (2012). Pseudo-synesthesia through reading books with colored letters. *PloS One, 7*, e39799. doi: 10.1371/journal.pone.0039799.

Colizoli, O., Murre, J. M., & Rouw, R. (2014). Defining (trained) grapheme-color synesthesia. *Frontiers in Human Neuroscience, 8*, 368. doi: 10.3389/fnhum.2014.00368.

Colizoli, O., Murre, J. M., Scholte, H. S., van Es, D. M., Knapen, T., & Rouw, R. (2016). Visual cortex activity predicts subjective experience after reading books with colored letters. *Neuropsychologia, 88*, 15–27. doi: 10.1016/j.neuropsychologia.2015.07.006.

Cytowic, R. E. (1993). *The man who tasted shapes: A bizarre medical mystery offers revolutionary insights into emotions, reasoning, and consciousness.* New York: Tarcher/Putnam.

Cytowic, R. E. (2002). *Synesthesia: A union of the senses.* Cambridge, MA: MIT Press.

Cytowic, R. E., & Eagleman, D. M. (2009). *Wednesday is indigo blue: Discovering the brain of synesthesia.* Cambridge, MA: MIT Press.

Deroy, O., & Spence, C. (2013). Why we are not all synesthetes (not even weakly so). *Psychonomic Bulletin & Review, 20*, 643–64. doi: 10.3758/s13423-013-0387-2.

Dienes, Z., & Hutton, S. (2013). Understanding hypnosis metacognitively: rTMS applied to DLPFC increases hypnotic suggestibility. *Cortex, 49*, 386–92. doi: 10.1016/j.cortex.2012.07.009.

Dittrich, A., & Scharfetter, C. (Eds.). (1987). *Ethnopsychotherapie: Psychotherapie mittels außergewöhnlicher Bewußtseinszustände in westlichen und indigenen Kulturen.* Stuttgart: Enke.

Dixon, M. J., Smilek, D., Cudahy, C., & Merikle, P. M. (2000). Five plus two equals yellow. *Nature, 406*, 365. doi: 10.1038/35019148.

Dixon, M. J., Smilek, D., & Merikle, P. M. (2004). Not all synaesthetes are created equal: Projector versus associator synaesthetes. *Cognitive Affective and Behavioral Neuroscience, 4*, 335–43.

Eagleman, D. M., & Goodale, M. A. (2009). Why color synesthesia involves more than color. *Trends in Cognitive Sciences, 13*, 288–92.

Egner, T., Jamieson, G., & Gruzelier, J. (2005). Hypnosis decouples cognitive control from conflict monitoring processes of the frontal lobe. *Neuroimage, 27*, 969–78.

Egner, T., & Raz, A. (2007). Cognitive control processes and hypnosis. In G. A. Jamieson (Ed.), *Hypnosis and conscious states: The cognitive neuroscience perspective* (pp. 29–50). Oxford, UK: Oxford University Press.

Elias, L. J., Saucier, D. M., Hardie, C., & Sarty, G. E. (2003). Dissociating semantic and perceptual components of synaesthesia: Behavioural and functional neuroanatomical investigations. *Cognitive Brain Research, 16*, 232–7. doi: 10.1016/S0926-6410(02)00278-1.

Ellis, H. (1898). Mescal: A new artificial paradise. *The Contemporary Review, 73.*

Fertonani, A., Pirulli, C., & Miniussi, C. (2011). Random noise stimulation improves neuroplasticity in perceptual learning. *Journal of Neuroscience, 31*, rp. doi: 10.1523/JNEUROSCI.2002-11.2011.

Fornazzari, L., Fischer, C. E., Ringer, L., & Schweizer, T. A. (2012). "Blue is music to my ears": Multimodal synesthesias after a thalamic stroke. *Neurocase, 18*, 318–22. doi: 10.1080/13554794.2011.608362.

Gebuis, T., Nijboer, T. C., & Van der Smagt, M. J. (2009). Multiple dimensions in bi-directional synesthesia. *European Journal of Neuroscience, 29*, 1703–10.

Griffiths, R. R., Johnson, M. W., Richards, W. A., Richards, B. D., McCann, U., & Jesse, R. (2011). Psilocybin occasioned mystical-type experiences: Immediate and persisting dose-related effects. *Psychopharmacology, 218*, 649–65. doi: 10.1007/s00213-011-2358-5.

Grossenbacher, P. G. (1997). Perception and sensory information in synaesthetic experience. In S. Baron-Cohen & J. E. Harrison (Eds.), *Synaesthesia: Classic and contemporary readings* (pp. 148–72). Oxford: Blackwell.

Hancock, P. (2006). Monozygotic twins' colour-number association: A case study. *Cortex, 42*, 147–50.

Hartman, A. M., & Hollister, L. E. (1963). Effect of mescaline, lysergic acid diethylamide and psilocybin on color perception. *Psychopharmacologia, 4*, 441–51.

Hastings, A. (2006). An extended nondrug MDMA-like experience evoked through posthypnotic suggestion. *Journal of Psychoactive Drugs, 38*, 273–83. doi: 10.1080/02791072.2006.10399853.

Hilgard, E. R. (1965). *Hypnotic susceptibility*. New York: Harcourt, Brace & World.

Hochel, M., & Milán, E. G. (2008). Synaesthesia: The existing state of affairs. *Cognitive Neuropsychology, 25*, 93–117.

Hofmann, A. (1983). *LSD my problem child: Reflections on sacred drugs, mysticism, and science*. Los Angeles: Jeremy P. Tarcher.

Hubbard, E. M. (2007). A real red-letter day. *Nature Neuroscience, 10*, 671–2.

Hubbard, E. M. (2011). *The cross-activation theory at ten: Substantial growth, future challenge*. Paper presented at the UK Synaesthesia Association, London, UK.

Hubbard, E. M., Arman, A. C., Ramachandran, V. S., & Boynton, G. M. (2005). Individual differences among grapheme-color synesthetes: brain-behavior correlations. *Neuron, 45*, 975–85.

Hubbard, E. M., Brang, D., & Ramachandran, V. S. (2011). The cross-activation theory at 10. *Journal of Neuropsychology, 5*, 152–77. doi: 10.1111/j.1748-6653.2011.02014.x.

Hubbard, E. M., & Ramachandran, V. S. (2003). Refining the experimental lever: A reply to Shanon & Pribram. *Journal of Consciousness Studies, 9*, 77–84.

Hubbard, E. M., & Ramachandran, V. S. (2005). Neurocognitive mechanisms of synesthesia. *Neuron, 48*, 509–20.

Hupé, J. M., Bordier, C., & Dojat, M. (2011). The neural bases of grapheme-color synesthesia are not localized in real color-sensitive areas. *Cerebral Cortex*. doi: 10.1093/cercor/bhr236.

Klüver, H. (1966). *Mescal and mechanisms of hallucinations*. Chicago, IL: University of Chicago Press.

Kosslyn, S. M., Thompson, W. L., Costantini-Ferrando, M. F., Alpert, N. M., & Spiegel, D. (2000). Hypnotic visual illusion alters color processing in the brain. *American Journal of Psychiatry, 157*, 1279–84.

Krause, B., & Cohen Kadosh, R. (2013). Can transcranial electrical stimulation improve learning difficulties in atypical brain development? A future possibility for cognitive training. *Developmental Cognitive Neuroscience, 6*(0), 176–94. doi: http://dx.doi.org/10.1016/j.dcn.2013.04.001.

Kusnir, F., & Thut, G. (2012). Formation of automatic letter-colour associations in non-synaesthetes through likelihood manipulation of letter-colour pairings. *Neuropsychologia, 50*, 3641–52. doi: 10.1016/j.neuropsychologia.2012.09.032.

Laurence, J.-R., Beaulieu-Prévost, D., & du Chéné, T. (2008). Measuring and understanding individual differences in hypnotizability. In M. R. Nash & A. Barnier (Eds.), *The Oxford handbook of hypnosis* (pp. 225–53). Oxford: Oxford University Press.

Lee, H.-M., & Roth, B. L. (2012). Hallucinogen actions on human brain revealed. *Proceedings of the National Academy of Sciences of the United States of America, 109.*

Looi, C. Y., Duta, M., Brem, A. K., Huber, S., Nuerk, H. C., & Cohen Kadosh, R. (2016). Combining brain stimulation and video game to promote long-term transfer of learning and cognitive enhancement. *Scientific Reports, 6*, 22003. doi: 10.1038/srep22003.

Ludwig, V. U., Adachi, I., & Matsuzawa, T. (2011). Visuoauditory mappings between high luminance and high pitch are shared by chimpanzees (Pan troglodytes) and humans. *Proceedings of the National Academy of Sciences of the United States of America, 108*, 20661–5. doi: 10.1073/pnas.1112605108.

Luke, D. P., & Terhune, D.B. (2013). The induction of synaesthesia with chemical agents: A systematic review. *Frontiers in Psychology, 4*, 753. doi: 10.3389/fpsyg.2013.00753.

Luke, D., Terhune, D. B., & Friday, R. (2012). Psychedelic synaesthesia: Evidence for a serotonergic role in synaesthesia. *Seeing and Perceiving, S1*, 74.

Marcusson-Clavertz, D., Terhune, D. B., & Cardeña, E. (2012). Individual differences and state effects on mind-wandering: Hypnotizability, dissociation, and sensory homogenization. *Consciousness and Cognition, 21*, 1097–108. doi: 10.1016/j.concog.2012.04.002.

Mattingley, J. B. (2009). Attention, automaticity, and awareness in synesthesia. *Ann N Y Acad Sci, 1156*, 141–67.

Mattingley, J. B., Rich, A. N., Yelland, G., & Bradshaw, J. L. (2001). Unconscious priming eliminates automatic binding of colour and alphanumeric form in synaesthesia. *Nature, 410*, 580–2. doi: 10.1038/35069062.

McGeown, W. J., Venneri, A., Kirsch, I., Nocetti, L., Roberts, K., Foan, L., & Mazzoni, G. (2012). Suggested visual hallucination without hypnosis enhances activity in visual areas of the brain. *Consciousness and Cognition, 21*, 100–16. doi: 10.1016/j.concog.2011.10.015.

Meier, B., & Rothen, N. (2007). When conditioned responses “fire back”: Bidirectional cross-activation creates learning opportunities in synesthesia. *Neuroscience, 147*, 569–72.

Meier, B., & Rothen, N. (2009). Training grapheme-colour associations produces a synaesthetic Stroop effect, but not a conditioned synaesthetic response. *Neuropsychologia, 47*, 1208–11. doi: 10.1016/j.neuropsychologia.2009.01.009.

Mendelsohn, A., Chalamish, Y., Solomonovich, A., & Dudai, Y. (2008). Mesmerizing memories: Brain substrates of episodic memory suppression in posthypnotic amnesia. *Neuron, 57*, 159–70. doi: 10.1016/j.neuron.2007.11.022.

Nikolić, D., Jurgens, U. M., Rothen, N., Meier, B., & Mroczko, A. (2011). Swimming-style synesthesia. *Cortex, 47*, 874–9. doi: 10.1016/j.cortex.2011.02.008.

Nikolić, D., Lichti, P., & Singer, W. (2007). Color opponency in synaesthetic experiences. *Psychological Science, 18*, 481–6.

Nunn, J. A., Gregory, L. J., Brammer, M., Williams, S. C., Parslow, D. M., Morgan, M. J., Gray, J. A. et al. (2002). Functional magnetic resonance imaging of synesthesia: Activation of V4/V8 by spoken words. *Nature Neuroscience, 5*, 371–5.

Oakley, D. A., & Halligan, P. W. (2009). Hypnotic suggestion and cognitive neuroscience. *Trends in Cognitive Sciences, 13*, 264–70. doi: 10.1016/j.tics.2009.03.004.

Pahnke, W. N., & Richards, W. A. (1966). Implications of LSD and experimental mysticism. *Journal of Religion and Health, 5*, 175–208.

Raichle, M. E., MacLeod, A. M., Snyder, A. Z., Powers, W. J., Gusnard, D. A., & Shulman, G. L. (2001). A default mode of brain function. *Proceedings of the National Academy of Sciences of the United States of America, 98*, 676–82. doi: 10.1073/pnas.98.2.676.

Ray, T. S. (2010). Psychedelics and the human receptorome. *PLoS One, 5*, e9019. doi: 10.1371/journal.pone.0009019.

Reis, J., Schambra, H. M., Cohen, L. G., Buch, E. R., Fritsch, B., Zarahn, E., Celnik, P. A., & Krakauer, J. W. (2009). Noninvasive cortical stimulation enhances motor skill acquisition over multiple days through an effect on consolidation. *Proceedings of the National Academy of Sciences of the United States of America, 106*, 1590–5. doi: 10.1073/pnas.0805413106.

Rhue, J. W., & Lynn, S. J. (1989). Fantasy proneness, hypnotizability, and absorption—a re-examination: A brief communication. *International Journal of Clinical and Experimental Hypnosis, 37*, 100–6.

Riba, J., Anderer, P., Jane, F., Saletu, B., & Barbanoj, M. J. (2004). Effects of the South American psychoactive beverage ayahuasca on regional brain electrical activity in humans: A functional neuroimaging study using low-resolution electromagnetic tomography. *Neuropsychobiology, 50*, 89–101. doi: 10.1159/000077946.

Ro, T., Farne, A., Johnson, R. M., Wedeen, V., Chu, Z., Wang, Z. J., Beauchamp, M. S. et al. (2007). Feeling sounds after a thalamic lesion. *Annals of Neurology, 62*, 433–41. doi: 10.1002/ana.21219.

Rothen, N., & Meier, B. (2014). Acquiring synaesthesia: Insights from training studies. *Frontiers in Human Neuroscience, 8*, 109. doi: 10.3389/fnhum.2014.00109.

Rothen, N., Meier, B., & Ward, J. (2012). Enhanced memory ability: Insights from synaesthesia. *Neuroscience and Biobehavioral Reviews, 36*, 1952–63. doi: 10.1016/j.neubiorev.2012.05.004.

Rothen, N., Seth, A. K., Witzel, C., & Ward, J. (2013). Diagnosing synaesthesia with online colour pickers: Maximising sensitivity and specificity. *Journal of Neuroscience Methods, 215*, 156–60. doi: 10.1016/j.jneumeth.2013.02.009.

Rothen, N., Wantz, A. L., & Meier, B. (2011). Training synaesthesia. *Perception, 40*, 1248–50.

Rouw, R., & Scholte, H. S. (2010). Neural basis of individual differences in synesthetic experiences. *Journal of Neuroscience, 30*, 6205–13. doi: 10.1523/JNEUROSCI.3444-09.2010.

Simner, J. (2012). Defining synaesthesia. *British Journal of Psychology, 103*, 1–15. doi: 10.1348/000712610X528305.

Simner, J., Harrold, J., Creed, H., Monro, L., & Foulkes, L. (2009). Early detection of markers for synaesthesia in childhood populations. *Brain, 132*, 57–64.

Simner, J., & Holenstein, E. (2007). Ordinal linguistic personification as a variant of synesthesia. *Journal of Cognitive Neuroscience, 19*, 694–703. doi: 10.1162/jocn.2007.19.4.694.

Simner, J., Mulvenna, C., Sagiv, N., Tsakanikos, E., Witherby, S. A., Fraser, C., Ward, J. et al. (2006). Synaesthesia: The prevalence of atypical cross-modal experiences. *Perception, 35*, 1024–33. doi: 10.1068/p5469.

Simpson, L., & McKellar, P. (1955). Types of synaesthesia. *Journal of Mental Science, 101*, 141–7.

Sinke, C., Halpern, J. H., Zedler, M., Neufeld, J., Emrich, H. M., & Passie, T. (2012). Genuine and drug-induced synesthesia: A comparison. *Consciousness and Cognition, 21*, 1419–34. doi: 10.1016/j.concog.2012.03.009.

Sjoberg, B. M. J., & Hollister, L. E. (1965). The effects of psychotomimetic drugs on primary suggestibility. *Psychopharmacologia, 8*, 251–62.

Smilek, D., Dixon, M. J., Cudahy, C., & Merikle, P. M. (2001). Synaesthetic photisms influence visual perception. *Journal of Cognitive Neuroscience, 13*, 930–6. doi: 10.1162/089892901753165845.

Snowball, A., Tachtsidis, I., Popescu, T., Thompson, J., Delazer, M., Zamarian, L., Zhu, T., & Cohen Kadosh, R. (2013). Long-term enhancement of brain function and cognition using cognitive training and brain stimulation. *Current Biology, 23*, 987–92. doi: 10.1016/j.cub.2013.04.045.

Spanos, N. P., & Gorassini, D. R. (1984). Structure of hypnotic test suggestions and attributions of responding involuntarily. *Journal of Personality and Social Psychology, 46*, 688–96.

Studerus, E. (2013). *Psilocybin-induced altered states of consciousness: Tolerability, assessment, and prediction*. Saarbrücken, Germany: Südwestdeutscher Verlag für Hochschulschriften.

Studerus, E., Gamma, A., & Vollenweider, F. X. (2010). Psychometric evaluation of the altered states of consciousness rating scale (OAV). *PLoS One, 5*, e12412. doi: 10.1371/journal.pone.0012412.

Szechtman, H., Woody, E., Bowers, K. S., & Nahmias, C. (1998). Where the imaginal appears real: A positron emission tomography study of auditory hallucinations. *Proceedings of the National Academy of Sciences of the United States of America, 95*, 1956–60.

Tart, C. T. (1975). *States of consciousness*. New York: E. P. Dutton.

Tellegen, A., & Atkinson, G. (1974). Openness to absorbing and self-altering experiences ("absorption"), a trait related to hypnotic susceptibility. *Journal of Abnormal Psychology, 83*, 268–77.

Terhune, D. B., Cardeña, E., & Lindgren, M. (2010). Disruption of synaesthesia by posthypnotic suggestion: An ERP study. *Neuropsychologia, 48*, 3360–4. doi: 10.1016/j.neuropsychologia.2010.07.004.

Terhune, D. B., Cardeña, E., & Lindgren, M. (2011a). Differential frontal-parietal phase synchrony during hypnosis as a function of hypnotic suggestibility. *Psychophysiology, 48*, 1444–7. doi: 10.1111/j.1469-8986.2011.01211.x.

Terhune, D. B., Cardeña, E., & Lindgren, M. (2011b). Dissociated control as a signature of typological variability in high hypnotic suggestibility. *Consciousness and Cognition, 20*, 727–36. doi: 10.1016/j.concog.2010.11.005.

Terhune, D. B., & Cohen Kadosh, R. (2012a). The emerging neuroscience of hypnosis. *Cortex, 48*, 382–6. doi: 10.1016/j.cortex.2011.08.007.

Terhune, D. B., & Cohen Kadosh, R. (2012b). *Posthypnotic manipulation of the visuospatial phenomenology of colour photisms modulates selective attention in synaesthesia*. Poster presented at the Association for the Scientific Study of Consciousness, Brighton, UK.

Terhune, D. B., Luke, D. P., Kaelen, M., Bolstridge, M., Feilding, A., Nutt, D., Carhart-Harris, R., & Ward, J. (2016). A placebo-controlled investigation of synaesthesia-like experiences under LSD. *Neuropsychologia, 88*, 28–34. doi: 10.1016/j.neuropsychologia.2016.04.005.

Terhune, D. B., Murray, E., Near, J., Stagg, C. J., Cowey, A., and Cohen Kadosh, R. (2015). Phosphene perception relates to visual cortex glutamate levels and covaries with atypical visuospatial awareness. *Cerebral Cortex, 25*, 4341–50. doi: 10.1093/cercor/bhv015.

Terhune, D. B., Rothen, N., & Cohen Kadosh, R. (2013). Correcting misconceptions about synaesthesia. *Neurobiology of Learning and Memory, 103*, 1–2. doi: 10.1016/j.nlm.2013.02.004.

Terhune, D. B., Song, S. M., Duta, M. D., & Cohen Kadosh, R. (2014). Probing the neurochemical basis of synaesthesia using psychophysics. *Frontiers in Human Neuroscience, 8*, 89. doi: 10.3389/fnhum.2014.00089.

Terhune, D. B., Tai, S., Cowey, A., Popescu, T., & Cohen Kadosh, R. (2011). Enhanced cortical excitability in grapheme-color synesthesia and its modulation. *Current Biology, 21*, 2006–9. doi: 10.1016/j.cub.2011.10.032.

van Leeuwen, T. M., den Ouden, H. E., & Hagoort, P. (2011). Effective connectivity determines the nature of subjective experience in grapheme-color synesthesia. *Journal of Neuroscience, 31*, 9879–84. doi: 10.1523/JNEUROSCI.0569-11.2011.

Wallach, J. V. (2009). Endogenous hallucinogens as ligands of the trace amine receptors: A possible role in sensory perception. *Medical Hypotheses, 72*(1), 91–4.

Ward, J. (2013). Synesthesia. *Annual Review of Psychology, 64*, 49–75. doi: 10.1146/annurev-psych-113011-143840.

Ward, J., Jonas, C., Dienes, Z., & Seth, A. (2010). Grapheme-colour synaesthesia improves detection of embedded shapes, but without pre-attentive 'pop-out' of synaesthetic colour. *Proceedings of the Royal Society of London. Series B: Biological Sciences, 277*, 1021–6.

Ward, J., Li, R., Salih, S., & Sagiv, N. (2007). Varieties of grapheme-colour synaesthesia: A new theory of phenomenological and behavioural differences. *Consciousness and Cognition, 16*, 913–31.

Ward, J., & Mattingley, J. B. (2006). Synaesthesia: An overview of contemporary findings and controversies. *Cortex, 42*, 129–36.

Ward, J., & Wright, T. (2012). Sensory substitution as an artificially acquired synaesthesia. *Neuroscience and Biobehavioral Reviews*. doi: 10.1016/j.neubiorev.2012.07.007.

Wasson, R. G. (1978). *The road to Eleusis: Unveiling the secret of the mysteries*. New York: Harcourt.

Witthoft, N., & Winawer, J. (2006). Synesthetic colors determined by having colored refrigerator magnets in childhood. *Cortex, 42*, 175–83.

Witthoft, N., & Winawer, J. (2013). Learning, memory, and synesthesia. *Psychological Science, 24*, 258–65. doi: 10.1177/0956797612452573.

Woody, E. Z., & Barnier, A. J. (2008). Hypnosis scales for the twenty-first century: What do we need and how should be use them? In M. R. Nash & A. Barnier (Eds.), *Oxford handbook of hypnosis* (pp. 255–81). Oxford, UK: Oxford University Press.

Yaro, C., & Ward, J. (2007). Searching for Shereshevskii: What is superior about the memory of synaesthetes? *Quarterly Journal of Experimental Psychology, 60*, 681–95.

Zeki, S. (1980). The representation of colours in the cerebral cortex. *Nature, 284*, 412–18.

12

Patrolling the Boundaries of Synaesthesia

A Critical Appraisal of Transient and Artificially Induced Forms of Synaesthetic Experiences

Malika Auvray and Mirko Farina[1]

12.1 Synaesthesia: an introduction

The first documented case of synaesthesia dates back to 1812 when Georg Sachs, an Austrian doctor, submitted within his doctoral dissertation an account of himself as synaesthete, giving detailed explanations of color perception for both numbers and letters (for an English translation of Sachs' report, see Jewanski et al., 2009). After Sachs' pioneering account, it took synaesthesia almost seventy years to enter mainstream science, and to be recognized as a genuine phenomenon of scientific relevance (Chabalier, 1864; Galton, 1880; Nussbaumer, 1873). By the end of the 1890s synaesthesia had nevertheless achieved a fully fledged scientific status, and its study had acquired a strong medical character (see Jewanski et al., 2011; Ward, 2013, for an in-depth historical analysis of synaesthesia).

The beginning of the twentieth century, however, took the study of synaesthesia far away from its earlier scientific tradition. With the emergence of expressionism and abstract art (Kandinsky and his synaesthetic paintings), dodecaphony in music (for instance, the Optophonic Piano built by Vladimir Rossine in 1916), and futurism in literature (Marinetti, 1911), the term gradually but progressively came to be associated with these artistic movements. Consequently, synaesthesia began to be studied more as a cultural metaphor for the expression of intersensory correspondence than as a biological, psychological, and medical phenomenon deeply and profoundly rooted in scientific practice. With the emergence of behaviorism in psychology (e.g., Skinner, 1938; Watson, 1930), the fate of research into synaesthesia changed again. Synaesthesia

[1] The two authors contributed equally to this work.

lost its surrealistic aura, its magical appeal, and ceased to puzzle psychologists, who started seeing it as nothing more than a learned association (see Howells, 1944), a rather trivial phenomenon of dubious scientific importance.

In recent decades, however (especially since the late 1980s), with the advent of cognitive neuroscience, synaesthesia has experienced a tremendous resurgence of interest (e.g., Baron-Cohen, 1996; Steven and Blakemore, 2004; Hubbard and Ramachandran, 2005; Rouw et al., 2011; Ward, 2013). This major modern revival has provided a new platform for a broad range of interdisciplinary collaborations (between neuroscientists, psychologists, and philosophers) that are now trying to better understand the neurological and psychological mechanisms underlying this peculiar form of experiencing the world. Even though this resurgence of interest has triggered important improvements in our general understanding of the phenomenon, bringing to light many new important findings, we still know very little about the neurological causes of synaesthesia and about the way it develops and progresses.

Synaesthesia is a condition in which people make unusual associations between various sensations. The stimulus triggering the unusual association can be sensory (such as a printed 2, e.g., see Grossenbacher and Lovelace, 2001), conceptual (such as the result of an arithmetic operation, e.g., see Dixon et al., 2000), or emotional (e.g., Ward, 2004). Such stimuli give rise to so-called canonical or developmental forms of synaesthesia, which are either innate or developed early in infancy (e.g., Baron-Cohen, 1996; Maurer, 1993) and remain constant throughout the lifetime. In recent years, a number of non-developmental cases, including post-hypnotic suggestion (e.g., Cohen Kadosh et al., 2009), drug habits (e.g., Friedrichs, 2009; Shanon, 2002), flavor perception (e.g., Stevenson and Boakes, 2004), and use of sensory substitution devices (e.g., Farina, 2013; Proulx and Stoerig, 2006; Ward and Meijer, 2010), have been linked or directly associated with the emergence of particular types of synaesthetic experiences. These borderline cases have been associated with cases of proper synaesthesia because they either induce some form of conscious, concurrent experience or show patterns of crossmodal interference that characterize canonical cases of synaesthesia (such as the Stroop interference effect, e.g. Mills et al., 1999; see Eagleman et al., 2007, for a review of the existing tests). Our purpose in this chapter is to investigate conceptually whether it is possible to count the abovementioned borderline cases as genuine synaesthetic experiences.

In section 12.2, we provide a number of definitions of synaesthesia in terms of its core definitional aspects (e.g., inducer-concurrent pairing, idiosyncrasy, consistency over time, and automaticity). The analysis of these criteria helps us in setting the benchmark for what ought to be counted as proper synaesthesia and therefore allows us to explore theoretically the question of whether borderline cases can be explained in light of these definitions. Having introduced such criteria, we then turn, in section 12.3, to the empirical analysis of two temporary forms of synaesthesia: those induced by post-hypnotic suggestion and drug-use. We review evidence for these cases and discuss whether it is appropriate to treat them as genuine forms of the condition.

In section 12.4, we analyze two alleged forms of learned synaesthesia. We first address the case of flavor perception, where certain odor-taste interactions have been claimed to correspond to a learned synaesthesia that would be common to us all (e.g., Stevenson and Boakes, 2004). We then turn to sensory substitution, tackling the idea of artificially acquired synaesthesia. We report preliminary evidence for this claim (Proulx and Stoerig, 2006; Ward and Meijer, 2010, Farina, 2013; Ward and Wright, 2012) and then critically discuss it. In section 12.5, drawing on the lessons learned from the analysis of transient and acquired cases of synaesthesia, we highlight the implications of their inclusion on the unity or plurality of the condition (e.g., Terhune and Cohen Kadosh, 2012). Counting such a wide range of phenomena as genuine synaesthetic experiences does indeed raise the question of whether it still makes sense to describe synaesthesia as a unitary event, or whether we should interpret it as an umbrella term that encompasses several different domains with independent probabilities of expression.

12.2 Definitions of synaesthesia

Synaesthesia is a condition in which "stimulation in one sensory or cognitive stream leads to associated experiences in a second, unstimulated stream" (Hubbard, 2007: 193; see also Cytowic, 2003). Synaesthesia is thus normally described as a "startling sensory blending" (Cytowic, 1997: 17) "not experienced by most people under comparable conditions" (Grossenbacher and Lovelace, 2001: 36). In synaesthesia, in fact, sensory experiences (such as tastes) or concepts (such as numbers) automatically evoke additional percepts, such as colors (Cohen Kadosh and Walsh, 2006: R963). For example, a grapheme-color synaesthete can experience color when reading a digit or a letter. Analogously, a hearing-color synaesthete can see colors when she hears particular sounds (Baron-Cohen et al., 1987), and a lexical-gustatory synaesthete can experience tastes when she hears or reads certain words (Ward and Simner, 2003). Thus, synaesthetic occurrences can be elicited by the visual appearance of a printed item, or by certain sounds, when spoken aloud. In other cases, just thinking about a particular letter, digit, or word can induce color experiences (Dixon et al., 2000; Smilek et al., 2001) and someone can have a synaesthetic experience by imagining the meaning of certain words (Rich et al., 2005).

To date, more than sixty-five different types of synaesthesia have been reported (Day, 2009; see http://www.daysyn.com/Types-of-Syn.html for a complete list), each with its own set of triggering stimuli and its correlated synaesthetic occurrences. Because of the intrinsic diversity and complexity of the phenomenon, a comprehensive and universally accepted definition of synaesthesia is yet to be formulated. The broad range of occurrences usually classified as synaesthetic presents a challenge for any researcher who wants to arrive at a shared understanding. Yet there are four criteria that can be used to get started. We would like to note here that none of these criteria should be taken as being individually necessary. We will argue instead that they are jointly sufficient, i.e., their joint combination allows us to distinguish between synaesthesia and other related phenomena. This point will be further detailed in the discussion.

First, synaesthesia is characterized by the existence of what Grossenbacher and Lovelace (2001) have called an inducer-concurrent pairing. The term "inducer", on their account, refers to the experience of the triggering stimulus that causes the correlated synaesthetic experience to emerge. The term "concurrent" denotes the associations being experienced by the synaesthete. Since this distinction was established in the literature at the onset of the 2000s, every type of synaesthesia is now minimally described in terms of this pairing (see Auvray and Deroy, 2015, for an in-depth discussion). This helpful distinction certainly provides a good starting point for a characterization of genuine forms of synaesthesia. However, there is an aspect of the concurrent that seems crucial in addition to its being paired with an inducer: this is the fact that the inducer is always consciously experienced. This requirement is central in many definitions that emphasize that synaesthesia is "a conscious experience of systematically induced sensory attributes" (Grossenbacher and Lovelace, 2001: 36). As Deroy and Spence (2013a) have recently noted, there are, among others, two related differences between synaesthesia and crossmodal correspondences. First, in the former, the concurrent is necessarily conscious, whereas in the latter the crossmodal matching is not. Second, in synaesthesia the concurrent is determined in an *absolute* way (i.e., a particular sound associated with a shape), while in crossmodal correspondences it functions in a *relative* way (a higher-pitched sound associated with a higher position in space; see Marks, 1987; Pedley and Harper, 1959). These two differences are directly linked as we are more conscious of absolute experiences than of relative ones. Thus, the first criterion to define synaesthesia must be the existence of a pairing between an inducer and a *conscious* concurrent.

A second important characteristic of synaesthesia is its relative idiosyncrasy. It has often been emphasized that in synaesthesia, the induced sensory attributes "are *not experienced* by most people under comparable conditions" (Grossenbacher and Lovelace, 2001: 36). In addition, there is not always a one-to-one correspondence between one type of concurrent and one type of inducer. For instance, D reports having the experience of a "pretty yellow-green" when she hears a Bb and of a "dirty yellow-green" when hearing a D# (Ortmann, 1933). Another synaesthete can nevertheless experience the contrary without anyone being entitled to question his synaesthetic associations. The possibility of generalization has also been investigated with letters, where As tend to be mainly seen as red and Bs as blue (Simner et al., 2005). Yet genuine synaesthetes can have very different associations (such as seeing a green A). Thus, even if certain regularities or tendencies can be observed, the inducer-concurrent pairing cannot be reduced to a learned association between regularities to which people have been exposed (Hubbard and Ramachandran, 2003). Rather, the set of observed concurrent pairings is broad and varies, even within the same family and between twins (Barnett et al., 2008). The atypical character of synaesthetic experiences thus seems to be another important aspect of synaesthetic occurrences.

A third important feature of synaesthetic experiences is their automaticity, i.e. the fact that the concurrent is experienced as an inevitable and involuntary consequence of the synaesthete coming across a specific inducer. The automaticity criterion has been extensively used in experimental tests (such as with a variant of the Stroop task, e.g. Dixon et al., 2000). For example, a person with grapheme-color synaesthesia should be able to determine unequivocally and automatically what color certain letters trigger in her mind. If the person needs mental effort or extra time to recall the colors she previously attributed to those letters, then she is most likely not a synaesthete and she is probably associating the two experiences at another level (e.g., semantic associations). It should be noted that in synaesthesia, the automaticity at stake is not pre-attentional. It is only after the inducer has been attended that the concurrent is elicited (e.g., see Sagiv et al., 2006; Deroy and Spence, 2013a). Nonetheless, the concurrent is elicited without voluntary control, and it cannot be recalled or dismissed at will. In recent years, a number of functional neuroimaging studies have further highlighted the automaticity of synaesthesia (MacLeod and Dunbar 1988; Nunn et al., 2002) and its crucial role in processes of attention, saliency, perceptual judgment, and awareness (for an interesting discussion of this topic see Mattingley, 2009). For all these reasons, the automaticity criterion has become increasingly important in the characterization of synaesthetic experiences and we include it in ours.

A fourth condition is consistency, which refers to the fact that the same inducer always triggers the same concurrent. To give an example, if the letter 'b' is perceived by the synaesthete as green, that letter should be consistently perceived as green even if the synaesthete is asked about it on multiple occasions over the course of her lifetime. In many articles in the contemporary literature, consistency has been described as the most fundamental characteristic of synaesthesia (Ward et al., 2010) and the test of consistency has come to be referred as the behavioral 'gold standard' for determining the authenticity of the condition (Rich et al., 2005). Synaesthetes are in fact normally included in empirical studies only after having passed the consistency test (Baron-Cohen et al., 1987), in which they first have to provide a set of their synaesthetic associations and then, after a long period of time (e.g., after six months; Ward and Simner, 2003), they are given a surprise retest. The consistency between their initial and re-tested scores is compared to a control group of non-synaesthetes. This control group is requested to invent analogous associations and recall them by memory alone in a shorter period of time (e.g., 2 weeks, Ward and Simner, 2003). Only those synaesthetes who clearly outperform control participants are considered as genuine synaesthetes, and therefore assessed by means of further studies (Ward and Simner, 2003). Typically, only one in six people who initially report synaesthesia are ultimately classified as synaesthetes (Simner, Glover, et al., 2006; Simner, Mulvenna, et al., 2006). While this rigorous approach seems to be effective to identify genuine cases of synaesthesia, it has been recently questioned for its circularity and somewhat biased nature (for more details see Proulx and Stoerig, 2006; Rich and Mattingley, forthcoming; Simner, 2012).

What should we make of those people who fail the consistency test but still report having synaesthetic experiences? There are, at least, two possibilities here; the first one is to consider that those persons are intentionally misreporting or inventing experiences they do not have. The second possibility is to acknowledge that they could also be genuine synaesthetes, and that they possess a type of synaesthesia that is not fully captured by the consistency requirement. If we accept the second possibility, we must consider whether consistency over time should be a definitional criterion, or whether, instead, it should merely characterizes a subset of synaesthetes only (Simner 2012: 7). To date there is no hard evidence available to settle this question. If anything, the opposite is true and many researchers have begun investigating the relevance of consistency, highlighting its potential circularity (Eagleman, 2009; Rich and Mattingley, forthcoming; Simner, 2012). They pointed out that almost all synaesthetes reported in the literature are synaesthetes who display consistency, but this is because these synaesthetes have been recruited for empirical studies on the basis of the consistency criterion. This was the test used for defining what ought to be counted as proper synaesthesia. Thus, there is theoretical room for arguing that the consistency criterion ends up being circular. Given this possibility, rather than seeing the requirement of consistency as a gold standard to assess the significance of any synaesthetic experience, we would like to call for a more careful assessment of its role in defining synaesthesia. Consequently, while we believe that consistency can offer a pretty reliable tool for singling out proper forms of synaesthesia, our characterization of the condition is not bounded to it, and rather envisages the need to complement consistency with other hallmark traits, namely inducer-concurrent pairing, idiosyncrasy, and automaticity.

It is worth mentioning here that there are several other features that have been considered as definitional aspects of synaesthesia, but we have not included them as jointly sufficient requirements, either because they can be considered as consequences of other criteria or because they do not seem to be applicable to the vast majority of the standard cases. In what follows we briefly discuss spatial extension and affect. Some researchers (e.g., Cytowic and Eagleman, 2009) have argued that spatial extension qualifies as a defining aspect of synaesthesia. According to these authors the synaesthetic occurrence experienced by the synaesthete is perceived as being localized in the world. This requirement, however, remains highly controversial as certain synaesthetes do experience the concurrent as being external, while others experience it in an internal space (for an in-depth analysis of the divide between associators and projectors, see Dixon et al., 2004). Note that the argument of spatial extension would not hold for the inducer either as it need not always be spatially extended for the synaesthetic percept to arise. Indeed some people do have synaesthetic experiences by simply imagining the meaning of words. We therefore believe that the requirement of spatial extension is not a defining character of any synaesthetic occurrence. Cytowic (1997) has also argued that synaesthesia is always affect laden. We believe that not all forms of synaesthesia manifest this feature. For instance, it is unlikely that spatial sequence synaesthesia—where people see all numerical sequences they come across as points in space—is necessarily affect laden. Hence, we believe that the requirement of being affect laden is not strictly necessary for genuine forms of synaesthesia and therefore we did not take it as a definitional aspect of the condition.

In summary, there are four fundamental criteria that we believe are jointly sufficient for individuating genuine forms of synaesthesia. These are: 1. the existence of pairing between an inducer and a conscious concurrent; 2. the relative idiosyncrasy of the pairings; 3. the automaticity of the process; 4. the consistency of the occurrence over time. In recent years, a number of researchers have hypothesized that synaesthesia can also be experienced in a more or less intermittent way and that it can be acquired. It has indeed been suggested that synaesthesia-like experiences can be induced by post-hypnotic suggestions (e.g., Kadosh et al., 2009), drug-use (e.g., Friedrichs, 2009; Shanon, 2002), flavor perception (e.g., Stevenson and Boakes, 2004), and extensive training with sensory substitution devices (e.g., Farina, 2013; Proulx and Stoerig, 2006; Ward and Wright, 2012; Ward and Meijer, 2010). In the next two sections we turn to these cases and assess whether they count as examples of synaesthesia in the light of the conditions we have just identified.

12.3 Transient forms of synaesthetic experiences: post-hypnotic suggestion and drug-use

12.3.1 Synaesthetic experiences triggered by post-hypnotic suggestion

Post-hypnotic suggestion has been used to trigger synaesthetic-type experiences. During post-hypnotic suggestion, the experimenter administers suggestions to their participants which consist of verbal statements that are intended to trigger various kinds of responses, i.e., affective, cognitive, or motor. It is worth noting here that this method works well only with highly suggestible persons, which comprise approximately 10–15 percent of the total population tested (see Laurence, Beaulieu-Prévost, and du Chéné, 2008; see also Terhune et al., Chapter 11 of this volume). Consequently, only this subset of people was involved in the studies described below.

In one study by Cohen Kadosh et al. (2009), four highly suggestible non-synaesthetes were hypnotized and instructed to associate six digit-color pairs. These participants were subsequently presented with black inked digits on a colored background and asked to detect the grapheme presented. The background could be in a color that is congruent with the one associated with the grapheme (e.g., if the N is perceived as yellow, a black N on a yellow background) or it could be inconsistent with it (e.g., a black N on a blue background). The participants displayed the same pattern of responses as congenital synaesthetes (as reported in Smilek et al., 2001, for instance); that is, they made more errors in the congruent condition than in the incongruent one. There was no such difference in the control group. These results suggest a form of automaticity in the associations. But did the participants show consistency? Only two participants in the study were re-tested; immediately after the experiment took place and then again one week after it. These two participants, unlike two control ones, displayed a consistency effect in the sense that they made more errors in the congruent condition than in the incongruent one.

Terhune and Cohen Kadosh (2012) investigated whether a post-hypnotically induced synaesthesia would display, as with its congenital counterpart, a divide between projectors (the concurrent is experienced as being located externally) and associators (the concurrent is experienced mentally, i.e. as being located in the mind's eye). Terhune and Cohen Kadosh first differentiated the participants who were responsive to hypnotic suggestions for either associator or projector grapheme-color synaesthesia. They subsequently administered post-hypnotic suggestions to associate four numbers with four colors and to experience the colors as either being spatially co-localized with graphemes (for the subgroup of projectors) or as mental images (for the subgroup of associators). The participants then underwent two versions of the Stroop color-naming task: one in which they had to name the colors *of* the digits and one in which they had to name the color *associated with* the digit. Researchers found similar results to those previously obtained with congenital synaesthetes (e.g., Dixon et al., 2004): projectors had larger congruency effects (i.e., faster responses for graphemes in the same color as that used for this pairing during the post-hypnotic suggestion than for graphemes in a different color) than associators in the first experimental conditions and there was no difference between the two in the second condition. Phenomenologically, participants reported an involuntary and vivid character of the induced color during the Stroop task, as congenital synaesthetes do.

It should be mentioned that, so far, no studies have been conducted on the neural mechanisms underlying post-hypnotically induced synaesthesia. Terhune (Chapter 11 of this volume) argues that the very possibility of inducing synaesthesia with post-hypnotic suggestion is at odds with the theory of greater anatomical connectivity. Indeed, it is highly unlikely that a corresponding hyper-connectivity could be induced in such a short amount of time, i.e. the few minutes of hypnotic suggestions. Post-hypnotic suggestion does seem sufficient to elicit similar behavioral and phenomenological markers as are found in congenital synaesthesia. More precisely, it appears to be sufficient to produce a pairing between an inducer and a concurrent. It should be noted, however, that a much-debated question in the literature concerns the extent to which a conscious status can be achieved in cases of post-hypnotic suggestion (Cohen Kadosh et al., 2009). In addition, in the current state of data, it can be equally argued that, rather than having the experience of synaesthetic concurrents, the participants engage in a vivid form of mental imagery (see Deroy and Spence, 2013a, see also Spence and Deroy, 2013b for an analysis of the difference between mental imagery and synaesthesia). Thus, further empirical investigation is needed to confirm the possibility of post-hypnotically elicited conscious concurrents. With respect to the second criterion of our characterization, the obtained pairing seems relatively idiosyncratic, as reflected by individual differences. Behavioral tests also suggest a high degree of automaticity in the process. The consistency criterion needs further empirical testing, as only two participants in Cohen Kadosh et al.'s (2009) study showed a positive result.

12.3.2 Drug-induced synaesthesia

Administration of pharmacological agents has long been used to induce abnormal crossmodal experiences that can be thought of as resembling synaesthetic experiences. Notable cases involve the use of mescaline (Ellis, 1898), LSD (Hofmann, 1983), and psilocybin (Luke et al., 2012; Wasson, 1978). It is hypothesized that these pharmacological agents trigger synaesthetic experiences over short periods of time and can potentially work with a great number of people (around 60 percent; see Luke et al., 2012; Tart, 1975), as opposed to post-hypnotic suggestion that is effective only with highly suggestible individuals.

Despite these potentialities, only a few early studies (Hartman and Hollister, 1963; Simpson and McKellar, 1955) have investigated the possibility of triggering synaesthetic experiences through drug-use, mostly because this kind of research started to be prohibited in the 1960s. In one of these studies, two congenital synaesthetes and two controls (the two authors of the article) reported their synaesthetic impressions after ingesting mescaline when presented with a range of possible inducers (Simpson and McKellar, 1955). The participants reported eight different types of synaesthetic experiences that for the synaesthetes were not the variant they previously possessed. This study therefore suggests the possibility of inducing synaesthetic experiences in non-synaesthetes and of triggering novel synaesthetic experiences in synaesthetes. In a similar vein, another early study by Hartman and Hollister (1963) showed that when the eighteen participants involved in the experiment were presented with different sounds, they experienced more visual concurrents (colors, brightening of the visual field, and other visual effects) when they were under the influence of LSD and mescaline than when they were not.

Other studies have used questionnaires and surveys to ascertain the possibility of drug-induced synaesthesia. Most of these surveys and questionnaires were, however, part of other studies investigating different topics and were only subsequently used for understanding the phenomenon of drug-induced synaesthesia. These surveys nevertheless revealed that synaesthetic experiences can be obtained with a broad set of different substances (that will not be further described here; the interested reader can consult Luke et al., 2012, for a review) and that they elicited a broad range of inducer-concurrent associations, with a greater variability in the inducer than in the concurrent. With regard to the former, although sounds are the most frequently reported, tactile, gustatory, olfactory, and pain also act as inducers (Leuner, 1962; Shanon, 2002). As for the latter, the most common concurrents are visual and can consist of abstract geometric imagery or more complex scenes (Friedrichs, 2009; Grof, 1975; Leuner, 1962; Siegel, 1975).

From the results mentioned above it seems possible to produce an inducer-concurrent pairing through drug-use. These pairings can be consciously reported, although—as was noted by Hubbard and Ramachandran (2003)—there is a difficulty in identifying experiences that are produced by drug-use. With respect to the pairing itself, Sinke et al. (2012), building on previous results by Mayer-Gross (1931), notice that the inducer and concurrents are experienced as an integrated unified entity. The experience can be so confusing in certain individuals that some people might even find it difficult to describe the modalities in which the stimuli occur. Thus, the inducer and concurrent seems to be experienced as less demarcated than in congenital synaesthesia. In addition, it should be mentioned that no study conducted so far has investigated whether the experience is genuinely perceptual as opposed to a mere vivid association (Aghajanian and Marek, 1999).

The described studies revealed variability among the inducer-concurrent pairing across people, satisfying the idiosyncrasy criterion. However, so far, no work has investigated systematically and experimentally automaticity in drug-use (see also Terhune, Chapter 11 of this volume). Sinke et al. (2012) suggest, based on previous verbal reports, that the experience of a synaesthetic concurrent is not necessarily triggered, which raises doubts about whether the automaticity criterion can be fulfilled. Indeed, sometimes, under the influence of drugs, one inducer can elicit a synaesthetic concurrent; however, in other occasions, the same inducer does not elicit anything (Studerus, Kometer, Hasler, and Vollenweider, 2011). Furthermore, even in cases of experienced synaesthesia, a stimulus does not always elicit its expected concurrent (Delay, Gérad, and Racamier, 1951; Leuner, 1962; Masters and Houston, 1966). For example, when a synaesthete perceives a letter (e.g., A), she always experience it with the same color (e.g., red). In drug-induced synaesthesia, one person can sometimes experience one letter (an A) as red and sometimes perceive the same letter with no color.

Consistency is also very problematic: preliminary research by Brang and Ramachandran (2008) suggested that pairings obtained through drugs could be consistent. Using a texture segregation test, Brang and Ramachandran in fact showed that one grapheme-color synaesthetic experience could be consistent. On the other hand, Sinke et al. (2012), referring to an old study by Beringer (1927) investigating mescaline-induced synaesthetic experiences, claims that there are no consistent inducer-concurrent couplings. For instance, the same tone might be red, but when repeated, it may be experienced as another color, and it can even be translated into another sensory modality. The authors nonetheless emphasize the possibility that some stimuli that are considered to be more associative may produce more consistent pairings. In this case they would display lower intra-personal and inter-personal variance; in our terminology, they would better satisfy the consistency criterion while counting as weaker cases of idiosyncrasy. In summary, there is no wide agreement on whether the synaesthetic experiences obtained through pharmacological agents satisfy the consistency and automaticity criteria.

12.4 Acquired synaesthesia: flavor perception and use of sensory substitution

We now turn to forms of synaesthesia that are induced less intermittently, i.e. the case of acquired synaesthesia. We first address the case of flavor perception and then turn to sensory substitution.

12.4.1 Flavor perception

Recent psychophysical research on flavor perception has investigated the possibility of odors eliciting changes in the perceived sweetness (i.e., taste) of liquid solutions (e.g., Stevenson, Prescott, and Boakes, 1999). This phenomenon, known as sweetness enhancement, led Stevenson and Boakes (2004; see also Stevenson and Tomiczek, 2007) to suggest that odors can induce a synaesthetic experience of taste that is common to us all.

Sweetness enhancement consists in adding 'sweet' odors, which have no taste (they cannot be detected by the taste receptors), as flavorings to solutions. When participants have to taste such solutions, they perceive them as being sweeter than the same solution deprived of the added odors (Cliff and Noble, 1990; Frank and Byram, 1988; Frank, Shaffer, and Smith, 1991; Schifferstein and Verlegh, 1996). For example, when caramel odor is added to a sucrose solution, the taste of the resulting mixture is perceived as being sweeter than the pure sucrose solution if tasted alone. It should be mentioned that the odors that typically induce sweet tastes appear to be related to previous instances of co-exposure with a sweet taste, such as might naturally occur during eating (e.g., Prescott, 2004; Stevenson, Prescott, and Boakes, 1995; Stevenson, Boakes, and Prescott, 1998). For example, the odors of vanilla, caramel, strawberry, and mint induce sweetness enhancement in western countries where people often experience those odors with sucrose. On the other hand, non-western participants do not describe some of these odors as sweet, probably due to a less frequent pairing of these odors with sweetness in their food culture (Nguyen, Valentin, Ly, Chrea, and Sauvageot, 2002). The modifications of the attribution of taste qualities to odors can also be obtained in laboratory settings, thanks to the repeated pairing of novel odors with a particular tastant. For example, novel odors (such as lychee or water chestnut) repeatedly paired with sucrose are later reported to be sweeter than their initial ratings (Yeomans and Mobini, 2006; Yeomans et al., 2006). Similarly, novel odors are reported to be sourer than their initial ratings if they are repeatedly paired with citric acid (Stevenson, Boakes, and Wilson, 2000a, 2000b), or more bitter if paired with bitter tastes such as sucrose octa-acetate (Yeomans et al., 2006; for the difficulty of distinguishing between tastes and flavors, see Spence et al., forthcoming).

The idea that odors can induce a synaesthetic experience of taste that is common to us all (Stevenson and Boakes, 2004; Stevenson and Tomiczek, 2007) could be central to the field of synaesthesia. Indeed, if it was possible to acquire synaesthetic experiences through repeated co-exposure to stimuli, this would provide an excellent model system for the study of synaesthesia, as every one of us experiences flavor. We believe, however, that two main arguments question the appropriateness of considering flavor perception as a ubiquitous example of synaesthetic experience between the senses of smell and taste. First, sweetness enhancement does not fulfill the second criterion, idiosyncrasy, as the addition of the same flavorants gives rise to the same effect within a given culture (e.g., mint increases the perception of sweetness in all westerners) or, in laboratory settings, through the same repeated pairings.

In addition, there are reasons to believe that sweetness enhancement does not satisfy our first criterion either, i.e. the existence of distinct inducer and consciously perceived concurrents. In particular, it has been shown that the results depend on the task given to the participants: the adoption of an analytic versus synthetic approach to the perception of flavor strongly influences the extent to which odor-taste integration is observed. Indeed, on the one hand, when the participants are encouraged to adopt a strategy of analyzing the individual elements in the mixtures, this results in a decrease in sweetness enhancement (Prescott, Johnstone, and Francis, 2004). On the other hand, it is when the participants are encouraged to adopt a synthetic approach, by being required to attend only to the overall flavor intensity, that a sweetness enhancement effect is obtained. However, it can then be argued that, in this latter case, attending only to the overall percept does not allow disentangling the relative contributions of the senses of taste and smell to the overall flavor. In other words, it encourages the blurring of the senses of taste and smell. In summary, in this case the stimuli in the two sensory modalities are not both consciously perceived at the same time (rather it is the synthesis of the two that is attended to); thus this does not count as inducer-concurrent pairings. In addition, a study by Frank, van der Klaauw, and Schifferstein (1993) has shown that sweetness enhancement crucially depends on the responses allowed to participants. Their study revealed that the sweetness enhancement of a sucrose solution that can be elicited by adding strawberry odor only occurs when the participants are asked to rate sweetness, and nothing else. However, when they are also asked to judge other qualities, such as sweetness, saltiness, sourness, and bitterness, the sweetness enhancement effect disappears. In summary, if the occurrence of sweetness enhancement is a function of the task requirements, this would undermine the very idea of a learned synaesthesia between the senses of taste and smell.

It should be mentioned that the same line of reasoning applies to other cases in the field of flavor where other types of interactions could be, at a first glance, similarly interpreted as a synaesthetic experience. But it will appear that mostly what is obtained is not an additional and distinct perceptual experience, but rather the replacement of one sensory experience with another. For example, in a study by Davidson and colleagues (1999), participants had to continuously rate the perceived intensity of flavor in their mouths while chewing a piece of mint-flavored gum. The taste of the mint-flavored gum comes from the sugar contained in it, while the menthol gives rise to the olfactory and trigeminal components. The perceived intensity of the menthol odor was shown to increase very rapidly when people initially started to chew the gum. Then, while the actual intensity of the menthol odor stayed fairly constant over the course of 4–5 minutes of chewing, its perceived intensity declined rapidly (tracking the decline in the sugar taste in the mouth), and could only be brought back up again by the release of additional sugar (i.e., by the addition of a tastant which has no smell). Davidson et al.'s results therefore show that people's perception of the intensity of the menthol flavor was actually being driven by the release of sugar in their mouths (and detected on their tongues). But in this case, the participants should not be considered as having a synaesthetic experience either because what they perceived was not the original sensory impression (that of sweetness) plus the individuated sensory impression of menthol odor, but instead one sensory impression replaced by the other. In other words, in this case, the sensory impression of sweetness was replaced by the sensory impression of the menthol odor and not added to it.

To conclude, sweetness enhancement (along with other phenomena in the field of flavor) surely is, once acquired, consistent over time, thus fulfilling our fourth criterion. The third criterion, automaticity of the process, however, remains controversial. Furthermore, sweetness enhancement does not satisfy the first criterion (i.e., inducer-concurrent pairing) in that it does not involve distinct concurrents and inducers that are consciously perceived at the same time. In addition, it does not involve idiosyncrasy, at least intra-culturally.

12.4.2 Sensory substitution

Sensory substitution devices (SSDs) aim at replacing the functions of an impaired sensory modality (e.g. sight) by providing the environmental information normally gathered by another sensory modality (e.g. touch or audition). To do so, these systems typically convert visual images, obtained through a video camera, into patterns of either auditory (e.g., the vOICe: see Meijer, 1992; Vibe: see Hanneton et al., 2010) or tactile (e.g., the Tongue Display Unit: see Bach-y-Rita and Kercel, 2003) stimulation. The translation code for visual-to-tactile devices is analogical; for instance, a visual circle is translated into a circular pattern of tactile stimuli. The code used in visual-to-auditory devices translates several dimensions of the visual signal into dimensions of the auditory signal. For instance, the vOICe translates vertical position into frequency, horizontal position into time scanning, and visual brightness into auditory loudness. Through training with sensory substitution devices, users gradually develop the ability to perform localization tasks (e.g., Levy-Tzedek et al., 2012; Proulx et al., 2008; Renier et al., 2005) and simple form, as well as complex shape recognition (e.g., Arno et al., 2001; Auvray et al., 2007; Pollok et al., 2005; see also Auvray and Myin, 2009; Deroy and Auvray, 2012b, Kiverstein et al., 2015, for reviews).

Proulx and Stoerig (2006) speculated that the long-term use of SSDs may induce, in practiced users, the emergence of forms of synaesthesia (for an analogous claim see also Farina, 2013; Proulx, 2010, Renier and De Volder, 2013; Ward and Wright, 2012). Ward and Meijer (2010) defended this view based on the phenomenological reports gathered on two persons who became blind later in life and have been using the vOICe for more than ten years. One of these practiced users (PF) describes her experiences as analogous to a form of:

> Monochrome artificially induced synaesthesia only in certain frequencies of sound. It is almost as if you had a computer with two monitors running simultaneously different pictures, one was a very grey blurred version of the real world, and the other was a pure grey background with a big semi-circular light grey arc on it, and sometimes you switched your attention between both.
> (Ward and Meijer, 2010: 497–8).

PF also affirms that the sounds generated by the device elicited visual experiences, caused forms of depth perception to emerge, and even triggered the experience of colors (Ward and Meijer 2010: 497). Another interesting thing that PF reported was that her experiences of images, color, or motion when hearing sounds do not change as a function of other parameters such as her mood, the time, or environmental factors. This has been taken to suggest a form of consistency of her "synaesthetic percepts" over time (quoted in Ward and Meijer 2010: 498).

Is the claim that SSD-use is comparable to the synaesthetic experiences enjoyed by colored-hearing synaesthetes (e.g., Ward and Meijer, 2010; Ward and Wright, 2012) tenable? To answer this question, we need to be specific and carefully define the level of users' experience and the different processes that are involved in SSD-use. This has not been done clearly so far. In SSD-use there is the information that is provided to the users in their intact sensory modality (audition in the case of visual-to-auditory devices), which we label here as the 'substituting information'. This information corresponds to the conversion of a signal from another sensory modality (i.e., vision in the case of visual-to-auditory sensory substitution devices), which we define as the 'substituted information'. The substituted information can be understood at the level of information processing; that is, it can be inferred from the substituting information and the knowledge of the translation code (e.g., understanding that there is a visual diagonal line from a sound increasing in pitch). Note that this also involves specific knowledge of our movements. For instance, the distance of an object, although not given by the translation code, can be deduced from triangulation, i.e. two points of view on the object. Then, there could be a phenomenology associated with the process of perceiving, that we will label 'associated phenomenology'. This corresponds to phosphenes or impressions of colors that blind persons reported while using the device, and can be considered as an 'extra', an addition to the level of pure information processing. The associated phenomenology thus does not necessarily follow from the translation code but is joined to the sensory occurrence experienced through the coupling with the device.

When researchers argue that SSD-use is a form of acquired synaesthesia, they identify the inducer with the substituting information. The concurrent is linked to either the substituted information or to the associated phenomenology. There is therefore a trap into which one can easily fall by confusing these two levels. In what remains of this section, we will disentangle the two claims and analyze them separately to establish the extent to which each fulfills the four criteria for genuine forms of synaesthesia that we listed in section 12.2.[2] Note, a potential difficulty comes from the fact that there are many results gathered at the level of information processing, whereas the claims on the associated phenomenology are based only on the verbal reports from two late blind persons.

The first criterion we discussed for identifying genuine forms of synaesthesia is the existence of a pairing between an inducer and a conscious concurrent. This involves both the inducer and the concurrent consciously perceiving at the same time. According to O'Regan and Noë (2001), for instance, in trained users, access to the substituting information fades away). In this case, the inducer and the concurrent cannot be perceived at the same time. On the other hand, Ward and Wright (2012) defend that both keep on being perceived while acknowledging that there are actually no data to confirm or disconfirm this point. What can be said for now is that, if the concurrent is the substituted information only, additional data will shed light on the question of whether, after training, both the inducer and the concurrent are consciously perceived at the same time. Similarly, if the concurrent is the associated phenomenology, more data is clearly needed. Let's just note here that many of the claims equating SSD-use and synaesthesia re-occurring in the literature mention the verbal report from one of the two participants in Ward and Meijer's (2010) study who describes her experiences as analogous to a form of "monochrome artificially induced synaesthesia" (see the complete quote at the beginning of the section). However, while she describes her experience as being akin to synaesthesia, her report underlines that she switched her attention between the different impressions that the sounds give rise to, which is at odds with congenital synaesthetic experiences.

The second criterion that we listed for characterizing proper forms of synaesthesia is idiosyncrasy. This involves two levels: first, that synaesthetes have an experience that is additional to what the rest of the population experiences; second, that this additional experience greatly differs among them. While saying that SSD-users have

[2] Besides an in-depth analysis of the four criteria we discussed in this entry, Farina (2013) also reported two other interesting analogies between developmental forms of synaesthesia and SSD-use. According to him, both SSD-perception and developmental forms of synaesthesia exploit cross-modal plasticity and both could be characterized by analogous neural mechanisms. In other words, both these forms of perceiving (on his account) are cross-modal and both exhibit "disinhibited feedback", or a reduction in the amount of inhibition along feedback pathways—a phenomenon known as cortical unmasking.

an experience that is not shared with non-users is not problematic; saying that this experience differs among users proves to be far more controversial. Here again, let's dissociate the substituted information from the associated phenomenology. With respect to the former, there is nothing idiosyncratic about the users' experience. This is obvious from the fact that SSDs are based on a determined translation code, which is the same for each user. Given specific visual information recorded by the camera, this information will be translated into auditory information in the same way. Thus, for a given visual image, every user will obtain the same auditory information. From that information, users are then given the same possibility to have experiences of shapes, size, and so on with the device. The extent to which they do reach these abilities then only depends on the amount of training they had. But here there is no qualitative difference between them; only quantitative ones correlated with training. With respect to the associated phenomenology, there is again a crucial lack of data to confirm idiosyncrasy, as only two persons reported some forms of colors and light. One important thing we would like to emphasize is that any supposed idiosyncrasy of associated phenomenology would remain very limited (merely colors and light) and it is hard to imagine it reaching the wide set of pairings occurring in congenital synaesthesia.

With respect to the third criterion, there are actually no data to assess if SSD-use becomes automatic or not. It seems that the argument could be problematic in the case of the substituted information. Several authors, such as O'Regan and Noë (2001), have claimed that after training, SSD-use becomes automatic and that at this moment the device and the sensory processing becomes transparent. Similarly, Farina (2013) hypothesized that "after extensive practice, the device gets increasingly transparent, its boundaries progressively fade away, and the perception experienced through the coupling with it becomes involuntary" (652). However, it should be noted that while the experience of the concurrent becomes automatized, the fact that the inducer remains consciously perceived (first criterion) might be lost correspondingly. It thus might be the case that before training the experience lacks automaticity, whereas after training it lacks conscious attention to the inducer. Of course, users could regress to the substituting modality but then this could reflect breaks of transparency (thereby losing the automaticity criterion) or an attentional displacement. The question is: in this case, would the user still have access to the substituted information? Note that in opposition to this idea that after experience, while the device becomes transparent the inducing modality is lost, Ward and Wright (2012) have argued that it remains a complicated dual experience. These two opposite views remain purely speculative and any scientific claim about automaticity will have to await further empirical investigation (such as Stroop tests run on expert users).

Finally, with respect to the fourth criterion—the consistency of the occurrence over time—there are similarly no data to confirm or disconfirm this position. With regard to the associated phenomenology, there is only one verbal report (an e-mail from PF) that was quoted at the beginning of this section saying that mood, time, and environmental factors do not change the images, color, and motion effects she experienced. Thus, much more evidence is needed to build a case for consistency. With regard to the substituted information, even with a lack of data, the argument to say that it fulfills consistency is not very strong: through the same translation code the same inducer will give rise to the same concurrent. Along the same lines as the first criterion (the presence of an inducer-concurrent pairing), it is not hard to see how the consistency criterion is fulfilled exactly to the extent to which it does not fulfill the idiosyncrasy criterion. The same inducer might give rise to the same concurrent, but this will also be the same for all of the users in a way that negates idiosyncrasy.

To summarize, the aim of this section was to clarify the debate on SSD-use being akin to synaesthesia, by dissociating the substituted information from the associated phenomenology. When considering the associated phenomenology, the genuine existence of a concurrent that would be different from visual imagery is currently lacking empirical support. In addition, this concurrent would not be absolute (as in synaesthesia) but rather relative (for instance, the louder, the brighter). The idiosyncrasy of the pairing, although limited to a narrow set, is still an option, and there is currently no substantial evidence for automaticity and consistency, although these cannot be ruled out either. This suggests that the idea that the associated phenomenology involved in SSD-use is a form of artificially induced synaesthesia is not yet scientifically established. It can be either provisionally endorsed, conditional on further scientific evidence (as Farina, 2013 suggests), or rejected as scientifically unfounded (as Deroy and Auvray, 2012a, 2012b have previously argued). When considering the substituted information, there is no problem in considering that the experience is consistent, and the presence of a concurrent is not questionable either. However, the extent to which both the concurrent and the inducer are consciously perceived remains unclear. The question of automaticity remains open, and there cannot be any idiosyncrasy involved. Thus, anyone defending SSD-use at the level of the substituted information will have to give up this last criterion.

12.5 Conclusions

12.5.1 Summary of the analyses

The aim of this chapter was to examine the extent to which alleged cases of transient and acquired forms of synaesthetic experiences can be considered as genuine cases of synaesthesia.

Table 12.1 gives an overview of the analyses. To summarize them, in post-hypnotic suggestion, the concurrent is consciously reported during the experiment although the extent to which a conscious status can be achieved in such cases remains highly controversial. There is idiosyncrasy and automaticity; however, the question of consistency remains open to further empirical confirmation (although preliminary

Table 12.1. Summary of the criteria fulfilled by four alleged cases of synaesthetic experiences: post-hypnotic suggestion, drug-use, flavor perception, and use of sensory substitution devices. In the table we also added congenital synaesthesia and crossmodal correspondences. The terms yes and no are used when the claim is not controversial, debated is added when there are existing data but their interpretation is subject to controversy, and lack of data is used when more empirical data are needed.

Criteria cases	Inducer-concurrent pairing	Idiosyncrasy	Automaticity of the process	Consistency over time
Congenital synaesthesia	Yes	Yes	Yes	Yes
Post-hypnotic suggestions	Debated	Yes	Yes	Lack of data
Drug-use	Debated	Yes	Lack of data	Lack of data
Sweetness enhancement	No	No	Debated	Yes
SSD: associated phenomenology	Debated	Yes (narrow set)	Lack of data	Lack of data
SSD: substituted information	Lack of data	No	Lack of data	Yes
Crossmodal correspondences	No	No	Yes	Yes

results by Cohen Kadosh et al., 2009 point in this direction). With respect to drug-use, there is an inducer-concurrent pairing, although the inducer and concurrent seem to be experienced as less demarcated than in congenital synaesthesia. As for post-hypnotic suggestions, these pairings can be consciously reported, although there is a difficulty in identifying experiences that are induced while being under the influence of drugs, and it remains unclear whether the concurrent is different from vivid hallucinations. There is idiosyncrasy. However, there are no studies investigating automaticity experimentally. Furthermore, there are reports suggesting it is unlikely to be the case as under the influence of drugs someone can report a pairing one time and not the other. Consistency also remains controversial with preliminary studies pointing in different directions.

With regard to sweetness enhancement, the inducer and concurrent are not both consciously perceived at the same time, as the phenomenon occurs when the participants adopt a synthetic strategy and when they are not provided with the scales that allow them to disentangle their perception from different sensory modalities. There is no idiosyncrasy (at least intra-culturally), the automaticity remains controversial, and there is consistency. With respect to sensory substitution, when the concurrent is considered to be the associated phenomenology, there is a crucial lack of empirical data, as the hypothesis arises from only two verbal reports. These preliminary reports suggest there might be a consciously perceived concurrent (but without certainty of its perceptual status, i.e. differences from added visual imagery). There can be idiosyncrasy, although narrower than congenital synaesthesia, and there are no substantial data to show if there can be automaticity and consistency. When the concurrent is considered to be the substituted information, the existence of an inducer-concurrent pairing can be acknowledged; however, the extent to which both the concurrent and the inducer are consciously perceived awaits further empirical data. In addition, the concurrent is linked to the inducer more in a relative than in an absolute way (which is closer to crossmodal correspondences than synaesthesia; see Deroy and Spence, 2013a) and there is no idiosyncrasy. In summary, it appears that none of the alleged cases of synaesthesia we considered can be claimed to match the criteria we established to single out genuine forms of synaesthesia.

12.5.2 Borderline cases: closer to crossmodal correspondences than synaesthetic experiences?

Table 12.1 also shows that the alleged cases of transient and acquired synaesthesia are not closer to congenital synaesthesia than they are to crossmodal correspondences. Indeed, two main criteria distinguish synaesthesia from crossmodal correspondences: pairing and idiosyncrasy, whereas they both share automaticity and consistency. We will first discuss the shared criteria and then move on to analyze the non-shared ones. Many of the claims that link borderline cases to synaesthesia emphasize their automaticity and consistency; however, these two criteria alone do not allow these cases to be distinguished from crossmodal correspondences. Thus, obtaining a Stroop effect or any measure of automaticity allows the strength of an association to be assessed, but it does not allow assessing if this association occurs at a semantic level or at a perceptual level. The same is true for any measure of consistency. To repeat it again, only further empirical data will confirm that there is a strong association of the pairings. However, in the absence of the two remaining criteria (i.e. pairing and idiosyncrasy), this will not help in disentangling whether these associations resemble synaesthesia, crossmodal correspondences, or associations occurring at an even higher level of processing (such as conceptual or semantic associations).

Thus, for us to say that the borderline cases resemble more synaesthesia than crossmodal correspondences, the other two criteria must be fulfilled. Idiosyncrasy is the easiest to discuss as the extent to which each of the borderline cases fulfills it is less subject to debate. This criterion rules out sweetness enhancement and SSD-use with substituted information as concurrent. The first criterion is less straightforward to discuss as it involves taking into account different levels of associations. Many articles discuss the nature of synaesthetic experiences (see Auvray and Deroy, 2015, for a review), but there seems to be a consensus on the idea that it has to involve a process close to a perceptual one, otherwise it would be impossible to say that synaesthesia is different from hallucination, from visual imagery, and from semantic and conceptual associations. So far, none of the mentioned borderline cases can be affirmed with certainty to be genuinely perceptual. To reiterate, this is not the case of sweetness enhancement and SSD-use with substituted information as concurrent. In the case of SSD-use with associate phenomenology as concurrent, as well as with post-hypnotic suggestions, there are no data so far to distinguish the associated experience from mental imagery. As for drug-use, there are no data either to distinguish the associations that are made from hallucinations.

In light of these considerations, we would like to conclude this chapter with an appeal for cautiousness. If anything, these borderline cases crucially show that it is false to think of sensory modalities as being non-overlapping and discrete (see Haigh et al., 2013 for this claim in the context of SSD-use). This claim is already crucial in the fields of psychology and philosophy of perception. Going one step further and linking borderline cases to synaesthesia can be interesting as a working hypothesis, as it gave rise to studies using the experimental methodologies from synaesthesia that in return allow us to better document and hence understand these cases. However, it can prove highly misleading to go beyond the limits of a working hypothesis and have strong affirmations that do not rest on firm empirical grounds. There are two main reasons for resisting the fashionable phenomenon of synaesthesia and applying this term to any phenomena that share a vague resemblance (thereby avoiding terminological confusion). First, to fully understand different phenomena, we have to keep their study separate. It is thus important to bear in mind what these borderline cases do not share with synaesthesia to allow research into these differences, which might prove to be the specificity of each of these borderline cases. Second, keeping different phenomena distinct is specifically what allows a unified vision of each of these phenomena. It is by considering as synaesthetic only the cases that were identified as fulfilling the definitions that the study of synaesthesia can preserve a scientific robustness. Furthermore, treating such a wide range of phenomena as genuine synaesthetic experiences does threaten an understanding of synaesthesia as a unitary event. It additionally prevents treating synaesthesia as a natural kind of its own. Anyone defending a broad acceptance of the term synaesthesia will have to give an account of why one or several criteria to define synaesthesia can be loosened in some cases without weakening the understanding and definitions given to congenital synaesthesia.

Acknowledgements

We would like to thank Ophelia Deroy, Julian Kiverstein, John Sutton, and the two anonymous reviewers for their helpful and stimulating feedback on earlier drafts of this manuscript. MF is funded by a grant from the British Academy and by King's College, London.

References

Arno, P., Vanlierde, A., Streel, E., Wanet-Defalque, M. C., Sanabria-Bohorquez, S., & Veraart, C. (2001). Auditory substitution of vision: Pattern recognition by the blind. *Applied Cognitive Psychology, 15*(5), 509–19.

Aghajanian, G. K., & Marek, G. J. (1999). Serotonin and hallucinogens. *Neuropsychopharmacology, 21*, 16S–23S.

Auvray, M., & Deroy, O. (2015). How do synesthetes experience the world? In M. Matthen (Ed.), *Oxford Handbook of Philosophy of Perception* (pp. 640–58). Oxford: Oxford University Press.

Auvray, M., Hanneton, S., & O'Regan, J. K. (2007). Learning to perceive with a visuo-auditory substitution system: Localization and object recognition with The Voice. *Perception, 36*, 416–30.

Auvray, M., & Myin, E. (2009). Perception with compensatory devices: From sensory substitution to sensorimotor extension. *Cognitive Science, 33*, 1036–58.

Auvray, M., & Spence, C. (2008). The multisensory perception of flavor. *Consciousness & Cognition, 17*, 1016–31.

Bach-y-Rita, P., & Kercel, S. W. (2003). Sensory substitution and the human-machine interface. *Trends in Cognitive Sciences, 7*, 541–6.

Barnett, K. J., Foxe, J. J., Molholm, S., Kelly, S. P., Shalgi, S., Mitchell, K. J., & Newell, F. N. (2008). Differences in early sensory-perceptual processing in synesthesia: A visual evoked potential study. *NeuroImage, 43*, 605–13.

Baron-Cohen, S. (1996). Is there a normal phase of synaesthesia in development? *Psyche, 2*, 2–27.

Baron-Cohen, S., Wyke, M. A., & Binnie, C. (1987). Hearing words and seeing colours: An experimental investigation of a case of synaesthesia. *Perception, 16*, 761–7.

Beringer, K. (1927). Der Meskalinrausch, seine Geschichte und Erscheinungsweise, S. 1–315. Berlin: J.

Brang, D., McGeoch, P. D., & Ramachandran, V. S. (2008). Apotemnophilia: A neurological disorder. *Neuroreport, 19*(13), 1305–6.

Brang, D., Hubbard, E. M., Coulson, S., Huang, M., & Ramachandran, V. S. (2010). Magnetoencephalography reveals early activation of V4 in grapheme-color synesthesia. *NeuroImage, 53*, 268–74.

Chabalier, E. (1864). De la pseudochromesthesie [About pseudochromestesia]. *Journal de Medecine de Lyon, 1*, 92–102.

Cliff, M., & Noble, A. C. (1990). Time–intensity evaluation of sweetness and fruitiness and their interaction in a model solution. *Journal of Food Science, 55*, 450–4.

Cohen Kadosh, R, Henik, A., Catena, A., Walsh, V., & Fuentes, L. J. (2009). Induced cross-modal synaesthetic experience without abnormal neuronal connections. *Psychological Science, 20*, 258–65.

Cytowic, R. (1989). *Synaesthesia: A union of the senses*. New York, USA: Springer.

Cytowic, R. (1997). Synaesthesia: Phenomenology and neuropsychology—A review of current knowledge. In S. Baron-Cohen, & E. Harrison (Eds.), *Synaesthesia: Classic and Contemporary Readings* (pp. 17–42). Oxford: Oxford Blackwell.

Cytowic, R. (2003). *The man who tasted shapes*. Cambridge, MA: MIT Press.

Cytowic, R., & Eagleman, D. M. (2009). *Wednesday is indigo blue: Discovering the brain of synesthesia*. Cambridge, MA: MIT Press.

Day, S. (2009). Types of synesthesia. In Synesthesia. Retrieved from <http://www.daysyn.com/Types-of-Syn.html> [last accessed April 2013].

Delay, J., Gérad, H. P., & Racamier, P. C. (1951). Les synesthésies dans l'intoxication Mescalinique [Synaesthesias with mescalinic intoxication]. *L'Encephale, 40*, 1–10.

Deroy, O., & Auvray, M. (2012a). Reading the world through the skin and ears: A new perspective on sensory substitution. *Frontiers in Theoretical and Philosophical Psychology, 3*, 457. doi: 10.3389/fpsyg.2012.00457.

Deroy, O., & Auvray, M. (2012b). Reading the world through the skin and ears: A new perspective on sensory substitution. *Frontiers in Psychology, 3*, 457.

Deroy, O., & Auvray, M. (2014). A crossmodal perspective on sensory substitution. In S. Biggs, M. Matthen, & D. Stokes (Eds.), *Perception and Its Modalities* (pp. 327–49). Oxford: Oxford University Press.

Deroy, O., & Spence, C. (2013a). Why we are not all synesthetes (not even weakly so). *Psychonomic Bulletin & Review, 20*, 643–64.

Deroy, O., & Spence, C. (2013b). Training, drugs, and hypnosis: Artificial synaesthesia, or artificial paradises? *Frontiers in Psychology, 4*, 660. doi:10.3389/fpsyg.2013.00660.

Davidson, J. M., Linforth, R. S. T., Hollowood, T. A., & Taylor, A. J. (1999). Effect of sucrose on the perceived flavor intensity of chewing gum. *Journal of Agriculture and Food Chemistry, 47*, 4336–40.

Dixon, M. J., Smilek, D., Cudahy, C., & Merikle, P. M. (2000). Five plus two equals yellow. *Nature, 406*, 365.

Dixon, M. J., Smilek, D., & Merikle, P. M. (2004). Not all synaesthetes are created equal: Projector versus associator synesthetes. *Cognitive, Affective and Behavioral Neuroscience, 4*, 335–43.

Eagleman, D. M. (2009). The objectification of overlearned sequences: A new view of spatial sequence synesthesia. *Cortex, 45*, 1266–7.

Eagleman, D. M., Kagan, A. D., Nelson, S. S., Sagaram, D., & Sarma, A. K. (2007). A standardized test battery for the study of synesthesia. *Journal of Neuroscientific Methods, 159*, 139–45.

Ellis, H. (1898). Mescal: A new artificial paradise. *The Contemporary Review, 73*, 130–41.

Farina, M. (2013). Neither touch nor vision: Sensory substitution as artificial synaesthesia? *Biology and Philosophy, 28*, 639–55.

Frank, R. A., & Byram, J. (1988). Taste-smell interactions are tastant and odorant dependent. *Chemical Senses, 13*, 445–55.

Frank, R. A., Shaffer, G., & Smith, D. V. (1991). Taste-odor similarities predict taste enhancement and suppression in taste-odor mixtures. *Chemical Senses, 16*, 523.

Frank, R. A., van der Klaauw, N. J., & Schifferstein, H. N. J. (1993). Both perceptual and conceptual factors influence taste-odor and taste-taste interactions. *Perception & Psychophysics, 54*, 343–54.

Friedrichs, H. (2009). *Die Psychologie des Meskalinrausches [The Psychology of Mescaline Intoxications]*. Berlin: VWB—Verlag für Wissenschaft und Bildung.

Galton, F. (1880). Visualised numerals. *Nature, 21*, 252–6.

Grof, S. (1975). *Realms of the human unconsciousness*. New York, USA: Viking Press.

Grossenbacher, P. G., & Lovelace, C. T. (2001). Mechanisms of synesthesia: Cognitive and physiological constraints. *Trends in Cognitive Sciences, 5*, 36–41.

Haigh, A., Brown, D. J., Meijer, P., Proulx, M. J. (2013). How well do you see what you hear? The acuity of visual-to-auditory sensory substitution. *Frontiers in Psychology, 4*, 330. doi: 10.3389/fpsyg.2013.00330.

Hanneton, S., Auvray, M., & Durette, B. (2010). The Vibe: A versatile vision-to-audition sensory substitution device. *Applied Bionics and Biomechanics, 7*, 269–76.

Hartman, A. M., & Hollister, L. E. (1963). Effect of mescaline, lysergic acid diethylamide and psilocybin on color perception. *Psychopharmacolgia, 4*, 441–51.

Hofmann, A. (1983). *LSD my problem child: Reflections on sacred drugs, mysticism, and science.* Los Angeles, USA: Jeremy P. Tarcher.

Howells, T. (1944). The experimental development of color-tone synesthesia. *Journal of Experimental Psychology, 34*, 87–103.

Hubbard, E. M. (2007). Neurophysiology of synesthesia. *Current Psychiatry Reports, 9*, 193–9.

Hubbard, E., & Ramachandran, V. S. (2003). The phenomenology of synaesthesia. *Journal of Consciousness Studies, 10*, 49–57.

Hubbard, E. M., & Ramachandran, V. S. (2005). Neurocognitive mechanisms of synesthesia. *Neuron, 48*, 509–20.

Jewanski, J., Day, S. A., Simner, J., & Ward, J. (2011). The development of a scientific understanding of synesthesia during the mid-nineteenth century (1849–1873). *Journal of the History of the Neurosciences, 20*, 284–305.

Jewanski, J., Day, S. A., Ward, J. (2009). A colorful albino: The first documented case of synaesthesia, by Georg Tobias Ludwig Sachs in 1812. *Journal of the History of the Neurosciences, 18*, 293–303.

Kadosh, R. C., & Walsh, V. (2006). Cognitive neuroscience: Rewired or crosswired brains?. *Current Biology, 16*, R962–R963.

Kiverstein, J., Farina, M., & Clark, A. (2015). Substituting the senses". In M. Matthen (Ed.), *The Oxford Handbook of the Philosophy of Perception* (pp. 659–78). Oxford: Oxford University Press.

Laurence, J. R., Beaulieu-Prévost, D., & Du Chéné, T. (2008). Measuring and understanding individual differences. In M. Nash & A. Barnier (Eds.), *The Oxford Handbook of Hypnosis: Theory, Research, and Practice* (pp. 225–53). Oxford, UK: Oxford University Press.

Leuner, H. (1962). *Die experimentelle psychose [The experimental psychosis].* Berlin, Germany: Springer.

Levy-Tzedek, S., Hanassy, S., Abboud, S., Maidenbaum, S., & Amedi, A. (2012). Fast, accurate reaching movements with a visual-to-auditory sensory substitution device. *Restorative Neurology and Neuroscience, 30*, 313–23.

Loomis, J. M. (2010). Sensory substitution for orientation and mobility: What progress are we making? Sidebar 1.1 (pp. 7–10) to Chapter 1, *Perceiving to Move and Moving to Perceive: Control of Locomotion by Students with Vision Loss* by D. A. Guth, J. J. Rieser, & D. H. Ashmead (pp. 3–44). In: R. William, R. Wiener, R. L. Welsh, & B. B. Blasch (Eds.), *Foundations of Orientation and Mobility, Third Edition, Volume 1 (History and Theory).* New York: AFB Press.

Luke, D., Terhune, D. B., & Friday, R. (2012). Psychedelic synaesthesia: Evidence for a serotonergic role in synaesthesia. *Seeing and Perceiving, S1*, 74.

MacLeod, C. M., & Dunbar, K. (1988). Training and Stroop-like interference: Evidence for a continuum of automaticity. *Journal of Experimental Psychology: Human Perception and Performance, 14*, 126–35.

Marinetti, F. T. (1911). *Distruzione: Poema Futurista [Destruction: Futuristic Poem]*. Milano, Italy: Edizioni futuriste di Poesia.

Marks, L. E. (1987). On cross-modal similarity: Auditory–visual interactions in speeded discrimination. *Journal of Experimental Psychology: Human Perception and Performance, 13*, 384–94.

Masters, R. E. L., & Houston, J. (1966). *The varieties of psychedelic experience*. New York/ Chicago: Holt, Rinehart & Winston.

Mattingley, J. B. (2009). Attention, automaticity, and awareness in synesthesia. *Annals of the New York Academy of Sciences, 1156*, 141–67.

Maurer, D. (1993). Neonatal synesthesia: Implications for the processing of speech and faces. In B. de Boysson-Bardies, S. de Schonen, P. Jusczyk, P. McNeilage, & J. Morton (Eds.), *Developmental Neurocognition: Speech and Face Processing in the First Year of Life* (pp. 109–24). Kluwer Academic: Dordrecht, The Netherlands.

Mayer-Gross, W. (1931). Über synästhesien im meskalinrausch [About synaesthesia in mescaline intoxication]. In: G. Anschütz (Ed.), *Farbe-Ton-Forschungen Bd. III* (pp. 266–77). Hamburg: Psychologischästhetische Forschungsgesellschaft.

Meijer, P. B. L. (1992). An experimental system for auditory image representations. *IEEE Transactions on Biomedical Engineering, 39*, 112–21.

Mills, C. B., Boteler, E. H., Howell, O., & Glenda K. (1999). Digit synaesthesia: A case study using a Stroop-type test. *Cognitive Neuropsychology, 16*, 181–91.

Nguyen, D. H., Valentin, D., Ly, M. H., Chrea, C., & Sauvageot, F. (2002). When does smell enhance taste? Effect of culture and odorant/tastant relationship. Paper presented at the European Chemoreception Research Organisation conference, Erlangen, Germany.

Nunn, J. A., Gregory, L. J., Brammer, M., Williams, S. C. R., Parslow, D. M., Morgan, M. J., Morris, R. G., Bullmore, E. T., Baron-Cohen, S., & Gray, J. A. (2002). Functional magnetic resonance imaging of synesthesia: Activation of V4/V8 by spoken words. *Nature Neuroscience, 5*, 371–5.

Nussbaumer, F. A. (1873). Über subjektive Farbempfindungen, die durch objektive Gehörempfindungen erzeugt werden [About subjective colour sensations, caused by objective auditory sensations]. *Wiener Medizinishe Wochenschrift, 1*, 4–7.

O'Regan, J. K., & Noë, A. (2001). A sensorimotor account of vision and visual consciousness. *Behavioral and Brain Sciences, 24*, 939–1031.

Ortmann, O. (1933). Theories of synesthesia in the light of a case of colored hearing. *Human Biology, 5*, 155–211.

Pedley, P. E., & Harper, R. S. (1959). Pitch and the vertical localization of sound. *The American Journal of Psychology, 72*, 447–9.

Pollok, B., Schnitzler, I., Mierdorf, T., Stoerig, P., & Schnitzler, A. (2005). Image-to-sound conversion: Experience-induced plasticity in auditory cortex of blindfolded adults. *Experimental Brain Research, 167*, 287–91.

Prescott, J. (2004). Psychological processes in flavour perception. In A. J. Taylor & D. D. Roberts (Eds.), *Flavor Perception* (pp. 257–77). Oxford, UK: Blackwell.

Prescott, J., Johnstone, V., & Francis, J. (2004). Odor-taste interactions: Effects of attentional strategies during exposure. *Chemical Senses, 29*, 331–40.

Proulx, M. J. (2010). Synthetic synaesthesia and sensory substitution. *Consciousness and Cognition, 19*, 501–3.

Proulx, M. J., & Stoerig, P. (2006). Seeing sounds and tingling tongues: Qualia in synaesthesia and sensory substitution. *Anthropology & Philosophy, 7*, 135–51.

Proulx, M. J., Stoerig, P., Ludowig, E., & Knoll, I. (2008). Seeing 'where' through the ears: effects of learning-by-doing and long-term sensory deprivation on localization based on image-to-sound substitution. *PLoS One, 3*(3), e1840.

Renier, L., Collignon, O., Poirier, C., Tranduy, D., Vanlierde, A., Bol, A., . . . & De Volder, A. G. (2005). Cross-modal activation of visual cortex during depth perception using auditory substitution of vision. *Neuroimage, 26*, 573–80.

Renier, L., & De Volder, A. G. (2013). Sensory substitution devices: Creating "artificial synaesthesias". In: J. Simner & E. Hubbard (Eds), *The Oxford Handbook of Synaesthesia* (pp. 853–68). Oxford, UK: Oxford University Press.

Rich, A. N., Bradshaw, J. L., & Mattingley, J. B. (2005). A systematic, large-scale study of synaesthesia: Implications for the role of early experience in lexical colour associations. *Cognition, 98*, 53–84.

Rich, A. N., & Mattingley, J. B. (in press). The role of attention in synaesthesia. In: J. Simner & E. Hubbard (Eds), *The Oxford Handbook of Synaesthesia*. Oxford, UK: Oxford University Press.

Robertson, L. C., & Sagiv, N. (2005). *Synesthesia: Perspectives from Cognitive Neuroscience*. New York, USA: Oxford University Press.

Rouw, R., Scholte, H. S., & Colizoli, O. (2011). Brain areas involved in synaesthesia: A review. *Journal of Neuropsychology, 5*, 214–42.

Sachs, G. T. L. (1812). Historiae naturalis duorum leucaetiopum: Auctoris ipsius et sororis eius. *Solisbaci [Natural history of two albinos, the author and his sister]*. Germany: Sumptibus Bibliopoli Seideliani.

Sagiv, N., Heer, J., & Robertson, L. (2006). Does binding of synesthetic color to the evoking grapheme require attention? *Cortex, 42*, 232–42.

Schifferstein, H. N. J., & Verlegh, P. W. J. (1996). The role of congruency and pleasantness in odor-induced taste enhancement. *Acta Psychologica, 94*, 87–105.

Shanon, B. (2002). Ayahuasca visualizations: A structural typology. *Journal of Consciousness Studies, 9*, 3–30.

Siegel, R. K. (1975). *Hallucinations—Behavior, Experience, and Theory*. New York, USA: John Wiley & Sons.

Simner, J. (2012). Defining synaesthesia. *British Journal of Psychology, 103*, 1–15.

Simner, J., Glover, L., & Mowat, A. (2006). Linguistic determinants of word colouring in grapheme-colour synaesthesia. *Cortex, 42*, 281–9.

Simner, J., Mulvenna, C., Sagiv, N., Tsakanikos, E., Witherby, S. A., Fraser, C., Kirsten, S., & Ward, J. (2006). Synaesthesia: The prevalence of atypical cross-modal experiences. *Perception, 35*, 1024–33.

Simner, J., & Ward, J. (2008). Synaesthesia, color terms, and color space: Color claims came from color names in Beeli, Esslen, and Jancke. *Psychological Science, 19*, 412–14.

Simner, J., Ward, J., Lanz, M., Jansari, A., Noonan, K., Glover, L., & Oakley, D. A. (2005). Non-random associations of graphemes to colours in synaesthetic and non-synaesthetic populations. *Cognitive Neuropsychology, 22*, 1069–85.

Simpson, L., & McKellar, P. (1955). Types of synaesthesia. *Journal of Mental Science, 101*, 141–7.

Sinke, C., Halpern, J. H., Zedler, M., Neufeld, J., Emrich, H. M., & Passie, T. (2012). Genuine and drug-induced synesthesia: A comparison. *Consciousness and Cognition, 21*, 1419–34.

Skinner, B. F. (1938). *The behavior of organisms: An experimental analysis.* Oxford, UK: Appleton-Century-Crofts.

Smilek, D., Dixon, M. J., Cudahy, C., & Merikle, P. M. (2001). Synaesthetic photisms influence visual perception. *Journal of Cognitive Neuroscience, 13*, 930–6.

Spence, C., & Deroy, O. (2012). Crossmodal correspondences: Innate or learned? *Perception, 3*, 316–8.

Spence, C., & Deroy, O. (2013a). Crossmodal mental imagery. In S. Lacey and R. Lawson (Eds), *Multisensory imagery: Theory and applications* (pp. 157–83). Philadelphia, USA: Springer.

Spence, C., & Deroy, O. (2013b). How automatic are crossmodal correspondences?. *Consciousness and Cognition, 22*, 245–60.

Spence, C., Auvray, M., & Smith, B. (2014). Confusing tastes and flavours. In S. Biggs, M. Matthen, & D. Stokes (Eds.), *Perception and Its Modalities* (pp. 247–76). Oxford: Oxford University Press.

Steven, M. S., & Blakemore, C. (2004). Visual synaesthesia in the blind. *Perception, 33*, 855–68.

Stevenson, R. J., & Boakes, R. A. (2004). Sweet and sour smells: Learned synaesthesia between the senses of taste and smell. In G. A. Calvert, C. Spence, & B. E. Stein (Eds.), *The Handbook of Multisensory Processing* (pp. 69–83). Cambridge, MA: MIT Press.

Stevenson, R. J, Boakes, R. A., & Prescott, J. (1998). Changes in odor sweetness resulting from implicit learning of a simultaneous odor-sweetness association: An example of learned synesthesia. *Learning and Motivation, 29*, 113–32.

Stevenson, R. J., Boakes, R. A., & Wilson, J. P. (2000a). Counter-conditioning following human odor-taste and color-taste learning. *Learning and Motivation, 31*, 114–27.

Stevenson, R. J., Boakes, R. A. & Wilson, J. P. (2000b). The persistence of conditioned odor perceptions: Evaluative conditioning is not unique. *Journal of Experimental Psychology: Learning, Memory and Cognition, 26*, 423–40.

Stevenson, R. J., Prescott, J., & Boakes, R. A. (1995). The acquisition of taste properties by odors. *Learning and Motivation, 26*, 433–55.

Stevenson, R. J., Prescott, J., & Boakes, R. A. (1999). Confusing tastes and smells: How odours can influence the perception of sweet and sour tastes. *Chemical Senses, 24*, 627–35.

Stevenson, R. J., & Tomiczek, C. M. (2007). Olfactory induced synesthesias: A review and model. *Psychological Bulletin, 133*, 294–309.

Studerus, E., Kometer, M., Hasler, F., & Vollenweider, F. X. (2011). Acute, subacute and long-term subjective effects of psilocybin in healthy humans: A pooled analysis of experimental studies. *Journal of Psychopharmacology, 25*, 1434–52.

Tart, C. T. (1975). *States of consciousness.* New York, USA: E. P. Dutton.

Terhune, D. B., & Cohen Kadosh, R. (2012). Synaesthesias. In: J. D. Blom, & I. Sommer (Eds.), *Hallucinations. Research and Practice* (pp. 91–104). New York, USA: Springer.

Ward, J. (2004). Emotionally mediated synaesthesia. *Cognitive Neuropsychology, 21*, 761–72.

Ward, J. (2013). Synaesthesia. *Annual Review of Psychology, 64*, 2–27.

Ward, J., Jonas, C., Dienes, Z., & Seth, A. (2010). Grapheme-colour synaesthesia improves detection of embedded shapes, but without pre-attentive "pop-out" of synaesthetic colour. *Proceeding of the Royal Society London B Biological Sciences, 277*, 1021–6.

Ward, J., & Meijer, P. (2010). Visual experiences in the blind induced by an auditory sensory substitution device. *Consciousness and Cognition, 19*, 492–500.

Ward, J., & Simner, J. (2003). Lexical-gustatory synaesthesia: Linguistic and conceptual factors. *Cognition, 89*, 237–61.

Wasson, R. G. (1978). *The road to Eleusis: Unveiling the secret of the mysteries.* New York, USA: Harcourt.

Watson, J. B. (1930). *Behaviorism* (Revised edition). Chicago, USA: University of Chicago Press.

Ward, J., & Wright, T. (2012). Sensory substitution as an artificially acquired synaesthesia. *Neuroscience and Biobehavioral Review*, doi: 10.1016/j.neubiorev.2012.07.007.

Yeomans, M. R., & Mobini, S. (2006). Hunger alters the expression of acquired hedonic but not sensory qualities of food-paired odors in humans. *Journal of Experimental Psychology: Animal Behavior Processes, 32*, 460–6.

Yeomans, M. R., Mobini, S., Elliman, T. D., Walker, H. C., & Stevenson, R. J. (2006). Hedonic and sensory characteristics of odors conditioned by pairing with tastants in humans. *Journal of Experimental Psychology: Animal Behavior Processes, 32*, 215–28.

13

Mirror-Touch Synaesthesia

Intersubjective or Intermodal Fusion?

Frédérique de Vignemont

Watching someone eating, I would taste and feel their food in my mouth, and I struggled with weight loss because I always felt full.

(*The Guardian*, Saturday 19 March 2011)

Fiona Torrance describes here how she feels what other people feel. She catches, so to speak, other people's experiences. She presents an extreme version of what is known as *mirror-touch synaesthesia* (MTS). Typically, individuals with MTS report consciously feeling tactile sensations on their own body when they see another person being touched. In other words, they have what may be called vicarious tactile sensations.[1] Vicarious tactile sensations may almost seem unbelievable. How could one feel from the inside someone else's sensations? Interestingly, it has been repeatedly shown that in any individual (with MTS or not), part of the same brain areas are activated when one experiences tactile sensations and when one observes another individual receiving a tactile stimulus (Keysers et al., 2004; Ebish et al., 2008; Wood et al., 2010). Hence, vicarious touch is not limited to individuals with MTS. It happens to any of us. It just does not normally reach the threshold of consciousness.

MTS is thus more than a marginal—though puzzling—condition. But what is its explanation? It can be considered from two distinct perspectives, which are already revealed in the very name of mirror-touch synaesthesia. On the one hand, it is qualified as a kind of *mirror* phenomenon. As such, it should be understood in the same way as action mirroring. It results from the fusion between self and others. On the other hand, it is qualified as a kind of *synaesthesia*. As such, it should be understood in the same way as coloured audition, for example. It results from the fusion between the senses, and more specifically between vision and touch.

[1] A state is vicarious if (i) it is caused by another person undergoing a specific mental state and (ii) it is isomorphic to some extent to the other person's state.

In this chapter, I will consider both interpretations. First, I will focus on the intersubjective dimension of vicarious touch. In particular, I will examine whether it constitutes a kind of empathy. I will then argue that vicarious touch cannot be taken as evidence in favour of embodied social cognition. Second, I will focus on the intermodal dimension of vicarious touch. I will show how it differs from standard cases of idiosyncratic synaesthesia. I will then argue that it is a by-product of the multimodal nature of non-vicarious bodily experiences.

13.1 An intersubjective account of vicarious touch

> These systems may be crucial for empathy because they enable the observer to simulate another's experience by activating the same brain areas that are active when the observer experiences the same emotion or state.
>
> (Banissy and Ward, 2007: 815)

> Vicarious somatosensory activity has a crucial role in empathy and social perception.
>
> (Keyser et al., 2010: 426)

Individuals with MTS feel touch on their body although they are not touched and it is someone else who is touched. If they are simultaneously touched, then they can make mistakes in reporting where they were touched. For instance, if they are touched on their left cheek and they see another individual being touched on her right cheek, they report feeling touch either on both sides or on the right cheek, the side of their face that was not touched (Banissy and Ward, 2007). These results cannot be explained away by a mere effect of attention. They make no errors if they see a visual flash on the other person's face. Nor do they make any error if they see an object or a dummy being stroked (Holle et al., 2011). MTS is thus clearly related to perceiving another subject experiencing tactile sensations.

Interestingly, individuals who have MTS also display distinctive features in social cognition. They have a higher empathetic score in questionnaires than non-MTS subjects (Banissy and Ward, 2007). They are better in recognition of facial expression (Banissy et al., 2011). Finally, they are more prone to confusion between self and others in the enfacement illusion (Maister et al., 2013). In the standard version of the enfacement illusion, the participant is seated in front of another individual and both faces are synchronously stroked. Then the participant looks at the picture of her face morphed at various degrees with the picture of the other individual's face. She has to judge when it is her face and when it is the other's face. The illusion leads to a significant increase in self-attribution of the morphed images (Tsakiris, 2008). The experiment was done with individuals with MTS with a slightly different paradigm. Only the face of the individual seated in front was stroked, and not the participant's own face. Yet, like in the standard enfacement illusion, it led to a significant increase in self-attribution of the morphed images of the two faces (Maister et al., 2013). The observation of the other face being touched thus sufficed to induce the illusion in

MTS. Consequently, it has been suggested that MTS results from abnormal self-other processing, which facilitates some social skills, including empathy (Banissy and Ward, 2013). More generally, it has been argued that vicarious touch "is naturally described as empathy for touch" (Goldman, 2011).

At first sight, the notion of empathy in the context of tactile sensations may seem more surprising than 'natural'. The folk notion of empathy classically refers to *affective* sharing; that is, feeling other people's emotions such as grief, happiness, or fear. It is true that one talks of empathy for pain, which is a bodily sensation. But pain has a distinctive affective dimension, and evidence shows that empathetic pain is primarily driven by the affective component of pain (de Vignemont and Jacob, 2012). It is true also that there can be affective touch but it relies on a different neural network than touch. Interestingly, brain areas activated in affective touch are not activated in vicarious touch (Keysers et al., 2010).

However, the main issue is not so much the lack of affectivity in vicarious touch. Rather, what is at stake here is the distinction between *empathy* and *emotional contagion*. Only some vicarious experiences qualify as empathy. Other vicarious experiences can merely be contagious states. Both contagious states and empathetic states are isomorphic to some extent to the target state and both are caused by the observation (or imagination) of signs indicating that another individual is undergoing the target state. But a contagious experience is a *self-centred* vicarious experience. Typically, when I yawn because I see you yawning, I might think that I am tired or bored, but my yawning does not inform me about your sleepiness. Most of the time, I do not even realize that I yawn because you did. By contrast, an empathetic experience is an *other-directed* vicarious experience. It contributes to the understanding of the target's original experience. When I empathize with your distress, I understand what you are feeling in virtue of sharing your emotion. Empathy is intimately related to third-person mindreading. Now the question is: is vicarious touch a case of contagion or of empathy? In other words, is vicarious touch crucial for understanding other people's tactile experiences?

13.2 Tactile empathy

> The somatosensory mirror system, which matches observed and felt touch, is involved in understanding the effect of tactile stimulation on others.
>
> (Blakemore et al., 2005: 1581)

> The capacity to understand the tactile experience of others... thus appears to depend on the re-use of mechanisms that mediate our capacity to interact with the world of objects.
>
> (Wood et al., 2010: 30)

As illustrated by these quotations, there seems to be little doubt in the literature that understanding other people's tactile experiences (hereafter tactile mindreading) depends on vicarious touch. It is then of no surprise that embodied theorists have taken the discovery of a shared neural network for touch and touch observation as evidence for the embodied view of social cognition. Embodied theorists try to elevate the importance of the body in explaining cognitive activities. They claim that the body has a crucial significance in how and what the organism thinks and feels. In particular, in the domain of social cognition, they reject excessive cognitive sophistication. On their view, mindreading does not require a highly cognitive and interpretative strategy of understanding other people's mental states. Access to others' mental states can be direct and non-propositional. Such access seems to be provided by vicarious touch.

> Our capacity to experience and directly understand the tactile experience of others could be mediated by *embodied* simulation, that is, by the externally triggered activation of some of the same neural network underpinning our own tactile sensations.
>
> (Gallese, 2007: 9, my emphasis)

> These findings suggest the existence of a visuotactile mirroring mechanism, and that the understanding of an observed touch . . . could be mediated by *embodied* simulation.
>
> (Ebisch et al., 2008: 1612, my emphasis)

In many cases reported in the literature of so-called embodied processes, it is not clear in what sense those processes are related to the body (Goldman and de Vignemont, 2009), but there is no such problem in the case of vicarious touch. Instead, as I shall argue, the problem is that vicarious touch plays no crucial role in social cognition.

Ascribing tactile sensations to other people seems indeed of little interest for our general understanding of them. In the case of pain mindreading, you can learn that what causes the pain is to be avoided. You can also predict how people will react. You can finally help them. But in the case of touch, what do you learn and what can you predict? Let us imagine that you see me being stroked by a paintbrush. You then understand that I feel touch. So what? What kind of prediction can you make on the basis of this newly acquired knowledge? If we assume that the tactile stimulus is affectively neutral (neither painful or disgusting nor especially pleasant), then it is hard to see what consequences it will have on my behaviour. Therefore, you cannot anticipate my next action on the basis of tactile mindreading.

The second source of puzzlement directly concerns vicarious touch. I will assume here that when you experience vicarious touch, you imagine feeling a tactile sensation on your body.[2] It is then not clear what you specifically gain in your understanding of my tactile experience by imagining what I feel. In a nutshell, it seems that one gains more information about the content of the other individual's tactile experience via

[2] I take imagination here as a kind of simulation that makes an off-line use of the tactile system (Goldman, 2006; de Vignemont and Jacob, 2012).

visual analysis of the tactile event than via vicarious touch. Let us compare in more detail the information respectively carried by a standard tactile experience, by a vicarious experience, and by a visual experience of the tactile event. The content of a standard tactile experience carries information about (i) the relation of pressure of an object with one's body, (ii) the location on a specific part of one's body, (iii) some of the properties of the object, including temperature, shape, texture, and so forth. What about vicarious touch? Unfortunately, no study has been done to investigate how fine-grained the content of vicarious tactile experience is. However, on the basis of the brain activity in the somatosensory cortex, it seems that it mainly represents the pressure of the object on the body. It also sometimes represents its location, but not always: "What is being touched does not matter as long as touch occurs" (Keysers et al., 2004: 339). Several brain imaging studies indeed found activity only in SII, and not in SI, when participants observed another person being touched (Keysers et al., 2004; Ebisch et al., 2008).[3] Finally, one does not vicariously feel whether the object is hot or cold, rough or smooth, big or small. By contrast, the visual experience of the tactile event is highly informative. Not only does it represent the fact that an object is in contact with someone's body and where it is located, but it also represents some of the properties of the object. Hence, one learns more about what the other feels by mere vision than by vicarious touch. Since vision is anyway the necessary intermediary for vicarious touch, it is hard to see why one should add the additional cost to imagine the other person's tactile experience. There is no information that one learns that is not already carried by one's visual experience.

This is not to say that vicarious tactile experience is only an impoverished version of the visual experience of touch. Seeing a tactile event and vicariously feeling touch differ in one important respect. They have different modes of presentation, or format. One may then argue that vicarious touch plays a major role for understanding other people, not so much because of the information its content carries, but because of its specific tactile *format*. Interestingly, it has been recently proposed that the most promising path for embodied social cognition is the hypothesis that social cognition is embodied because it exploits representations with bodily format (Goldman and de Vignemont, 2009; Gallese and Sinigaglia, 2011). Bodily format is a class of representational code that characterizes somatosensory, interoceptive, affective, and motor representations. It has to be distinguished from bodily content; that is, representations that carry information about the body. Some representations can have both a bodily content and a bodily format (for example, tactile representations). But one can envisage dissociations. For instance, the visual representation of one's body has a bodily content, but it is not encoded in a bodily format. Conversely, affective states are endowed with a bodily format, but they do not have a spatial bodily content. I shall now consider three potential roles that the bodily format of vicarious touch

[3] But this analysis does not apply to MTS. Clearly, the body part that is touched does matter and activity is found in SI.

can play. Thanks to vicarious touch, one may grasp the objectivity of the world, the subjectivity of other people, or intersubjectivity.

Touch is traditionally assumed as the only sensory modality that gives direct access to the objectivity of the external world through feelings of resistance. One may then suggest that vicarious tactile experience differs from visual experience of a tactile event in offering a first-person experience of the objectivity of whatever is in contact with the other individual's skin. But does one need vicarious experience of objectivity? It seems that one could easily dispense with it since one is already in almost constant contact with the external world. Furthermore, even if vicarious touch does afford this supplementary grasp of objectivity, this will have nothing to do with mindreading and empathy.

Alternatively, one may argue that vicarious touch is not so much about objectivity as it is about subjectivity. It grounds "the capacity to understand the tactile experience of others, and by extension to understand others as experiencing selves" (Wood et al., 2010). One may even extend this view and claim that one vicariously experiences the intersubjective relation that occurs between the person who is touched and the person who is touching her. However, vicarious touch can be elicited in non-social situations. Brain activity corresponding to vicarious touch was found even when participants observed paper rolls being stroked (Keysers et al., 2004). Arguably, one does not experience the "experiencing self" of the paper rolls. It is important at this point to distinguish between two aspects of touch: the active side (*touchant*) and the passive side (*touché*). Results such as those with the paper rolls indicate that in some circumstances, vicarious touch is not induced by seeing the person receiving the tactile stimulation, but rather by seeing the *stroking movement* itself. As such, it constitutes a vicarious touchant experience rather than a vicarious touché experience. Keyser et al. (2010) conclude that vicarious touch corresponds to the mirroring of tactile consequences of the touching movement. Meanwhile, another study found that vicarious touch could be induced by observing the wind stroking another individual's arm (Ebisch et al., 2008). The only difference with voluntary touch was that there was no activity in SI, and the activity in SII was less intense. These results seem hardly compatible with the interpretation of vicarious touch in terms of empathy.

To conclude, vicarious touch, and more specifically MTS, have been—wrongly—conceived in terms of tactile empathy. Vicarious touch suffers from two main flaws: its lack of predictive power and its informational poverty. First, it is not clear in what sense it is useful to empathize with someone's tactile experiences. Unlike pain, touch has almost no direct implication for action. Hence, vicarious touch cannot be used to make specific predictions about the person who is touched. Nor does it have any function for prosocial behaviour. Second, the role of vicarious touch for mindreading, and more generally for social cognition, is minimal. This is not to say that MTS does not result from the disruption of self-other distinction, as argued by Banissy and Ward (2013). This is rather to say that the collapse of self-other distinction is more characteristic of emotional contagion than of empathy. One catches other people's tactile experiences. But one can as well remain ignorant of the source of one's vicarious tactile experience. Vicarious touch is a self-centred experience with almost no bearing on the understanding of other people. Sharing another's tactile experience is of little interest for mindreading, and more generally for social cognition.

13.3 An intermodal account of vicarious touch

At this stage, one may want to turn to the other interpretation of MTS in terms of synaesthesia. There are, however, two ways the notion of synaesthesia can be interpreted. The current dominant model refers to supplementary sensations that some people experience for specific stimulations. Almost any combination of senses can be associated. For example, auditory stimuli can induce experiences of colour. Individuals with these peculiar subjective experiences may be as frequent as one in 100 (Simner et al., 2006). On this interpretation, synaesthesia is a condition in which a stimulus experience, which may be perceptual, emotional, or imaginative, is a sufficient automatic cause of an arbitrary, idiosyncratic experience in a sensory modality, which is the same as or different from the modality of the stimulus (Macpherson, 2007). As I will show soon, on this definition, MTS is a misnamed phenomenon. There is, however, another interpretation of the term of synaesthesia, which does not refer to the confusion between the senses, but rather to their collaboration to achieve the most reliable rendering of perceptual properties:

> It is not the case that the schema of the body has two different parts, the one optic and the other tactile. It is in essence a synaesthesia.... The synaesthesia, therefore, is the normal situation.
>
> (Schilder, 1935: 38)

Here I will suggest interpreting vicarious touch as a by-product of the multimodal (or synaesthetic) nature of tactile experiences. But I will first show that MTS should not be understood on the model of coloured audition.

As in coloured audition, MTS consists in an experience in one modality automatically caused by an experience in another modality. But the similarity ends there. First, it is not clear how idiosyncratic MTS is. It is true that only 1.6 per cent of the population report consciously feeling other people's tactile sensations (Banissy et al., 2009), but as said earlier, even non-MTS individuals partially activate the same brain areas when they experience tactile sensations and when they observe another individual receiving a tactile stimulus (Keysers et al., 2004; Ebish et al., 2008; Wood et al., 2010). The difference between vicarious touch and MTS may then be just a matter of intensity. It has been suggested that individuals with MTS consciously experience vicarious touch unlike other people because of a heightened activity in the somatosensory cortex (Blakemore et al., 2005).

The second peculiarity of MTS concerns the nature of the so-called synaesthetic experience. In coloured audition, a musical note can induce the experience of any colour. There is in principle nothing in common between the B flat you hear and the blue you see. But in MTS, seeing a tactile stimulus applied to another individual's body part induces you to experience it as if you were receiving the tactile stimulus on your own body on the same body part, either on the same side or on the other side (for example, seeing a left cheek being touched induces a vicarious sensation on the left or right cheek). The content of your experience is not arbitrary. You merely feel on your body what you see.

Hence, MTS differs on several points from classic cases of synaesthesia to such an extent that one may wonder whether the phenomenon is not mislabelled.[4] At least, it seems clear that one cannot shed light on MTS by appealing to current theories of synaesthesia. However, the notion of synaesthesia does not necessarily mean the specific condition that affects only 1.6 per cent of the population. It can also refer to the constant merging of the senses in bodily awareness, as suggested by Schilder (1935). I shall now argue that there is no major qualitative difference in the involvement of vision in touch, vicarious touch, and MTS. Instead, it should be understood as a continuum. The argument can be articulated into three steps:

(1) The multimodality thesis: Bodily experiences, including tactile experiences, result from the integration of vision and touch. They are constitutively multimodal.
(2) Vision can take many bodies as objects. It carries information not only about one's body, but also about other people's bodies (and other objects).
(3) Hence, visual information about other people can influence tactile experiences.

Put another way, the multimodal nature of bodily experiences opens the door to the influence of the vision of other bodies, thus enabling vicarious bodily experiences. I will now focus on non-vicarious tactile experience and show the essential contribution of vision (for a detailed account, see de Vignemont, 2014a). I will then conclude by explaining how the multimodality of tactile experiences can account for vicarious tactile experiences.

13.4 The multimodality thesis

For a long time, most research has studied each sensory modality in isolation. This is in line with a modular conception of perception according to which the first levels of

[4] One may also say that it has been an error to call it a 'mirror' phenomenon. There are important differences between action mirroring and vicarious sensations. For one thing, action has a physical counterpart, namely the bodily movement, which can be directly seen. By contrast, sensation is exclusively internal. Arguably, one cannot directly see a tactile sensation; all one can see is the tactile stimulus. It is possible for a touch to elicit no sensation if, for example, one is anaesthetized. For further discussion, see Jacob and de Vignemont (2017).

sensory processing are encapsulated, isolated from the influence of any other kind of information. However, not only do we experience the world through multiple senses at the same time, but those senses can influence each other. Information from one modality then affects information in another modality. The recent literature has thus emphasized the importance of multisensory interaction, which appears to be "beyond modularity" (Driver and Spence, 2000). Multisensory effects are often automatic and mandatory since they can occur very early on in sensory processing. It may even seem now that a purely unimodal experience (not affected one way or the other by information coming from a different modality) is more the exception than the rule. Multisensory effects are indeed pervasive. They can be found between most modalities, although I shall primarily analyse how touch is affected by vision.

This is well illustrated by the Rubber Hand Illusion. Participants sit with one arm resting on a table, hidden behind a screen. They are asked to visually fixate on a rubber hand presented in front of them, and the experimenter simultaneously strokes with two paintbrushes both the participants' hand and the fake hand. The illusion occurs after a couple of minutes, but only if the two hands are in a congruent position and synchronously stimulated (Botvinick and Cohen, 1998; Tsakiris and Haggard, 2005). Most participants then report feeling as if they were touched on the rubber hand and as if the rubber hand was their hand. After the stroking, they mislocate their hand towards the rubber hand. Furthermore, when they see the rubber hand hit by a hammer, subjects react vividly, as if their own hand was hit (Ehrsson et al., 2007). The link between bodily experiences and visual information can sometimes be so tight that the mere presence of the latter can automatically induce the former. For example, it was found that when participants saw the light from a laser pointer 'stroking' a rubber hand, more than half of them reported that they felt the touch of the laser on their skin (they said that it felt 'warm', for example), even though their own hand was not stroked (Durgin et al., 2007). The resolution of conflict between somatosensory information and visual information leads here to an illusory experience. But most of the time the presence of visual information improves the reliability and accuracy of bodily experiences. Vision is indeed characterized by its spatial richness and reliability. It is necessary to compensate for the flaws of the bodily senses.

To be aware that one is touched 'here' is one thing, and to locate 'here' is another thing. A cross indicating 'you are here' is of little interest if there is no reference point on the map. Likewise, tactile localization requires a spatial frame of reference, which cannot be provided by tactile information itself. More precisely, bodily senses (including the sense of touch, but also the sense of posture and the sense of balance) do not directly carry information about the shape of the various parts of the body, their size, and their spatial configuration. For example, the fact that we have two arms, that they are cylinder-shaped, that they are of such length, and that they are connected to the torso on one end and to the hands on the other cannot be easily derived from the bodily senses. It is true that one receives somatosensory feedback when acting, which can carry information about the size of the limbs. But this can give only a rough estimate. In particular, to know how far one can reach with one's hand does not indicate the respective size of one's fingers, palm, forearm, and upper arm. Active exploration of each body part by haptic touch seems to fare better and to be more specific. However, this involves complex tactile-proprioceptive processing, and that in turn requires taking into account the size of the exploratory body parts (e.g., fingers). Hence, the scope of information that the bodily senses directly carry is limited. For tactile sensations to get a relatively rich and accurate spatial content, raw spatial tactile signals thus need to be interpreted with the help of a topological and geometric mental map of the body.

This hypothesis can be traced back to Bonnier (1905), who first introduced the notion of schema of the body to refer to the spatial organization of bodily sensations. Head and Holmes (1911) also posited the existence of a model of the skin surface of the body used for localizing bodily sensations. But it is O'Shaughnessy (1980) who best argues in favour of a dual specification of the spatial content of bodily experiences. What he calls a long-term body image explains how the spatial contents of all bodily experiences share the same structural shape of the body over an extended period. The long-term body image plays a structural role in spatially shaping bodily experiences. For the sake of simplicity, I will use the term 'body map', which is less theoretically laden. It is thanks to the body map that sensations are experienced as being at more than an isolated body point. The body map is required to spatially organize bodily experiences, to give them a spatial frame of reference. It is the background on which bodily sensations are experienced. For example, one can experience sensations in a phantom limb thanks to the body map that still represents the amputated limb.

Now one question concerns the origin of the body map. And the answer is that it is partly visual. Let us go back to the Rubber Hand Illusion. I have argued that one feels sensations within the frame of reference provided by the body map. Thus, if one can feel sensations *in the rubber hand*, it must be because the rubber hand has been integrated into the body map. What is interesting here is that the body map has adjusted to incorporate a rubber hand that was only *seen*, and only for a couple of minutes. Other studies have found that the visual distortion of the size of body parts can affect tactile experiences. For instance, if you are touched on two spots on your finger after observing the image of a smaller version of your hand, you will experience the distance between the two tactile stimuli as relatively smaller (Taylor-Clarke et al., 2004). It is interesting to note that only vision can directly process size information (Longo and Haggard, 2010). Vision is thus needed to fill in the metric details of the body map.

More generally, vision offers more reliable information about spatial properties than touch and proprioception, and it often dominates them when in conflict. It is thus optimal to combine visual information with proprioceptive information to achieve the most accurate perceptual estimate of the bodily location (van Beers et al., 1999). This is well illustrated by prismatic adaptation (Welch and Warren,

1980). When participants wear prismatic goggles that displace the visual field laterally by a fixed amount (typically, 10–15°), the visual system carries information about the location of their hand that is incongruent with somatosensory information. After a while, the visual deviation affects not only where the participants see and judge their hand to be, but also where they feel their hand to be: the hand is usually localized closer to the visually perceived position than to the position perceived proprioceptively. The involvement of visual information in bodily experiences is not restricted to cases in which one is actually seeing one's body. It persists even after one can no longer see one's body and even after one has moved. For instance, in the Rubber Hand Illusion, we have seen that participants mislocalize their hand towards the rubber hand. Interestingly, they have no current visual experience of either hand when they are asked to make the report. Yet their bodily experience is determined by the *visual memory* of the location of the rubber hand. It has also been found that bodily experiences can result from the integration of current proprioceptive information and *visual prediction* of the hand location (Smeets et al., 2006). When moving in the dark, participants still used the visual estimate of their hand location, which was updated on the basis of their intention to move. It was only after several movements that participants relied less on their visual estimate because each movement of the unseen hand added uncertainty to their visual estimate. The results thus show that when one moves one's hand, one anticipates the sensory consequences of one's movements, including the expected visual location of the hand. Furthermore, they show that the bodily experience, which represents the location of the hand, can be updated on the basis of visual expectation, even when one is in the dark.

According to the multimodality thesis that I defend, those effects reveal the constitutive multimodal nature of bodily awareness. In a nutshell, bodily experiences evolved to reliably track bodily states. Their function is to afford a veridical rendering of bodily properties (O'Shaughnessy, 1980). It is fulfilled if and only if bodily experiences are reliably correlated with bodily states that they are designed to indicate. Vision is then necessary to the veridical rendering of bodily properties because of the limits of the body senses and because of the spatial 'expertise' of vision. As claimed by Stein and Meredith (1993: 6), "the sensory modalities have evolved to work in concert". The same can be said of vision and body senses. Their interaction improves the likelihood of detecting, localizing, and identifying bodily events and properties. It is thus beneficial to combine different sources of information to achieve the best perceptual judgements. In other words, the more information, the better. Consequently, vision has been selected by evolutionary pressure because it is required by the very nature of bodily experiences. The contribution of vision to bodily experiences is not a mere causal accident.

One may reply that bodily awareness in blind people shows that vision is *not* necessary to bodily awareness. But the fact is that blind individuals have bodily experiences of a different type than sighted individuals. There are fundamental differences between bodily experiences in those who see and in those who have never seen. First, blind individuals are not sensitive to the same bodily illusions, and in particular they are not sensitive to the non-visual version of the Rubber Hand Illusion (Petkova et al., 2012). Second, the metrics of their body map is impaired (Kinsbourne and Lempert, 1980). For instance, Helders (1986) reported that their torso appears to blind individuals long and very narrow with disproportionately big arms and hands. Third, even when asked to localize their body parts and their tactile sensations with their eyes closed, the performance of sighted subjects differs from that of blind subjects (Jones, 1972). There are two reasons for this. On the one hand, even in the absence of visual information, sighted individuals do not rely as much as they could on somatosensory information because their processing of bodily information has been shaped by the almost constant involvement of visual information. On the other hand, blind individuals compensate for the lack of vision by dedicating more resources to somatosensory processing, as revealed by large-scale cortical reorganization (for a review, see Merabet and Pascual-Leone, 2010). Fourth, congenitally blind individuals do not exploit the same spatial frames of reference. Close your eyes and cross your hands over your body midline. If your left hand is briefly touched, and then your right hand, you take longer and are less accurate in judging which hand was touched first than if your hands are uncrossed (Yamamoto and Kitazawa, 2001). This effect has been observed both in sighted adults who have their eyes closed and in non-congenitally blind adults. The effect can be explained by the conflict between two spatial frames of bodily experiences: the frame of the body (left hand) and the egocentric frame (on the right). But it is reduced when sighted adults cross their hands in a space that is not visually accessible like behind their back (Kobor et al., 2006). And it is absent in sighted young children and in congenitally blind adults (Röder et al., 2004; Pagel et al., 2009). This reveals that in their case there is no conflict between the two spatial frames. This is not to say that congenitally blind individuals and young children have no external reference frame in general. It only shows that in their case, tactile information is not automatically remapped into the frame in eye-centred coordinates because of the lack of visual experiences at crucial stages in development (Pagel et al., 2009).

To recapitulate, whether or not one is currently seeing one's body, vision plays an essential role in delineating the boundaries of the body, in locating our body parts in space, and in bridging the gap between what happens on the skin and what happens in the external world. Without vision, bodily experiences cannot fulfil their function to the same extent and in the same way. Now the question is how the multimodality thesis can account for vicarious touch.

13.5 A continuum

Vicarious touch is not radically different from touch. Both are influenced by vision. I will now argue that the involvement of vision in bodily experiences opens the door to the influence of other people. More precisely, there are two ways in which what happens on other people's bodies can invade us, so to speak. First, vicarious touch can find its origin in erroneous parsing of the relevant information to bind together in tactile experiences. Second, vicarious touch can find its origin in body representations shared between self and others.

Let me consider the parsing hypothesis first. Multimodal integration is of use only when the signals carry information about a particular property of the same object or event. In particular, visuo-tactile integration requires selecting the information that comes from one's body, and segregating that information from the information that concerns other bodies. This mechanism is reliable most of the time, but is not infallible, as shown by the Rubber Hand Illusion. This illusion results from the integration of visual information about the rubber hand with tactile and proprioceptive information. But this integration should not have occurred since the visual information was not about the same object as the object of somatosensory information, namely the participants' hands. We still know very little about the parsing mechanism that selects the relevant information for integration (for more details, see de Vignemont, 2014b). As noted by Shams (2012), this is a "difficult problem" for the perceptual system:

> The problem of whether to combine two signals involves an (implicit or explicit) inference about whether the two signals are caused by the same object or by different objects, i.e., causal inference. This is not a trivial problem.... The different senses have different precisions in all dimensions, including the temporal and spatial dimensions, and even if the two signals are derived from the same object/event, the noise in the environment and in the nervous system makes the sensory signals somewhat inconsistent with each other most of the time. Therefore, the nervous system needs to use as much information as possible to solve this difficult problem.

One hypothesis is then that vicarious touch is the consequence of the failure of the parsing mechanism. In a nutshell, what happens on someone else's body is taken to be relevant for visuo-tactile integration. In other words, vicarious touch results from a false-positive error. One may further suggest that in MTS, there are more false positives due to a parsing mechanism that is less reliable than in normal individuals. This hypothesis is compatible with Banissy and Ward's (2013) view that individuals with MTS have some abnormal self-other processing. What I suggest here is that those abnormalities interfere at the level of the parsing mechanism.

There is, however, a second possible explanation of vicarious touch, which does not assume the failure of the parsing process. Rather, it interprets vicarious touch as the collateral effect of a well-functioning process. A classic problem in the imitation literature is known as the correspondence problem: how does one map another person's movements to one's own movements (Goldenberg, 1995; Heyes, 2001)? The classic way to approach the correspondence problem has been in sensorimotor terms: how does one map visual information to motor commands (e.g., Brass and Heyes, 2005)? However, one may also conceive the correspondence problem in bodily terms: how does one map the movement of another body onto one's body?

Goldenberg (1995) defends an embodied approach to imitation, according to which one uses knowledge about the body to decode the other's movement and copy it. The special role of body representation in imitation is especially salient for some specific types of actions. This is the case, for instance, when one imitates meaningless gestures. Upon seeing a military salute, one can recognize it as such and use a stored motor schema of the salute to replicate it. But when one sees a person putting her thumb above her eyebrow, the only solution is to encode the movement in terms of the body parts that are seen and their spatial relations. To respect bodily congruency, one needs to exploit an interpersonal representation of the body, which indifferently represents one's body and other people's bodies. Arguably, the existence of shared body representations is not limited to the motor system, and can also be found in the sensory domain (for a review, see de Vignemont, 2014c). For instance, it is well known that viewing the body part that is touched (without viewing the touching object) enhances tactile acuity. Importantly, the effect of visual enhancement of touch is as effective when seeing one's own body part as when seeing another person's body part (Haggard, 2006). Likewise, Thomas et al. (2006) found that participants were faster in detecting touch when they saw a non-predictive visual cue on another person's body at the corresponding location. The authors concluded:

> We believe that our results provide the first behavioural evidence in normal subjects for interpersonal body representation based on a somatotopic spatial map, at the purely sensory level. (Thomas et al., 2006: 328)

Hence, vicarious touch is not the only phenomenon in which visual information about other people's bodies influences tactile experiences. This can be explained by the fact that vision of other people participates in shaping the body map that structures tactile sensation. For example, Price (2006) suggested that phantom limbs in aplastic patients with congenital limb deficiency could be explained by the fact that they constantly see other bodies with two arms and two legs. This enables them to generate a body template, which supplements their own body map. One may also conceive that visual information about other people's bodies may supplement the representation of the configuration of our own body for body parts that are not directly visually available, like the back.

It thus seems that bodily experiences, including tactile experiences, are partly based on visual information that is primarily about one's body, but that can also be about other bodies. It is then no surprise that one can experience vicarious touch.

To conclude, vicarious touch is often considered on a par with other phenomena such as action mirroring and empathy for pain within the general framework on embodied social cognition, but it is actually an oddball. Whereas action mirroring plays a role in imitation and empathy for pain in our understanding other people and in our helping them, it is not clear what role vicarious touch can play. Tactile mindreading is already of little interest but tactile mindreading via tactile sharing is even more puzzling. Why add the extra cost of imagining tactile sensations felt by others when one has all the information on the basis of visual analysis? Vicarious touch is just a case of contagion. More precisely, I have argued that vicarious touch is a collateral effect of the fundamental multimodal nature of bodily experiences. Any tactile experience is grounded in vision. Visual information is normally about one's body, but not always. Hence, vision of other people's bodies can interfere with touch. On this view, MTS is thus a case of both intermodal confusion and intersubjective confusion. These confusions are merely taking more extreme forms in MTS than in the normal population.

References

Banissy MJ, Cohen Kadosh R, Maus GW, Walsh V, Ward J. (2009). Prevalence, characteristics and a neurocognitive model of mirror-touch synaesthesia. *Exp Brain Res.* 198(2–3): 261–72.

Banissy MJ, Garrido L, Kusnir F, Duchaine B, Walsh V, Ward J. (2011). Superior facial expression, but not identity recognition, in mirror-touch synesthesia. *J Neurosci.* 31(5): 1820–4.

Banissy MJ, Ward J. (2007). Mirror-touch synesthesia is linked with empathy. *Nat Neurosci.* 10 (7): 815–16.

Banissy MJ, Ward J. (2013). Mechanisms of self-other representations and vicarious experiences of touch in mirror-touch synesthesia. *Front Hum Neurosci.* 7: 112.

Blakemore S-J, Bristow D, Bird G, Frith C, Ward J. (2005). Somatosensory activations during the observation of touch and a case of vision-touch synaesthesia. *Brain* 128: 1571–83.

Bonnier P. (1905). L'Aschématie. *Revue Neurologique* (Paris) 13: 605–9.

Botvinick, M, Cohen, J. (1998). Rubber hands 'feel' touch that eyes see. *Nature* 391: 756.

Brass M, Heyes, C. (2005). Imitation: Is cognitive neuroscience solving the correspondence problem? *Trends in Cognitive Sciences* 9: 489–95.

Driver J, Spence, C. (2000). Multisensory perception: Beyond modularity and convergence. *Curr Biol.* 10(20): R731–5.

Durgin FH, Evans L, Dunphy N, Klostermann S, Simmons K. (2007). Rubber hands feel the touch of light. *Psychol Sci.* 18(2): 152–7.

Ebisch SJ, Perrucci MG, Ferretti A, Del Gratta C, Romani GL, Gallese V. (2008). The sense of touch: Embodied simulation in a visuotactile mirroring mechanism for observed animate or inanimate touch. *J Cogn Neurosci.* 20(9): 1611–23.

Ehrsson HH, Wiech K, Weiskopf N, Dolan RJ, Passingham RE. (2007). Threatening a rubber hand that you feel is yours elicits a cortical anxiety response. *Proceedings of the National Academy of Sciences of the United States of America* 104(23): 9828–33.

Gallese V (2007). Embodied simulation: from mirror neuron systems to interpersonal relations. *Novartis Found Symp* 278: 3–12.

Gallese V, Sinigaglia C. (2011). What is so special about embodied simulation? *Trends Cogn Sci.* 15(11): 512–19.

Goldenberg G. (1995). Imitating gestures and manipulating a mannikin—the representation of the human body in ideomotor apraxia. *Neuropsychologia* 33(1): 63–72.

Goldman AI. (2006). *Simulating minds.* Oxford: Oxford University Press.

Goldman AI. (2011). Two routes to empathy: Insights from cognitive neuroscience. In A. Coplan and P. Goldie (eds.), *Empathy: Philosophical and Psychological Perspectives*, 31–44. Oxford: Oxford University Press.

Goldman AI and de Vignemont F. (2009). Is social cognition embodied? *Trends in Cognitive Sciences* 13(4): 154–9.

Haggard P. (2006). Just seeing you makes me feel better: Interpersonal enhancement of touch. *Soc Neurosci.* 1(2): 104–10.

Head H, Holmes G. (1911). Sensory disturbances from cerebral lesions. *Brain* 34: 102–254.

Helders PJM. (1986). Early motor signs of blindness or very low vision in very young children. *Early Intervention* 359–65.

Heyes C. (2001). Causes and consequences of imitation. *Trends Cogn Sci.* 5(6): 253–61.

Holle H, Banissy M, Wright T, Bowling N, Ward J. (2011). "That's not a real body": Identifying stimulus qualities that modulate synaesthetic experiences of touch. *Conscious Cogn.* 20(3): 720–6.

Jacob P, de Vignemont F. (2017). Vicarious pain: Imagination, mirroring or perception? In J. Kiverstein (ed), *Routledge handbook of social mind.* London: Routledge, 498–514.

Jones B. (1972). Development of Cutaneous and kinesthetic localization by blind and sighted children. *Developmental Psychology* 6(2): 349–52.

Keysers C, Kaas JH, Gazzola V. (2010). Somatosensation in social perception. *Nat Rev Neurosci.* 11(6): 417–28.

Keysers C, Wicker B, Gazzola V, Anton JL, Fogassi L, Gallese V. (2004). A touching sight: SII/PV Activation during the observation and experience of touch. *Neuron* 42: 335–46.

Kinsbourne M, Lempert H. (1980). Human figure representation by blind children. *J Gen Psychol.* 102: 33–7.

Kóbor I, Füredi L, Kovács G, Spence C, Vidnyánszky Z. (2006). Back-to-front: Improved tactile discrimination performance in the space you cannot see. *Neurosci Lett.* 400(1–2): 163–7.

Longo MR, Haggard P. (2010). An implicit body representation underlying human position sense. *Proc Natl Acad Sci USA* 107(26): 11727–32.

Macpherson F. (2007). Synaesthesia, functionalism and phenomenology. In De Caro M, Ferretti F, Marraffa M. (eds.) *Cartographies of the mind: Philosophy and psychology in intersection.* Series: Studies in Brain and Mind, 4.

Maister L, Banissy MJ, Tsakiris M. (2013). Mirror-touch synaesthesia changes representations of self-identity. *Neuropsychologia* 51(5): 802–8.

Merabet LB, Pascual-Leone A. (2010). Neural reorganization following sensory loss: The opportunity of change. *Nat Rev Neurosci.* 11(1): 44–52.

O'Shaughnessy B. (1980). *The Will.* Vol. 1. Cambridge: Cambridge University Press.

Pagel B, Heed T, Röder B. (2009). Change of reference frame for tactile localization during child development. *Dev Sci.* 12(6): 929–37.

Petkova VI, Zetterberg H, Ehrsson HH. (2012). Rubber hands feel touch, but not in blind individuals. *PLoS ONE* 7(4): e35912.

Price EH. (2006). A critical review of congenital phantom limb cases and a developmental theory for the basis of body image. *Conscious Cogn.* 15(2): 310–22.

Röder B, Rösler F, Spence C. (2004). Early vision impairs tactile perception in the blind. *Curr Biol.* 14(2): 121–4.

Schilder P. (1935). *The image and appearance of the human body*. New York: International Universities Press.

Shams L. (2012). Early integration and Bayesian causal inference in multisensory perception. In Murray MM, Wallace M (eds). *The neural bases of multisensory processes*. Boca Raton, FL: CRC Press.

Simner J, Mulvenna C, Sagiv N, Tsakanikos E, Witherby SA, Fraser C, Scott K, Ward J. (2006). Synaesthesia: The prevalence of atypical cross-modal experiences. *Perception* 35(8): 1024–33.

Smeets JB, van den Dobbelsteen JJ, de Grave DD, van Beers RJ, Brenner E. (2006). Sensory integration does not lead to sensory calibration. *Proc Natl Acad Sci USA* 103(49): 18781–6.

Stein BE, Meredith MA. (1993). *The merging of the senses*. Cambridge, MA: MIT Press.

Taylor-Clarke M, Jacobsen P, Haggard P. (2004). Keeping the world a constant size: Object constancy in human touch. *Nat Neurosci*. 7(3): 219–20.

Thomas R, Press C, Haggard P. (2006). Shared representations in body perception. *Acta Psychol (Amst)*. 121(3): 317–30.

Tsakiris M. (2008). Looking for myself: Current multisensory input alters self-face recognition. *PLoS One* 3(12): e4040.

Tsakiris M, Haggard P. (2005). The rubber hand illusion revisited: Visuotactile integration and self-attribution. *J Exp Psychol Hum Percept Perform* 31(1): 80–91.

van Beers RJ, Sittig AC, Denier van der Gon JJ. (1999). Integration of proprioceptive and visual position information: An experimentally supported model. *J Neurophysiol*. 81(3): 1355–64.

de Vignemont F. (2014a). A multimodal conception of bodily awareness. *Mind* 123: 492.

de Vignemont F. (2014b). Multimodal unity and multimodal binding. In *Sensory integration and the unity of consciousness*, edited by C. Hill and D. Bennett. Cambridge, MA: MIT Press.

de Vignemont F. (2014c). Shared body representations and the "Whose" system. *Neuropsychologia* 55: 128–36.

de Vignemont F, Jacob P. (2012). What it's like to feel another's pain. *Philosophy of Science* 79 (2): 295–316.

Welch RB, Warren DH. (1980). Immediate perceptual response to intersensory discrepancy. *Psychological Bulletin* 88: 638–67.

Wood R, Gallese V, Cattaneo L. (2010). Visuotactile empathy within the primary somatosensory cortex revealed by short-latency afferent inhibition. *Neurosci Lett*. 473(1): 28–31.

Yamamoto S, Kitazawa S. (2001). Reversal of subjective temporal order due to arm crossing. *Nat Neurosci*. 4(7): 759–65.

14

Personification, Synaesthesia, and Social Cognition

Noam Sagiv,[1] Monika Sobczak-Edmans, and Adrian L. Williams

Synaesthesia is traditionally defined as a condition in which stimulation in one sensory modality evokes an experience usually associated with other sensory modalities. Variations of this have often been cited by researchers throughout the literature (e.g., Marks, 1975; Baron-Cohen, Wyke, and Binnie, 1987; Cytowic, 1989; Paulesu et al., 1995; Martino and Marks, 2001; Mattingley, Rich, Yelland, and Bradshaw, 2001; Hubbard and Ramachandran, 2005; Sagiv and Ward, 2006; Jäncke and Langer, 2011). Considerable efforts have been made to demonstrate the perceptual reality of synaesthesia (e.g., Hubbard and Ramachandran, 2001; Smilek et al., 2001, Palmeri et al., 2002); i.e., to show that synaesthesia is a genuine perceptual phenomenon (rather than merely reflecting metaphorical speech or plain confabulation) with verifiable behavioural consequences (e.g., impacting visual search times, detection rates, and grouping).[2] This was deemed to serve as stronger evidence for the genuineness of synaesthesia compared with mere consistency of the reported synaesthetic correspondences (which, in principle, could be faked with superior memory and practice, however unlikely it is that someone would go through with such a scam). However, over the years, synaesthesia researchers have noticed that individuals with synaesthesia report additional experiences in which either the inducer or the concurrent experience is not necessarily a vivid perceptual experience; including, for example, number forms (in which number concepts cue specific spatial location with or without the visualization of a number line; e.g., Sagiv et al., 2006) or grapheme personification (a phenomenon in which letters and numbers are personified and endowed with gender, personalities, and other mental or biographical attributes;

[1] Address for correspondence: Noam Sagiv, Psychology Division, Department of Life Sciences, Brunel University, Uxbridge UB8 3PH, United Kingdom. E-mail: noam.sagiv@brunel.ac.uk.

[2] We use the term perceptual reality here as it was used in the psychological literature of the time. It should not be confused with the questions of perceptual presence or insight into whether the experience is shared by others.

e.g., Amin et al., 2001). Although in both cases it was suggested that the phenomena share much in common with synaesthesia and there may be a case for considering them to be types of synaesthesia in their own right, the status of such phenomena remains somewhat controversial.

It seems, however, that accepted wisdom about synaesthesia is gradually changing. The term is now used to refer to an ever growing number of phenomena—a trend that worries some scientists and scholars (e.g., Deroy and Spence, 2013; Rothen and Meier, 2013). Indeed, it has proved easier to discuss what certain specific phenomena share with canonical forms of synaesthesia than to provide a more inclusive definition that is not so liberal as to include any phenomenon involving two cognitive or perceptual domains. The first signs of change probably emerged when it became clear that one of the most studied and least controversial types of synaesthesia does not neatly fall within the limits of the traditional definition.

14.1 Relaxing the boundaries of synaesthesia: the curious case of coloured graphemes

Before we consider personification in synaesthesia, it may be instructive to examine the case of coloured graphemes. Even though it is now commonly given as an example of synaesthesia, it may come as a surprise to some readers that this is a relatively recent development. Shanon's (1982) study illustrates this well; in his paper titled 'Colour associates to semantic linear orders', he refrains from using the term synaesthesia to describe the phenomenon of coloured numbers and coloured weekdays. Furthermore, he states clearly that the phenomenon is distinct from synaesthesia where the perceptual experience is cross-modal. Instead, it seems to be the concept (say 7, or Tuesday) that elicits a colour experience rather than stimulation in any particular modality. This view of synaesthesia is indeed in line with typical dictionary definitions of synaesthesia that tend to emphasize the cross-modal nature of the experience.[3]

A decade later, Baron-Cohen, Harrison, Goldstein, and Wyke (1993) found that the associations reported by all nine cases of coloured hearing synaesthesia who took part in their study are in fact determined by the constituent graphemes of the colour-inducing word. These cases have been assumed to be variants of synaesthesia—a view that was adopted unchallenged in the years to follow. This

[3] For example, the Oxford English Dictionary defines synaesthesia as "Production, from a sense-impression of one kind, of an associated mental image of a sense-impression of another kind" (meaning 1c; www.oed.com), while the Merriam-Webster Dictionary defines it as "a concomitant sensation and especially a subjective sensation or image of a sense (as of color) other than the one (as of sound) being stimulated; also: the condition marked by the experience of such sensations" (http://www.merriam-webster.com). We should point out that the Oxford English Dictionary also endorses the term to describe a somatosensory experience in a different part of the body than the one stimulated (meaning 1a).

can be justified on the grounds that these individuals can *see* colours induced by words they *hear*, thereby fulfilling the conditions set in traditional definitions of synaesthesia (even if the same colours may also be induced by visual presentation of the graphemes/words).[4]

Coloured-grapheme synaesthesia soon became the focus of much of synaesthesia research in psychology, at which point most studies presented the inducing stimuli visually. Some researchers have not worried much about the fact that the inducer (grapheme shapes) and the concurrent (colours) belonged to the same sensory modality. Indeed, there is some degree of functional segregation in the processing of colour and shape (e.g., Zeki, 2003, but cf Gegenfurtner and Kiper, 2003). If one were to consider these to be different senses, then coloured graphemes could still be captured by the old definitions.[5] However, a number of authors felt it necessary to acknowledge that synaesthetic experiences may occur in the *same* modality as the inducer (e.g., Sagiv, 2005; Weiss, Zilles, and Fink, 2005; Sagiv and Ward, 2006).[6] However, more was to follow.

Simner (2007) emphasized the conceptual and linguistic nature of some common inducers, and urged us to think of synaesthesia as a psycholinguistic phenomenon as much as it is a perceptual one. Indeed, reflecting on the synaesthesia literature, Macpherson (2007) concluded that synaesthetic inducers may be sensory experiences, non-sensory experiences, or even mental images.

However, Hubbard (2007) may have offered the most radical reconceptualization of synaesthesia, declaring that it is "an experience in which stimulation in one sensory or cognitive stream leads to associated experiences in a second, unstimulated stream". By allowing that both inducers and concurrents may not be strictly sensory in nature, he opened the door for admission into the synaesthesia club of both spatial number forms and grapheme personification, and perhaps a whole host of phenomena that we do not currently consider to be synaesthesia variants (e.g., associative memory recall). Interestingly, it also allows for motoric concurrents, e.g., Devereux's unusual case of audio motor-synaesthesia (1966) and perhaps more mundane spontaneous movement to music. Since we will focus on personification in synaesthesia in much of the remainder of this chapter, the reader may expect by now that we will proceed to justify the inclusion of personification in the synaesthetic canon. However, we would first like to consider whether a precise synaesthesia definition is necessary or even possible.

[4] The key distinction between the mode of presentation of the inducer and the level of processing at which the colour correspondences are determined received little attention, with few exceptions (e.g., Ward and Sagiv, 2007; Ward, Li, Salih, and Sagiv, 2007).

[5] Clearly, debating any definition of synaesthesia will be informed by discussion on what counts as a sensory modality or how many senses we have.

[6] Note that such a definition also captures phenomena such as Mitempfindung (Burrack, Knoch, and Brugger, 2006) in which tactile stimulation in one location is also perceived in an additional one.

14.2 Definitions and their limitations

As the discussions on defining synaesthesia continue (Simner, 2012; Cohen Kadosh and Terhune, 2012; Eagleman, 2012), we have become increasingly convinced that the additional phenomena commonly reported by synaesthetes could provide us with valuable clues to cognitive mechanisms and brain function, whether or not one chooses to classify those as types of synaesthesia.

Definitions and labels can be valuable for facilitating effective communication and dissemination of knowledge, but there are several reasons not to be deterred from studying phenomena that do not neatly fall within the scope of a current definition. First, definitions are not set in stone. They always reflect our current understanding and evolve with our theories on the subject matter. When systems of classifications are introduced, reclassification may occur. This is not unique to psychology and examples can be found in zoology, botany, and astronomy, to name a few. For example, Pluto lost its planet status in 2006, nearly a century after its discovery (Schilling, 2006). The decision to demote Pluto was based on a vote on proposed alternatives to defining a planet brought before a few hundred astronomers. We may need to measure the size, shape, and orbit of candidate objects to establish whether they meet the agreed criteria for planets, but there is no set of observations that unequivocally determines what the threshold should be between planets, minor planets, and rocks. Admittedly, planet/rock sizes and orbits lie on a continuum (and might therefore be a matter of convention) while it is not clear that synaesthesia and related phenomena do too. However, presenting a precise set of criteria for any type of synaesthesia may involve at least some thresholds of certain continuous parameters: How reliably must synaesthetic colours be evoked? Is it sufficient if the experiences are reported, say, 62.8 per cent of the time? Similarly, one may set certain requirements with respect to the vividness rating of concurrent experience, or consistency measures.

We should therefore remember that even if we do manage to agree on a set of diagnostic criteria, such criteria are, in many cases, constructs of the human mind designed to help us think about problems and build on existing knowledge without having to start from scratch every time. They should not be regarded as tools for limiting the scope of research endeavours.[7]

A more fundamental challenge for defining synaesthesia on the basis of phenomenological and behavioural features is the possibility that different types of synaesthesia may have sets of features with partly overlapping distributions. If this is the case, then we cannot establish precise criteria because individual features may not be

[7] Cf the statements recently made by the National Institute of Mental Health (NIMH) Director, Thomas Insel, ahead of the publication of the latest edition of the Diagnostic and Statistical Manual of Mental Disorders (DSM-5) (NIMH Director's Blog published on 29 April 2013; http://www.nimh.nih.gov/about/director/2013/transforming-diagnosis.shtml).

present in some synaesthesia variants.[8] For example, synaesthesia is usually thought to involve an idiosyncratic perceptual experience, elicited in a consistent manner even after long periods of time; however, we seem to have exceptions to each rule/feature (e.g., mirror-touch synaesthesia may lack the feature of idiosyncrasy because the concurrents are rather predictable; grapheme personification may lack a distinct perceptual experience; and, for all we know, drug-induced coloured music synaesthesia may turn out to be less consistent than the naturally occurring variety of the same phenomenon, but we may still consider it a form of synaesthesia).

A related issue concerns the possibility that we are dealing with several clusters of phenomena rather than a single phenomenon. Novich, Cheng, and Eagleman (2011) looked at how different types of synaesthesia cluster in 19,133 individuals who have completed their Synaesthesia Battery (Eagleman, Kagan, Nelson, Sagaram, and Sarma, 2007). On the basis of the prevalence data of the various types they documented, they identified five clusters and suggested that types of synaesthesia in different clusters may have distinct mechanisms and possibly different genetic bases.

We must therefore recognize the heterogeneity in synaesthesia (Eagleman, 2012). The process of defining synaesthesia may be subject to the same difficulties we face when attempting to define less desirable conditions and diseases. As Lynall and Blakemore (2013) put it: "like schizophrenia and dementia, convenient terminology and minimal definition might hide a variety of conditions, with different aetiologies and manifestations". Indeed, scientists are trying to understand and distinguish between the various aetiologies. However, a rush to classify and label phenomena has the disadvantage of creating layers of overlapping and sometimes conflicting and misguided terminologies that impede progress rather than simplify scientific discussion.

While we agree that it is a good exercise to reflect on the nomenclature of one's field of study and ponder definitions, we suspect the boundaries between synaesthesia and several other phenomena cannot be as sharp as some researchers want them to be. We therefore propose to set the question of a definition aside for a while and consider the case of personification—itself a complex set of phenomena that, to different degrees, share some features with synaesthesia.

14.3 Different types of personification in synaesthesia

We first encountered personification in synaesthesia when one of our synaesthetes incidentally commented that besides colours he also associates gender and personality with the letters of the alphabet. He noted that these are stable properties of letters (as were his colours), and he was unable to indicate how exactly he came to know what these personal characteristics were. He just did. It soon became clear that

[8] This is reminiscent of the problems we encounter in categorizing objects or experiences more generally (for a discussion see Marks, Chapter 1 of this volume).

this is not uncommon among coloured-grapheme synaesthetes, although we did not formally study these reports until a few years later (Amin et al., 2011), despite initial warnings from some colleagues that this was too 'weird'. It also turned out that both Flournoy (1893) and Calkins (1893) described the phenomenon over a century before we learned about its existence, and before a few more recent anecdotal reports (e.g., Cytowic, 2002; Day, 2005).

As in synaesthesia, these personal characteristics were elicited by graphemes and other ordinal sequences (numbers, weekdays, months); they seemed to be automatically elicited, rather than the product of an intentional effort; the correspondences reported were most certainly idiosyncratic (admittedly, they often raise some eyebrows); and it was synaesthetes' impression that these properties of letters were relatively stable. In essence, this seemed to *resemble* synaesthesia in many ways, with one notable exception: No vivid perceptual experience is elicited here.[9] Synaesthetes become aware of these person-like properties of letters although they typically do not form a vivid visual mental image that they can inspect and describe. In other words, the concurrent experience seems to belong to the realm of social cognition rather than perception. Of course, we use visual, auditory, and sometime tactile inputs in everyday life to read other people's moods, attitudes, and intentions, but the end result of this process is that we attribute mental states and personal characteristics to the people we interact with. At first glance, it appears that synaesthetes somehow generate such characteristics without their usual stimulus and attribute them to concepts like graphemes and time units.

Simner and Holenstein (2007) offered the label "ordinal linguistic personification" (OLP) to describe the condition, later revising it to "sequence-personality synaesthesia" (Simner, Gartner, and Taylor, 2011). However, it has since transpired that personification in synaesthetes is not limited to sequences. For example, Smilek et al. (2007) described a case of a synaesthete who personified inanimate objects. The phenomenon bears some resemblance to grapheme personification in the sense that person-like characteristics are automatically and reliably attributed, but the inducers are common objects.[10] In that sense, it is admittedly removed one step further from canonical forms of synaesthesia since common objects are not so common as inducers. Nevertheless, we

[9] Note that we studied grapheme personification in individuals with coloured-grapheme synaesthesia as a matter of convenience (up to a third of the latter group also report the former). It could be said that in these individuals there was, at least, a vivid experience of colour. However, coloured-grapheme synaesthesia can exist without grapheme personification and vice versa (Simner and Holenstein, 2007). Hence we treat them here as distinct phenomena. In and of itself, grapheme personification does not appear to involve any vivid perceptual experience, but merely knowing what gender, mood, or personality are associated with a certain grapheme. Nevertheless, an associated affective component is not uncommon (Dael, Sierro, and Mohr, 2013); for example, liking or disliking certain letters (Simner and Holenstein, 2007; Amin et al., 2011).

[10] Object personification is common in individuals who personify graphemes (Amin et al., 2011); however, it also occurs in the general population without synaesthesia or grapheme personification. Thus it need not depend on other forms of personification.

have extended our investigations to this phenomenon to examine what it shares with grapheme personification. We advise against introducing additional labels to try to capture all instances of personification and we will not attempt further categorization at this point.

14.4 Empirical studies of grapheme personification

In our survey of 248 coloured-grapheme synaesthesia cases, 33 per cent also reported grapheme personification (Amin et al., 2011). As the prevalence of coloured-grapheme synaesthesia is thought to be 1.4 per cent (Simner et al., 2006), rising to 4.4 per cent if other types are included (notably, the more common coloured weekdays), this makes grapheme personification a relatively common phenomenon with a minimum prevalence of 0.5 per cent. Simner and Holenstein's (2007) survey (which included both synaesthetes and non-synaesthetes) resulted in a more generous estimate of 1.4 per cent. However, these estimates were obtained in English-speaking populations. Chun and Hupé (2013) found that nearly 12 per cent of the French-speaking population they surveyed reported personifying graphemes—an order of magnitude more common than in the English-speaking population. In line with our suggestion that there may be a link between grapheme personification and grammatical gender (Amin et al., 2011, Sobczak-Edmans and Sagiv, 2013), they attribute the gap between the English and French-speaking populations to grammatical gender (absent in English and prominent in French). It remains to be seen whether this will generalize to other populations and be validated.

As thirty-four individuals who personify graphemes filled out our questionnaire, we were able to describe the characteristics of the phenomenon in detail. They noted the genders and personalities they associated with graphemes; these were later used to assess the stability of these associations. The descriptions can be rather detailed and included not only personality and cognitive attributes like "likes to be at the centre of a crowd" and "very smart", but also moods, attitudes, interests, and even information on their social role and social life, such as "has lots of friends" or "P and Q hang out together quite often". Not all synaesthetes vividly visualize the graphemes as little figures, but some certainly comment on their appearance (cf, Luria, 1969: 31; Shereshevskii comments on seeing the number 87 as a "fat woman" next to "a man twirling his moustache").

Most participants personified both letters and numbers, and most attributed both gender and personality (although some synaesthete personified only a sub-set of graphemes). Interestingly, when one of our participants who only attributed gender to letters was asked to comment on the fact that unlike other synaesthetes, she does not attribute personalities as well, she commented: "well—I don't know them well enough". This anecdotal comment is interesting because it suggests that the process by which graphemes acquire their personalities is not the product of a deliberate mnemonic technique, but rather something that needs to be found out.

While we found synaesthetes to be generally consistent in their personality attributes, and more so than a control group, consistency was not as high as that for grapheme colours. This can partly be attributed to the different methodologies of assessing colour and personality consistency, and partly to the phenomenology of grapheme personification (Amin et al., 2011); some synaesthetes commented that graphemes' moods, for example, vary with their own.

The reliability and automaticity of gender and personality attributes can be tested using behavioural congruity paradigms often used in synaesthesia research (typically Stroop-like interference, or priming paradigms). For example, we measured reaction times to judgements of genders of target cartoon faces, which were preceded by irrelevant letter primes. Synaesthetes who personify graphemes were, as predicted, faster in determining that a face is male when primed with a letter that they personify as male, rather than female, and vice versa (Amin et al., 2011). A control group performing the same set of tasks did not show this effect; neither did a second group of control participants who were allowed to choose their own letter-gender pairing (rather then be assigned to one of the synaesthetes'; recall that these experiments are tailored to each synaesthete—their specific correspondences between letters and gender determine which trial is to be considered congruent or incongruent). Simner and Holenstein (2007) have shown, for example, that masculinity/femininity ratings of names are biased by the gender attributed to the first letter. Thus, grapheme gender influences both implicit and explicit measures. Furthermore, using Stroop tasks, Simner and Hubbard (2006) showed that grapheme gender and colour interact in synaesthesia. For example, colour Stroop slowdown of reaction times is limited to incongruent colours corresponding to other letters of the same gender.

The neural basis of grapheme personification was first assessed in a single case of a synaesthete who only attributes genders to half of the letters of the alphabet, but not personalities (Amin et al., 2011). We used a simple block-design fMRI study in which the synaesthete saw either a sequence of letters that she associates with gender or a sequence of letters without gender (while performing a letter repetition detection task; i.e., gender was task irrelevant). Comparing the two conditions revealed activation in the precuneus—an area in the medial parietal lobe associated with mental imagery and self-referential processing (e.g., Cavanna and Trimble, 2006). Interestingly, the precuneus lights up in other synaesthesia studies; although it is rarely in the limelight, it was recently suggested that activation in the precuneus may correlate with the intensity of synaesthetic experiences regardless of modality (Jones et al., 2011). We have now extended the study of the neural bases of grapheme personification to five additional synaesthetes (four of whom associate both gender and personality with graphemes; the fifth associates gender only). Since some of the synaesthetes personify most if not all the letters of the alphabet, we have had to modify the paradigm and contrast responses to letters of the Roman alphabet with responses to an unfamiliar alphabet (Hebrew) that they did not personify. Our preliminary results suggest that activations in this group (reporting richer grapheme personification) extend to the insula, precuneus, medial prefrontal cortex, and temporoparietal junction (Sobczak-Edmans, 2013; Sobczak-Edmans, Williams, and Sagiv, in preparation). These areas play a variety of roles in social cognition tasks. This activation of the social brain rather than the sensory cortices in synaesthetic personification suggests that personification could be considered a special class of synaesthesia-like phenomena, which we have tentatively labelled "social synaesthesia" (Amin et al., 2011, Sagiv, Sobczak, Ilbeigi, and Williams, 2012). We suspect that the synaesthesia purists will find this more palatable than admitting outright that grapheme personification should be regarded as a subtype of synaesthesia proper.

14.5 Empirical studies of inanimate object personification in synaesthesia

Though rare in non-synaesthete adults, we found inanimate object personification to be rather common among synaesthetes (Amin et al., 2011). Within the group of synaesthetes who personify graphemes and completed our survey, 82 per cent reported attributing *gender* and/or *personality* traits to objects (most frequently when it comes to fruits, vegetables, and computers). Seventy-one per cent attributed *feelings* to inanimate objects (with plants and household objects in the vanguard). The examples given by a number of synaesthetes suggested that the loneliness theme may be a relatively common inducement for considering the feelings of objects (e.g., feeling sorry for objects separated from their group for one reason or another). However, there were other examples, e.g. one synaesthete said after buying a new clothing item she first leaves it in the closet for a couple of weeks, so that it can get to know the others. Despite admitting to a number of eccentric habits resulting from personification, it generally did not impede everyday life (e.g., chopping previously personified vegetables to prepare a salad).

We used the prominence of the loneliness theme to create both a behavioural and a neuroimaging paradigm to assess the automaticity and neural mechanisms underlying inanimate object personification. Specifically, we created a stimulus set that includes images of a group of similar objects that are either uniformly distributed in space, or grouped together while excluding one object (see Figure 14.1). This sad social exclusion condition depicting a 'lonely object' was contrasted with the happier alternative object configuration. In the behavioural paradigm, these images were task-irrelevant primes presented before a target cartoon face. Synaesthetes were asked to judge the facial expression on the face. As we expected, whether objects were lonely (sad) or not (happier) primed our participants and modulated reaction times to happy/sad judgements of the target faces (Sobczak-Edmans, 2013). This is consistent with the claim that object personification is an automatic and rapid process, rather than a deliberate, active imagination/confabulation. In an earlier single case study Smilek et al. (2007) were able to verify the consistency of object

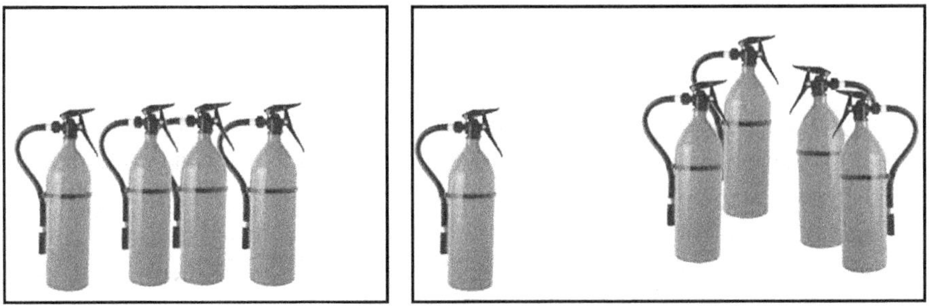

Figure 14.1. Stimuli used to induce object personification in synaesthetes. The right image resembles a social exclusion situation which typically causes those who regularly personify objects to pity the sad and lonely object. The left image represents the baseline condition.

personality associations reported by a synaesthete. They also showed that her eye movements were biased by the emotional associations she reported for graphemes (fewer but longer fixations on positive graphemes compared to negative graphemes in the synaesthete but not in a non-synaesthete matched control).

We recently piloted a simple fMRI paradigm based on the 'lonely object' paradigm on a synaesthete who reports personifying objects. Preliminary results indicate that personification of objects (presumed to be stronger in the lonely condition than in the baseline condition) activates a network of areas that partly overlaps with those found in our study of grapheme personification (including the precuneus and temporoparietal junction). We should point out that if some degree of personification is present in the baseline condition (in which the same objects are presented in a different configuration), then we may still be underestimating the extent to which considering the feelings of objects activates social brain networks in synaesthetes who personify. In sum, the evidence is mounting that object personification can be studied systematically in the lab, that it is automatically elicited and has predictable behavioural consequences, and that there is a neural basis suggestive of recruitment of a network of areas that ordinarily support social cognition.

14.6 Mechanisms of personification in synaesthesia and relationship to normal function

At present we do not know why some individuals are prone to personification and others are not. A related phenomenon—anthropomorphization of agents some of us interact with in everyday life (e.g., gadgets, pets, God)[11]—is stronger in lonelier

[11] The usage of personification and anthropomorphization in the literature overlaps to some extent. Here we are interested in the case of attributing mental states and/or personal characteristics (such as personality) where none exist. This is true for gods and gadgets. The case of pets is more problematic because they clearly do have a personality and a mind, even if less sophisticated. In this case, anthropomorphization manifests as attribution of higher-level mental states, assuming that they understand more than they do, etc.

individuals (Epley, Akalis, Waytz, and Cacioppo, 2008). Social isolation may be a contributing factor; however, given the similarities and strong association with other types of synaesthesia, it is likely that a genetic predisposition may be necessary.

Can grapheme personification be explained by individual differences in empathy? While this seemed like a plausible hypothesis that synaesthetic personification reflects a generally low threshold for considering the feelings of others, our data suggested that this was too simple (Amin et al., 2011): A sample of ten synaesthetes who were assessed using the Empathy Quotient (EQ; Baron-Cohen and Wheelwright, 2004) did not have a significantly higher average compared with the norm. What is more interesting is that two of the participants had extremely low scores (that should not normally be present in such a small sample). This suggested to us that it is possible to personify graphemes even with a low empathy score. We speculated that there may be two routes to personification; one may characterized by over-extension of mentalizing to objects; the other may be the outcome of difficulties in mentalizing resulting in an indiscriminate personification strategy (this could be the case if individuals use the wrong kind of cues for mentalizing, relying on, for example, lower-level physical features and ineffective heuristics).[12]

The cross-activation theory of synaesthesia (e.g., Hubbard, Brang, and Ramachandran, 2011), offered as a catch-all framework for explaining synaesthesia, could yield some testable predictions concerning the neural basis of personification. If synaesthesia is the result of cross-activation of sensory brain areas induced by the activation of sensory/language/number areas, then surely personification could be one of the outcomes we could expect if these were social brain areas that happened to cross-link with grapheme representations. Indeed, our preliminary findings suggest that personification is associated with activation within at least some areas implicated in social cognition.

While some progress has been made in understanding the neural basis of personification in synaesthesia, we have also proposed a more functional explanation of the emergence of grapheme and inanimate object personification, namely misattribution of self-referential processing (Sobczak-Edmans and Sagiv, 2013). We proposed that personification may be the result of an excessive manifestation of the tendency to perceive reality with the self as a model. The major clusters of activations we observed in our neuroimaging studies of both grapheme personification and object personification are consistent with this proposal, as many of the said areas—the insula, precuneus, posterior cingulate, and the inferior frontal cortex—have been implicated in self-referential processing. Further evidence for this comes from neuropsychology

[12] To illustrate the distinction between two hypothetical causes of personification, consider a signal detection theory analogy focused on discriminating animate from inanimate things: Personifying animate things would be a hit, failing to do so would be a miss, and personification of inanimate things is a false alarm. Two ways to increase the false alarm rates are (a) shift the criterion (lower the threshold) which is probably what most synaesthetes do; and (b) focus on poor discriminability which afflicts those with poor mentalizing skills.

and neuropsychiatry. Patients with parietal lesions sometimes exhibit personification of body parts. For example, somatoparaphrenia is the delusional misidentification of body parts—a subtype of asomatognosia which involves denial of limb ownership (Feinberg, Venneri, Simone, Fan, and Northoff, 2010); patients afflicted with the condition often attribute the limb to other people around them, and occasionally attribute to the limbs a name and personality traits (Critchley, 1955). Furthermore, some patients demonstrate misoplegia—hostility towards a limb they fail to recognize as their own (Loetscher, Regard, and Brugger, 2006); this seems to involve misattribution of agency. Personification may also occur in reduplicative misidentification syndromes (see Sobczak-Edmans and Sagiv, 2013). Incidentally, personification of body parts is not unheard of in the general population, particularly personification of the genitalia. However, it is unclear whether this reflects genuine personification or merely a strategy for diffusing the embarrassment associated with usage of the correct terminology (e.g., Cornog, 1986).

Nevertheless, there are additional examples of personification in the general population. First, it has been proposed that children tend to attribute consciousness to inanimate things (Piaget, 1929). Despite a long controversy citing immature language skills as a potential confound, it seems that genuine animistic thought is sometimes present (Smeets, 1973). Pretend play in early childhood may involve some forms of personification, e.g. while playing with dolls or interacting with imaginary friends (Taylor, Hulette, and Dishion, 2010). It seems, however, that there may be a regression to animistic thinking in old age and dementia (Zaitchik and Solomon, 2008).

While in modern society only a minority of well-adapted non-delusional adults spontaneously think about inanimate objects as if they had feelings, most of us do find object personification appealing in some restricted cases, e.g. in poetry, fiction, advertisement, and cartoons. Moreover, animistic thought is normative in some cultures (Guthrie, 1995); for example, the belief that spirits occupy physical objects. However, it may be necessary to distinguish between those who merely *accept* that belief, and those who actually *experience* this somehow, either in a weak form—knowing (as we often hear from synaesthetes with personified graphemes)—or in a strong form, as some sort of feeling of presence (Brugger, Regard, and Landis, 1997).

14.7 Summary and conclusion

We discussed here two types of personification found to be relatively common in synaesthetes, grapheme personification and inanimate object personification. The two share some key features with canonical forms of synaesthesia but usually lack a distinct vivid experience. The synaesthesia-like concurrents here are not colours, smells, etc., but rather feelings, attitudes, opinions, and other mental states (particularly in object personification), as well as rich biographical information (more so in grapheme personification). We propose that such phenomena could be classified as 'social synaesthesia', to distinguish it from more typical examples of synaesthesia, such as coloured graphemes and coloured music (Amin et al., 2011; Simner et al., 2016). One key feature of social synaesthesia may be unusual mapping between the self and others (rather than two different senses). We proposed that misattribution of self-referential processing may underlie these instances of personification. Synaesthetes' subjective reports are consistent with this (for example, some note that graphemes' moods vary with their own); however, if we are correct, it will be necessary to also explain why synaesthetes have limited insight into the self-referential aspect of grapheme/object personification and experience this as a passive observer. Investigating these extraordinary styles of social perception may provide us with a new point of view on the cognitive and neural basis of understanding others and oneself (Sagiv, Ilbeigi, and Ben-Tal, 2011). In the same way that visual illusions and hallucinations can be informative about ordinary visual perception, benign hyper-mentalizing in personification can shed more light on ordinary forms of mentalizing (Amin et al., 2011). The relationship to autoscopic phenomena, for example doppelgängers (Brugger, Regard, and Landis, 1997), is another interesting area for further investigation. Indeed, it has recently been proposed that synaesthesia in general, and personification in particular, could also play a useful role in the scientific study of consciousness (Sagiv and Frith, 2013).

We hope we have convinced readers that whether or not they embrace atypical forms of personification as a synaesthesia variant, at the very least these should be regarded as 'synaesthesia-like phenomena'. We suspect that a precise definition of synaesthesia with sharp category boundaries will remain difficult to agree upon. It may well be the case that advances in neurobiology and genetics will provide us with additional markers that could assist us in the classification of the variety of phenomena discussed here. Nevertheless, we suspect that if a similar mechanism, expressed in different parts of the brain, gives rise to the different types of synaesthesia, there is no good reason to believe that it will be restricted to the sensory cortices only. We urge the reader to consider the overlapping features of synaesthesia and synaesthesia-like phenomena and not to exclude from the discussion, a priori, grapheme personification or inanimate object personification. This may prove to be a more fruitful approach to making sense of the growing number of candidate synaesthesia variants.

References

Amin, M., Olu-Lafe, O., Claessen, L. E, Sobczak-Edmans, M., Ward, J., Williams, A. L., and Sagiv, N. (2011). Understanding grapheme personification: A social synaesthesia? *Journal of Neuropsychology*, 5(2):255–82.

Baron-Cohen, S. and Wheelwright, S. (2004). The empathy quotient: An investigation of adults with Asperger syndrome or high functioning autism, and normal sex differences. *Journal of Autism Developmental Disorders*, 34(2):163–75.

Baron-Cohen, S., Harrison, J., Goldstein, L. H., and Wyke, M. (1993). Coloured speech perception: Is synaesthesia what happens when modularity breaks down? *Perception*, 22(4):419–26.

Baron-Cohen, S., Wyke, M. A., and Binnie, C. (1987). Hearing words and seeing colours: An experimental investigation of a case of synaesthesia. *Perception*, 16(6):761–7.

Brugger, P., Regard, M., and Landis, T. (1997). Illusory reduplication of one's own body: Phenomenology and classification of autoscopic phenomena. *Cognitive Neuropsychiatry*, 2(1):19–38.

Burrack, A., Knoch, D., and Brugger, P. (2006). Mitempfindung in synaesthetes: Co-incidence or meaningful association? *Cortex*, 42(2):151–4.

Calkins, M. W. (1893). A statistical study of pseudochromesthesia and of mental-forms. *American Journal of Psychology*, 5(4):439–64.

Cavanna, A. E. and Trimble, M. R. (2006). The precuneus: A review of its functional anatomy and behavioural correlates. *Brain*, 129(3):564–83.

Chun, C. A. and Hupé, J-M. (2013). Mirror-touch and ticker tape experiences in synesthesia. *Frontiers in Psychology*, 4:776.

Cohen Kadosh, R. and Terhune, D. B. (2012). Redefining synaesthesia?. *British Journal of Psychology*, 103(1):20–3.

Cornog, M. (1986). Naming sexual body parts: Preliminary patterns and implications. *Journal of Sex Research*, 22(3):393–8.

Critchley, M. (1955). Personification of paralysed limbs in hemiplegics. *British Medical Journal*, 2:284–6.

Cytowic, R. E. (1989). *Synesthesia: A union of the senses*. Springer Verlag, New York.

Cytowic, R. E. (2002). *Synesthesia: A union of the senses*. MIT Press, Cambridge, MA, 2nd edition.

Dael, N., Sierro, G., and Mohr, C. (2013). Affect-related synesthesias: A prospective view on their existence, expression and underlying mechanisms. *Frontiers in Psychology*, 4:754.

Day, S. (2005). Some demographic and socio-cultural aspects of synaesthesia. In Robertson, L. C. and Sagiv, N., editors, *Synesthesia: Perspectives from cognitive neuroscience*, pp. 11–33. Oxford University Press, New York.

Deroy, O. and Spence, C. (2013). Why we are not all synesthetes (not even weakly so). *Psychonomic Bulletin & Review*, 20:1–22.

Devereux, G. (1966). An unusual audio-motor synesthesia in an adolescent. *Psychiatric Quarterly*, 40(1):459–71.

Eagleman, D. M. (2012). Synaesthesia in its protean guises. *British Journal of Psychology*, 103 (1):16–19.

Eagleman, D. M., Kagan, A. D., Nelson, S. S., Sagaram, D., and Sarma, A. K. (2007). A standardized test battery for the study of synesthesia. *Journal of Neuroscience Methods*, 159(1):139–45.

Epley, N., Akalis, S., Waytz, A., and Cacioppo, J. T. (2008). Creating social connection through inferential reproduction. *Psychological Science*, 19(2):114–20.

Feinberg, T. E., Venneri, A., Simone, A. M., Fan, Y., and Northoff, G. (2010). The neuroanatomy of asomatognosia and somatoparaphrenia. *Journal of Neurology, Neurosurgery & Psychiatry*, 81(3):276–81.

Flournoy, T. (1893). *Des phenomenes de synopsie* [Phenomena of Synopsia]. Felix Alcan, Paris.

Gegenfurtner, K. R. and Kiper, D. C. (2003). Color vision. *Annual Review of Neuroscience*, 26(1):181–206.

Guthrie, S. E. (1995). *Faces in the clouds: A new theory of religion*. Oxford University Press, New York.

Hubbard, E. (2007). Neurophysiology of synesthesia. *Current Psychiatry Reports*, 9(3):193–9.

Hubbard, E. M., Brang, D., and Ramachandran, V. S. (2011). The cross-activation theory at ten. *Journal of Neuropsychology*, 5(2):152–77.

Hubbard, E. M. and Ramachandran, V. S. (2005). Neurocognitive mechanisms of synesthesia. *Neuron*, 48(3):509–20.

Jäncke, L. and Langer, N. (2011). A strong parietal hub in the small-world network of coloured-hearing synaesthetes during resting state EEG. *Journal of Neuropsychology*, 5(2):178–202.

Jones, C. L., Gray, M. A., Minati, L., Simner, J., Critchley, H. D., and Ward, J. (2011). The neural basis of illusory gustatory sensations: Two rare cases of lexical-gustatory synaesthesia. *Journal of Neuropsychology*, 5(2):243–54.

Loetscher, T., Regard, M., and Brugger, P. (2006). Misoplegia: A review of the literature and a case without hemiplegia. *Journal of Neurology, Neurosurgery & Psychiatry*, 77(9):1099–100.

Luria, A. R. (1969). The mind of a mnemonist: A little book about a vast memory. Jonathan Cape, London.

Lynall, M. E. and Blakemore, C. (2013). What synesthesia isn't. In Simner, J. and Hubbard, E. M., editors, *The Oxford Handbook of Synesthesia*, pp. 959–98, Oxford University Press, Oxford.

Macpherson, F. (2007). Synaesthesia, functionalism and phenomenology. In Marraffa, M., de Caro, M., and Ferretti, F., editors, *Cartographies of the mind: Philosophy and psychology in intersection*, volume 4 of *Studies in Brain and Mind*, pp. 64–80. Springer, Dordrecht.

Marks, L. E. (1975). On colored-hearing synesthesia: Cross-modal translations of sensory dimensions. *Psychological Bulletin*, 82(3):303–31.

Martino, G. and Marks, L. E. (2001). Synesthesia: Strong and weak. *Current Directions in Psychological Science*, 10(2):61–5.

Mattingley, J. B., Rich, A. N., Yelland, G., and Bradshaw, J. L. (2001). Unconscious priming eliminates automatic binding of colour and alphanumeric form in synaesthesia. *Nature*, 410(6828):580–2.

Novich, S., Cheng, S., and Eagleman, D. M. (2011). Is synaesthesia one condition or many? A large-scale analysis reveals subgroups. *Journal of Neuropsychology*, 5(2):353–71.

Palmeri, T. J., Blake, R., Marois, R., Flanery, M. A., and Whetsell, W. (2002). The perceptual reality of synesthetic colors. *Proceedings of the National Academy of Sciences*, 99(6):4127–31.

Paulesu, E., Harrison, J., Baron-Cohen, S., Watson, J. D., Goldstein, L., Heather, J., Frackowiak, R. S., and Frith, C. D. (1995). The physiology of coloured hearing. A PET activation study of colour-word synaesthesia. *Brain*, 118(3):661–76.

Piaget, J. (1929/1960). *The child's conception of the world*. Littlefield Adams, New York.

Ramachandran, V. S. and Hubbard, E. M. (2001). Psychophysical investigations into the neural basis of synaesthesia. *Proceedings of the Royal Society of London B: Biological Sciences*, 268(1470):979–83.

Rothen, N. and Meier, B. (2013). Why vicarious experience is not an instance of synesthesia. *Frontiers in Human Neuroscience*, 7:128.

Sagiv, N. (2005). Synesthesia in perspective. In Robertson, L. C. and Sagiv, N., editors, *Synesthesia: Perspectives from cognitive neuroscience*, pp. 3–10. Oxford University Press, New York.

Sagiv, N. and Frith, C. D. (2013). Synesthesia and consciousness. In Simner, J. and Hubbard, E. M., editors, *The Oxford handbook of synesthesia*, pp. 924–40, Oxford University Press, Oxford.

Sagiv, N., Ilbeigi, A., and Ben-Tal, O. (2011). Reflections on synesthesia, perception, and cognition. *Intellectica*, 55(1):81–94.

Sagiv, N., Simner, J., Collins, J., Butterworth, B., and Ward, J. (2006). What is the relationship between synaesthesia and visuo-spatial number forms? *Cognition*, 101(1):114–28.

Sagiv, N., Sobczak, M., Ilbeigi, A., and Williams, S. (2012). Social synaesthesia. Presented at the Fourth International Congress on Synesthesia, Science and Art, University of Almeria, Spain, 16–19 February.

Sagiv, N. and Ward, J. (2006). Cross-modal interactions: Lessons from synesthesia. *Progress in Brain Research*, 155:263–75.

Schilling, G. (2006). Underworld character kicked out of planetary family. *Science*, 313(5791):1214–15.

Shanon, B. (1982). Colour associates to semantic linear orders. *Psychological Research*, 44(1):75–83.

Simner, J. (2007). Beyond perception: Synaesthesia as a psycholinguistic phenomenon. *Trends in Cognitive Sciences*, 11(1):23–9.

Simner, J. (2012). Defining synaesthesia. *British Journal of Psychology*, 103(1):1–15.

Simner, J., Gärtner, O., and Taylor, M. D. (2011). Cross-modal personality attributions in synaesthetes and non-synaesthetes. *Journal of Neuropsychology*, 5(2):283–301.

Simner, J. and Holenstein, E. (2007). Ordinal linguistic personification: The systematic attribution of animate qualities to the linguistic units of ordinal sequences. *Journal of Cognitive Neuroscience*, 19:694–703.

Simner, J. and Hubbard, E. M. (2006). Variants of synesthesia interact in cognitive tasks: Evidence for implicit associations and late connectivity in cross-talk theories. *Neuroscience*, 143(3):805–14.

Simner, J., Mulvenna, C., Sagiv, N., Tsakanikos, E., Witherby, S. A., Fraser, C., Scott, K., and Ward, J. (2006). Synaesthesia: The prevalence of atypical cross-modal experiences. *Perception*, 35(8):1024–33.

Simner, J., Rehme, M. K., Carmichael, D. A., Bastin, M. E., Sprooten, E., McIntosh, A. M., Lawrie, S. M., and Zedler, M. (2016). Social responsiveness to inanimate entities: Altered white matter in a 'social synaesthesia'. *Neuropsychologia*, 91:282–9.

Smeets, P. M. (1973). The animism controversy revisited: A probability analysis. *Journal of Genetic Psychology*, 123(2):219–25.

Smilek, D., Dixon, M. J., Cudahy, C., and Merikle, P. M. (2001). Synaesthetic photisms influence visual perception. *Journal of Cognitive Neuroscience*, 13(7):930–6.

Smilek, D., Malcolmson, K. A., Carriere, J. S., Eller, M., Kwan, D., and Reynolds, M. (2007). When '3' is a jerk and 'E' is a king: Personifying inanimate objects in synesthesia. *Journal of Cognitive Neuroscience*, 19(6):981–92.

Sobczak-Edmans, M. (2013). *A systematic study of personification in synaesthesia: Behavioural and neuroimaging studies* (Doctoral dissertation, Brunel University, School of Social Sciences Theses).

Sobczak-Edmans, M. and Sagiv, N. (2013). Synesthetic personification: The social world of graphemes. In Simner, J. and Hubbard, E. M., editors, *The Oxford handbook of synesthesia*, pp. 222–38, Oxford University Press, Oxford.

Sobczak-Edmans, M., Williams, A. L., and Sagiv, N. (in preparation). Personification in synaesthesia: Behavioural and fMRI studies.

Taylor, M., Hulette, A. C., and Dishion, T. J. (2010). Longitudinal outcomes of young high-risk adolescents with imaginary companions. *Developmental Psychology*, 46(6):1632–6.

Ward, J., Li, R., Salih, S., and Sagiv, N. (2007). Varieties of grapheme-colour synaesthesia: A new theory of phenomenological and behavioural differences. *Consciousness and Cognition*, 16(4):913–31.

Ward, J. and Sagiv, N. (2007). Synaesthesia for finger counting and dice patterns: A case of higher synaesthesia? *Neurocase*, 13(2):86–93.

Weiss, P. H., Zilles, K., and Fink, G. R. (2005). When visual perception causes feeling: Enhanced cross-modal processing in grapheme-color synesthesia. *Neuroimage*, 28(4):859–68.

Zaitchik, D. and Solomon, G. A. (2008). Animistic thinking in the elderly and in patients with Alzheimer's disease. *Cognitive Neuropsychology*, 25(1):27–37.

Zeki, S. (2003). The disunity of consciousness. *Trends in Cognitive Sciences*, 7(5):214–18.

Index

Note: 'n' following a page number refers to a footnote on that page, '*f*' refers to a figure and '*t*' refers to a table.

The manufacturer's authorised representative in the EU for product safety is Oxford University Press España S.A. of el Parque Empresarial San Fernando de Henares, Avenida de Castilla, 2 – 28830 Madrid (www.oup.es/en or product.safety@oup.com). OUP España S.A. also acts as importer into Spain of products made by the manufacturer.

www.ingramcontent.com/pod-product-compliance
Lightning Source LLC
LaVergne TN
LVHW011820200926
848484LV00005B/1262
9780199688289